RHINOPLASTY
An Expert Manual

RHINOPLASTY
An Expert Manual

Second Edition

Swapan Kumar Ghosh
MS DLO DNB
Professor
Department of ENT
Burdwan Medical College
Purba Bardhaman, West Bengal, India

Foreword
Ullas Raghavan

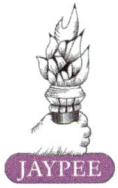

JAYPEE BROTHERS MEDICAL PUBLISHERS
The Health Sciences Publisher
New Delhi | London

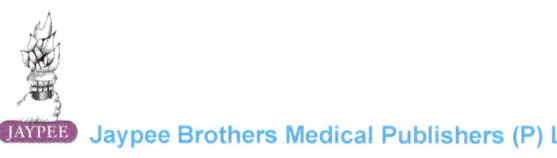
Jaypee Brothers Medical Publishers (P) Ltd

Headquarters
Jaypee Brothers Medical Publishers (P) Ltd
EMCA House, 23/23-B
Ansari Road, Daryaganj
New Delhi 110 002, India
Landline: +91-11-23272143, +91-11-23272703
+91-11-23282021, +91-11-23245672
Email: jaypee@jaypeebrothers.com

Corporate Office
Jaypee Brothers Medical Publishers (P) Ltd
4838/24, Ansari Road, Daryaganj
New Delhi 110 002, India
Phone: +91-11-43574357
Fax: +91-11-43574314
Email: jaypee@jaypeebrothers.com

Overseas Office
JP Medical Ltd
83 Victoria Street, London
SW1H 0HW (UK)
Phone: +44 20 3170 8910
Fax: +44 (0)20 3008 6180
Email: info@jpmedpub.com

Website: www.jaypeebrothers.com
Website: www.jaypeedigital.com

© 2024, Jaypee Brothers Medical Publishers

The views and opinions expressed in this book are solely those of the original contributor(s)/author(s) and do not necessarily represent those of editor(s) or publisher of the book.

All rights reserved. No part of this publication may be reproduced, stored or transmitted in any form or by any means, electronic, mechanical, photocopying, recording or otherwise, without the prior permission in writing of the publishers.

All brand names and product names used in this book are trade names, service marks, trademarks or registered trademarks of their respective owners. The publisher is not associated with any product or vendor mentioned in this book.

Medical knowledge and practice change constantly. This book is designed to provide accurate, authoritative information about the subject matter in question. However, readers are advised to check the most current information available on procedures included and check information from the manufacturer of each product to be administered, to verify the recommended dose, formula, method and duration of administration, adverse effects and contraindications. It is the responsibility of the practitioner to take all appropriate safety precautions. Neither the publisher nor the author(s)/editor(s) assume any liability for any injury and/or damage to persons or property arising from or related to use of material in this book.

This book is sold on the understanding that the publisher is not engaged in providing professional medical services. If such advice or services are required, the services of a competent medical professional should be sought.

Every effort has been made where necessary to contact holders of copyright to obtain permission to reproduce copyright material. If any have been inadvertently overlooked, the publisher will be pleased to make the necessary arrangements at the first opportunity.

Inquiries for bulk sales may be solicited at: jaypee@jaypeebrothers.com

Rhinoplasty: An Expert Manual

First Edition: 2017

Second Edition: 2024

ISBN: 978-93-5465-211-0

Dedicated to
My students
and
in loving memory of my parents

Foreword

Swapan Kumar Ghosh has correctly identified the need for a concise and clear manual for the rhinoplasty surgeon. Rhinoplasty is a surgery that has fascinated and mystified many surgeons. This leads to many confusing and contradictory teachings. This text does away with the mysticism and gives a clear instructional manual for the surgery. Helpfully illustrated and giving expert pointers. Even more importantly, it provides all these in a concise and direct manner. The text follows a logical manner from the history of the procedure to anesthetic considerations, operative steps, and postoperative care. For Indian surgeons, there is even a section on rhinoplasty in patients with atrophic rhinitis. A point of pride for Indian surgeons would be the origins of rhinoplasty with the work of Sushruta in 600 BC in India. This was built upon by many over the years and reminds us that we stand on the shoulders of giants. Swapan Kumar Ghosh and colleagues should be congratulated on their hard work in creating this manual.

Ullas Raghavan
MS FRCS (ORL-HNS) IBCFPRS EBCFPRS
Consultant ENT and Facial Plastic Surgeon
Department of Otorhinolaryngology and
Facial Plastic Surgery
Doncaster Royal Infirmary
South Yorkshire, England, UK

Preface to the Second Edition

The first edition of this book was published in 2017 and was designed to present the basic essential steps of rhinoplasty. It is a great satisfaction for me to bring out the completely revised, updated, and enlarged second edition of this book. Considering the development in the field of rhinoplasty and important feedback from the students and the physicians across the country, many new topics, diagrams, and photographs have been added. A new chapter on "Preservation Rhinoplasty" has been added. This book will guide surgeons, in a systematic manner, about the preoperative assessment and surgical techniques of rhinoplasty. The techniques have been described with the help of schematic drawings and clinical photographs. The description of the relevant anatomy and surgical techniques in this book is sufficiently clear so that the reader will be able to apply them in his or her practice. I am sure this book will set a new standard of teaching of rhinoplasty among the ENT surgeons and plastic surgeons in the country. I sincerely hope that the second edition of this book will be widely accepted and appreciated by the rhinoplasty surgeons in India and abroad.

Swapan Kumar Ghosh

Preface to the First Edition

The book is comprehensive and is designed for students of ENT and plastic surgery. Junior ENT surgeons and plastic surgeons will get interest in rhinoplasty by reading this book. Preoperative and postoperative photographs with short description of the procedure and illustrations will help in clear understanding of the subject. This book aims at providing guidance, in a systematic manner on preoperative assessment and surgical techniques of primary and secondary rhinoplasty to the ENT and plastic surgeons. The chapters have been primarily designed to present the basic essential steps of rhinoplasty operation. It will be very rewarding for me if this book becomes a resource of information for the doctors and helps in generating the interest to perform rhinoplasty surgery. I request all the students and doctors of ENT and plastic surgery to go through this book and send their comments, criticism and suggestions, so that I can enrich the book further with relevant materials in its next edition.

Swapan Kumar Ghosh

Acknowledgments

I take the privilege to express a profound sense of gratitude to my teachers, (Late) Professor SD Mukhopadhyay, Department of ENT, Calcutta National Medical College and (Late) Professor DK Banerjee, Department of ENT, RG Kar Medical College, Kolkata, West Bengal, India, who had a great influence during my early teaching period when I used to perform different types of rhinoplasty surgeries regularly at RG Kar Medical College, since 1995.

I wish to take the opportunity to express my sincere thanks to Dr Gilbert Nolst Trenité, Past President of European Academy of Facial Plastic Surgery and International Federation of Facial Plastic Surgery Societies for his guidance on many aspects of rhinoplasty during writing this book.

I would like to express my deep sense of gratitude to Dr Ullas Raghavan, Consultant ENT and Facial Plastic Surgeon, Doncaster Royal Infirmary, UK for writing the Foreword.

I am indebted to all my colleagues in the Department of ENT, Institute of Postgraduate Medical Education and Research (IPGMER) and Seth Sukhlal Karnani Memorial (SSKM) Hospital, Kolkata and Burdwan Medical College, Burdwan, West Bengal, India for their help and valuable comments. I gratefully acknowledge Dr Thang T Dinh, ENT Surgeon, Quang Ngai Provincial General Hospital, Vietnam for providing me with study materials.

I would like to thank Shri Jitendar P Vij (Group Chairman), Mr Ankit Vij (Managing Director), and production staff of M/s Jaypee Brothers Medical Publishers (P) Ltd, New Delhi, India, for their constant support and help. I sincerely acknowledge Mr Sabyasachi Hazra, M/s Jaypee Brothers Medical Publishers (P) Ltd, Kolkata branch for his assistance in publishing this book.

Finally, I shall be failing in my duties if I do not offer my heart-felt gratitude to my patients who so optimistically offered themselves to my surgeries.

Contents

1. History of Rhinoplasty 1
2. Anatomy and Physiology 4
3. Instruments and Preoperative Assessment 24
4. Anesthesia 32
5. Basic Technique 38
6. Incisions and Approaches 40
7. Mobilization of Soft Tissues (Skeletonization) 47
8. Nasal Spine 50
9. Removal of Hump 52
10. Septoplasty 62
11. Osteotomies 82
12. Shortening the Nose and Narrowing of Middle Third of Nose 90
13. Tip Plasty 92
14. Sutures and Dressing 118
15. Postoperative Care 120
16. Augmentation Rhinoplasty 122
17. Rhinoplasty in Atrophic Rhinitis 152
18. Surgery of the Crooked Nose 158
19. Surgery of Alar, Columellar Deformity, and Vestibular Stenosis 177
20. Nasal Reconstruction 193
21. Revision Rhinoplasty 211
22. Preservation Rhinoplasty 220

Index *227*

CHAPTER 1

History of Rhinoplasty

INTRODUCTION

The word rhinoplasty originates from two Greek words: rhinos and plastikos. Rhinos means "nose" in Greek and plastikos means "to shape." Plastic surgery for a deformed nose was first described in the Edwin Smith Papyrus,[1] a transcription of an ancient Egyptian medical text, the oldest known surgical treatise, dated to the Old Kingdom from 3000 to 2500 BC.[2] The first known cases of successful rhinoplasty were performed in India in 600 BC by the Ayurvedic doctor Sushruta, who gave an account of nasal reconstruction in the Sushruta Samhita, his medicosurgical compendium. Sushruta and his students performed plastic surgeries for deformities of noses, earlobes, etc., that were amputated as punishment at that time. Sushruta also pioneered the nasal reconstruction by forehead flap rhinoplasty.[3] Cutting of the nose or nose tip was a common way of punishing thieves in India during that period of time.[4]

The Arab physician Ibn Abi Usaibia (1203–1270) translated the Sushruta Samhita from Sanskrit to Arabic. Then Sushruta's medical compendium made a journey from Arabia to Persia to Egypt.

In 1794, British physicians traveled to India to see rhinoplasty being performed by native methods. In the Gentleman's Magazine (1794), Thomas Cruso and James Findlay published an article describing a rhinoplasty using forehead pedicle-flap that was a variation of the free-flap graft technique that Sushruta had described many years back.

In Great Britain, Joseph Constantine Carpue (1815) described two successful operations for correction of nasal deformity, which mentioned two rhinoplasties: the reconstruction of two damaged noses.[5] He spent 20 years in India studying local plastic surgery methods. In the mid-to-late 1800s, physicians in Europe and America experimented with different rhinoplasty techniques to enhance the shape, appearance, and nasal function.

In Germany, Karl Ferdinand von Grafe (1818) published an article wherein he described 55 rhinoplasty procedures. During World War I, thousands of troops suffered major facial injuries by bullets and sharp weapons leading to severe deformities. So, surgeons tried to develop reconstructive faciomaxillary procedures in a short and intense period of time. With these developments, related improvements also occurred in anesthesia and antiseptic techniques. Many surgeons around the western world worked hard for advancement of the technologies of plastic surgery and formed societies which later turned into organizations, such as the American Society of Plastic Surgeons. Rhinoplasty had major technological advancements through the dark times of the First and Second World War. Regarding modernizing techniques for aesthetic applications, in 1845, Joseph Dieffenbach introduced external incisions to the rhinoplasty surgeon community.

The American otolaryngologist, John Orlando Roe, entered history by performing the first, modern endonasal rhinoplasty and he was considered as the Father of Aesthetic Rhinoplasty after having reported a "simple operation" in 1887 describing the correction of a "pug nose" by an endonasal approach.[6]

In 1892, Robert F Weir, another American surgeon, also described his techniques for correction of the saddle nose.[7]

In 1898, Jacques Joseph, an orthopedic surgeon published his paper on reduction rhinoplasty, by external approach. Many budding rhinoplasty surgeons went to Germany to observe Joseph perform his rhinoplasties. Many of the basic techniques of rhinoplasty remain essentially the same today as when Joseph first described them. He is considered the father of modern rhinoplasty.[8] He classified various types of nasal deformities and described different procedures for the correction of the deformities. He also invented some operative instruments. Joseph's concepts were further disseminated by surgeons, such as Gustav Aufricht, Joseph Safian, and Samuel Fomon.[9]

In the early 20th century, Freer, in 1902, and Killian, in 1904, respectively, pioneered the submucous resection (SMR) technique for correction of deviated nasal septum. They performed SMR by raising mucoperichondrial flaps and excising parts of cartilaginous and bony septum, maintaining septal support by preserving 1-cm dorsal septal margin and 1-cm caudal septal margin.

In 1929, Peer and Metzenbaum performed the procedure to correct deviation of the caudal septum.

A Rethi (1934) introduced the external rhinoplasty approach with an incision to the columella to correct the deformed nasal tip.[10] Maurice H Cottle (1947) endonasally performed septoplasty with a hemitransfixion incision.[11] A Sercer (1957) described the "decortication of the nose" technique (open rhinoplasty) allowing greater exposure. Later, external rhinoplasty approach was advocated by Padovan (1970), Wilfred S Goodman (1970), and Jack P Gunter (1990).[12,13] Goodman (1973) mentioned his technical modifications in an article and popularized the external approach for rhinoplasty.[14] Jack Anderson (1982) described open approach in his article "Open Rhinoplasty: An Assessment".[15]

In 1984, Sheen first reported the use of spreader grafts in cases of primary and secondary rhinoplasty. In 1987, Jack P Guntur described the advantages of the external approach for performing a secondary rhinoplasty.[16]

From the 1950s to today, the history of rhinoplasty has seen advancements in technology and culture. Though once viewed as a luxury accessible only to the rich and famous, plastic surgery has now been recognized as an effective way for all types of people to beautify their physical form. Rhinoplasty operation has been among the most popular procedures sought by men and women in the last few decades.

REFERENCES

1. Shiffman M, Di Giuseppe A. Cosmetic surgery: Art and Techniques. Heidelberg: Springer Berlin; 2013. p. 20.
2. Brandt-Rauf PW, Brandt-Rauf SI. History of occupational medicine: Relevance of Imhotep and the Edwin Smith Papyrus. Br J Ind Med. 1987;44(1):68-70.
3. Sushruta. Sushruta Samhita. Calcutta, India: Kaviraj Kunjalal Publishing; 1998. pp. 1907-17.
4. Mazzola IC, Mazzola RF. History of reconstructive rhinoplasty. Facial Plast Surg. 2014;30(3):227-36.
5. Rinzler CA. The encyclopedia of cosmetic and plastic surgery, 1st edition. New York, USA: Facts on File; 2009. p. 151.
6. Roe JO. The deformity termed "Pug Nose" and its correction with a simple operation (Reprinted from the Medical Record. June 4, 1887). Plast Reconstr Surg. 1970;45(1):78-83.
7. Weir RF. On restoring sunken noses without scarring the face. New York: The Medical Record; 1892.
8. McDowell F, Valone JA, Brown JB. Bibliography and historical note on plastic surgery of the nose. Plast Reconstr Surg. 1952;10:149-85.
9. Vartanian AJ. Rhinoplasty, Basic closed technique. eMedicine Plastic Surgery; 2010.
10. Rethi A. Operation to shorten an excessively long nose. Revue de Chirurgie Plastique. 1934;2:85.
11. Arneja JS. Basic Open Rhinoplasty. emedicine.medscape.com. 2009.
12. Goodman WS, Charles DA. Technique of external rhinoplasty. J Otolaryngol. 1978;7(1):13-7.
13. Gunter JP. The merits of the open approach in rhinoplasty. Plast Reconstr Surg. 1997;99(3):863-7.
14. Goodman WS. External approach to rhinoplasty. Can J Otolaryngol. 1973;2(3):207-10.
15. Anderson JR, Johnson CM, Adamson P. Open rhinoplasty: An assessment. Otolaryngol Head Neck Surg. 1982;90(2):272-4.
16. Guntur JP, Rohrich RJ. External approach for secondary rhinoplasty. Plast Reconst Surg. 1987;80(2):161-74.

CHAPTER 2

Anatomy and Physiology

INTRODUCTION

Rhinoplasty can produce a dramatic improvement in one's appearance, but if not done properly, a permanent deformity results. Appearance-related surgery can damage a surgeon's professional reputation more than with other types of surgery. Knowledge of anatomy and physiology of the nose is needed, along with artistic skills. A surgeon performing rhinoplasty is considered proficient only after approximately 8 years of experience and continuing education.[1]

Understanding nasal anatomy in detail is important for successful rhinoplasty. Proper examination of the anatomic variations presented by a patient helps the surgeon to develop a rational and realistic surgical plan.[2]

TERMINOLOGY

- *Glabella:* Triangular area on frontal bone between the supraorbital ridges.
- *Nasion:* At the upper end of the suture between the nasal bones—The ideal nasion level is set between the lash and crease line of the upper eyelid.
- *Sellion:* It is the deepest point of the nasofrontal angle at the junction of forehead slope and the proximal nasal bridge. It is the soft tissue equivalent of the nasion.
- *Rhinion:* At the lower end of the suture between the nasal bones.
- *Radix:* The radix defines the nasal root. Centered at the nasion, the radix extends inferiorly to the level of the medial canthus and superiorly by an equivalent distance. At the nasion, the height of the radix is ideally between 9 and 14 mm as measured from the anterior corneal plane. Radix projection is one third the ideal nasal length **(Fig. 1)**.
- *Lobule:* It is the lower third of the nose bounded by the anterior nostril edge posteroinferiorly, the supratip area superiorly and the alar grooves laterally. Domes and lateral crura of the lower lateral cartilages form the lobule.
- *Dome:* Area of junction of medial and lateral crura.
- *Tip:* It is formed by domes of both lower lateral cartilages.
- *Limen nasi:* Nasal vestibule is bounded above and behind by a curved ridge, the limen nasi. It is formed by the lower margin of the upper lateral cartilage. Intercartilaginous incision is made here.
- *Internal nasal valve:* This slit-like segment is bounded by the nasal septum and the caudal margin of the upper lateral cartilage and is the location of

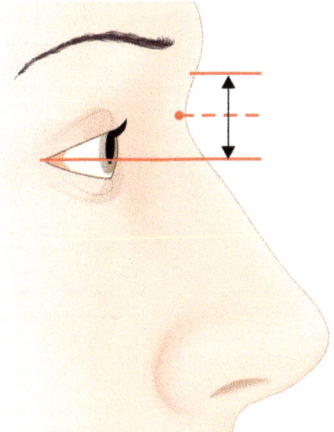

Fig. 1: Radix area.

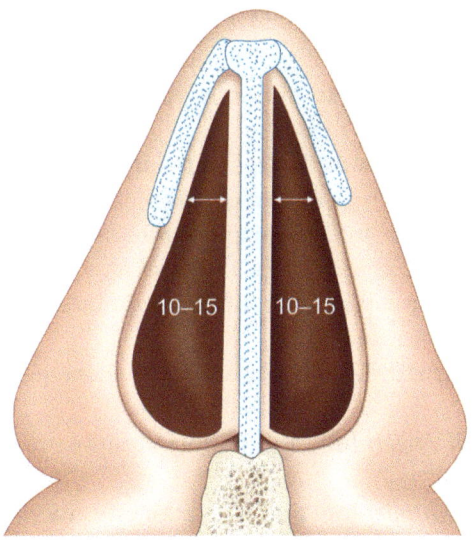

Fig. 2: The ideal angle between the caudal edge of the upper lateral cartilage and the septum is 10–15°.

the least cross-sectional area in the nose. The angle of the internal valve should be between 10° and 15° (**Fig. 2**).

- *Nasal valve area:* It is bounded by the anterior end of the inferior turbinate, the caudal septum, and the tissues surrounding the pyriform aperture. In lateral osteotomies, a small triangle of bone at the pyriform aperture (Webster triangle) is carefully preserved to prevent medialization of the inferior turbinate, which can reduce the cross-sectional area of the nasal valve area.

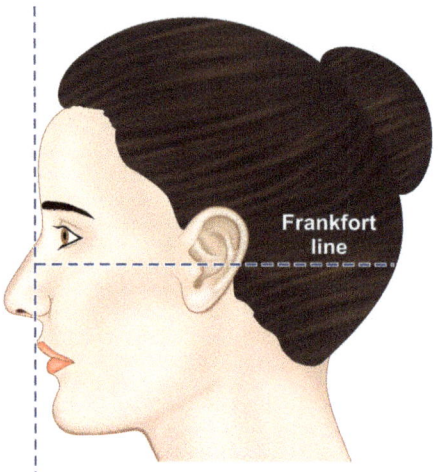

Fig. 3: Frankfort line touches the lower border of the infraorbital rim and the upper border of the external auditory canal.

- *Soft triangle:* Inferior to the dome, this is an area of lobule between external and vestibular skin devoid of cartilage. To prevent scarring, incision is avoided in this area.
- *Empty triangle:* It forms the lateral boundary of the nasal valve area and is the site where inspiratory collapse occurs most frequently. It is a triangular-shaped area devoid of cartilage and made up of dense fibrofatty tissue extending up to the margin of the pyriform aperture.
- *Frankfort line:* A line along the infraorbital margin and upper border of external auditory canal **(Fig. 3)**.
- *Subnasale:* Point at the anterior nasal spine where the nasal septum meets the upper lip.
- *Anterior septal angle:* Junction of dorsal and caudal borders of septal cartilage.
- *Posterior septal angle:* Junction of caudal and inferior borders of septal cartilage.
- *Gnathion:* This is the lowest point in the midline of chin.
- *Nasofrontal angle:* The angle between the dorsum of nose and glabellar part of the forehead. It is about 125° **(Fig. 4)**.
- *Nasolabial angle:* The angle between columella and upper lip. This should be about 90–100° in males and 100–110° in females **(Fig. 5)**.
- *Nasofacial angle (angle of nasal projection):* The angle between a line touching the nasion and chin (nasomental line) and dorsum of nose. This should be about 35° **(Fig. 6)**. A nasofacial angle of approximately 34° for females and 36° for males is the accepted standard.
- *Scroll region:* The lateral crus of the lower lateral cartilage is attached to the upper lateral cartilage with scroll, that is an outcurving of the

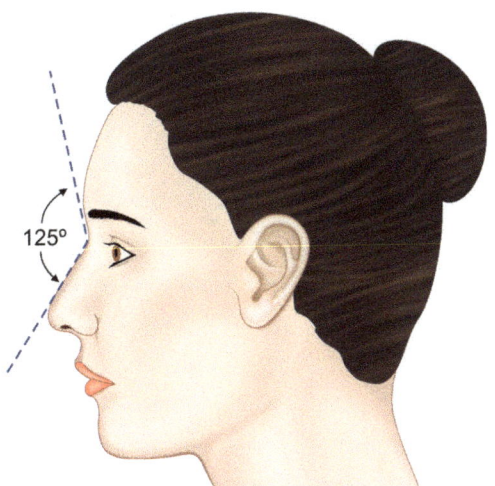

Fig. 4: Nasofrontal angle.

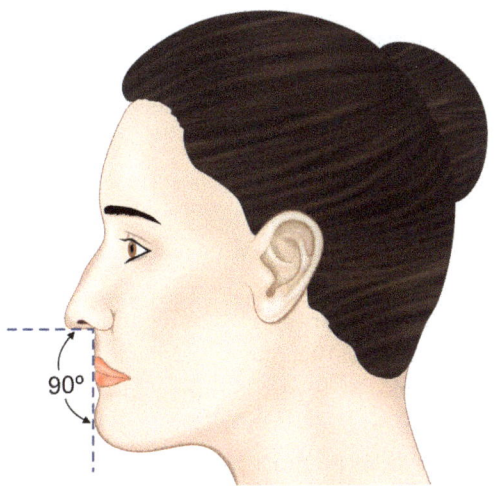

Fig. 5: Nasolabial angle.

caudal borders of the upper lateral cartilages and an incurving of the cephalic borders of the lower lateral cartilages. Several variations of the scrolls exist.

Less commonly, the cephalic border of the lower lateral cartilage abuts the caudal border of the upper lateral cartilage. Rarely, the caudal border of the upper lateral cartilage overlaps the cephalic border of the lower lateral cartilage.[3]

- *Alar lobule:* It is a portion of the lateral nasal sidewall. It contains fat and fibrous connective tissue and is devoid of cartilage. The lateral crus of the lower lateral cartilage runs in a more cephalic direction and is not found in the alar lobule.

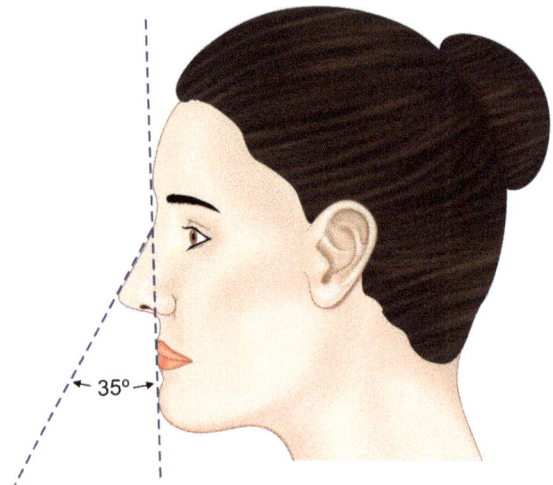

Fig. 6: Nasofacial angle.

- *Infratip lobule:* It is the portion of the lobule between the tip defining points and the columella.
- *Nostril sill:* It is the slight protuberance of soft tissue at the floor of the nostril at the entrance to the vestibule.
- *External nasal valve:* It is the alar rim composed of lower lateral cartilage and nasal floor.
- *Pyriform aperture:* It is the pear-shaped external bony opening of the nasal cavity.
- *Sesamoid cartilages:* These are small cartilages in the lateral space between the upper and lower lateral cartilages.
- *Supratip area:* It is the area just cephalic to the nasal tip at the caudal portion of the nasal dorsum.
- *Tip-defining points:* It is the most projecting area on each side of the tip producing external light reflection.
- *Weak triangle (converse):* It is the area immediately cephalic to the domes.
- *Keystone area:* The area is made by the junction of the nasal bones with the upper lateral cartilages and the septum, and is the widest part of the dorsum. The area should not be disturbed and the T-shaped contour of the nasal dorsum must be maintained during rhinoplasty.
- *Dorsal aesthetic lines:* These lines descend from the medial ends of the eyebrows vertically along the sidewalls of the nose and end at the sides of the nasal tip. Dorsal aesthetic lines do not go straight. They are wide at the keystone area and narrow at the radix and the supratip area.
- *Alar groove:* A depression that follows the caudal border of the lateral crus as it leaves the alar rim to take on a more cephalic position. The tip is separated from the thickened part of the ala by the alar groove.

- *Trichion:* Anterior hairline in the midline.
- *Menton:* Most inferior point on chin.
- *Nasal width:* The maximum distance between two alae.
- *Nasal height:* Height of the nose from nasion to subnasale.
- *Nasal index:* Nasal width/nasal height × 100. Leptorrhine (fine nose) has nasal index <70. Mesorrhine has nasal index between 70 and 84.90. Platyrrhine (broad nose) has nasal index >85.
- *Pronasale:* The most anterior midpoint of the nasal tip.
- *Nasal length:* From nasion to pronasale.
- *Tip projection:* Tip projection is the distance of the nasal tip from the vertical facial plane when measured from the level of the alar-facial groove. The ideal projection of the nasal tip is measured by using the Goode rule. Tip projection should be 55–60% of the distance between the nasion and tip-defining points.
- *Lobule projection:* It is the horizontal distance from the apex of the nostril to the highest point of the nasal tip. Lateral crural steal suture elongates the lobule and causes rotation of the tip. It should be supported with a columellar strut. Long lobule is corrected by medial crural overlap, usually done at the columella break point. For a 7–8 mm of overlap, resection and overlap can be combined.

Face is divided into three equal horizontal parts, limited by the lines intersecting four topographic points: Trichion (hairline in the midline), glabella, subnasale (nasal spine), and menton (lower edge of the chin) (**Fig. 7**).[4] Face is again divided into five vertical parts of equal width, limited by six vertical lines—two lines passing through the inner canthi, which includes the medial part of the face with nose, two lines crossing the lateral canthi, and two lines through the most outwardly situated point of the pinna on both sides (**Fig. 8**).[5] The nose is anatomically subdivided into three portions: The bony vault, the upper cartilaginous vault, and the lower cartilaginous vault.

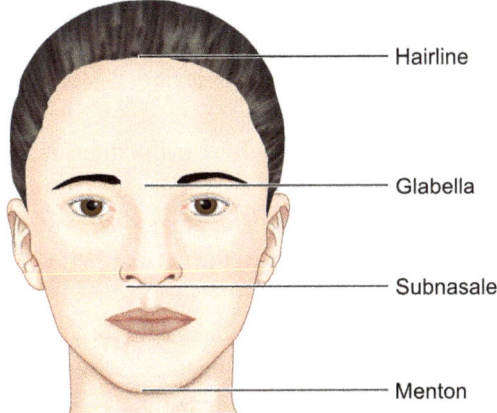

Fig. 7: The face is divided into three equal horizontal parts.

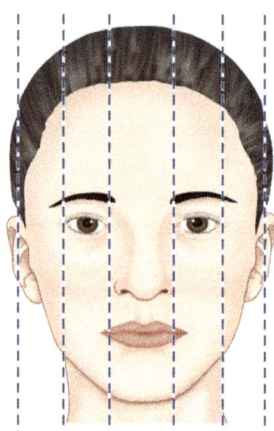

Fig. 8: Vertically the face is divided into five equal parts.

The nasal surface is made up of several concave and convex surfaces separated from one another by ridges. The topographic subunits of nose are the following: Tip, dorsum, sidewalls, alar lobules, soft triangles, and columella. When a large part of a subunit has been damaged, replacing the entire subunit rather than simply covering the defect often gives a better result.[6]

The skin of the upper third is fairly thick but becomes thinner in the mid-dorsal region. In the inferior third, the skin is thick and it contains large sebaceous glands. In the lower part of the nose, skin is adherent to the underlying structures.

The soft-tissue envelope at the rhinion is the thinnest because there is less subcutaneous fat, and the transverse nasalis muscle fibers become an aponeurosis here.

Muscles of the Nose

The muscles of the nose are situated deep to the skin and consist of four principal groups: The elevators, the depressors, the compressor, and the dilators. The elevators are the procerus and levator labii superioris alaeque nasi. The depressors are the alar nasalis and depressor septi nasi. The compressor of the nose is the transverse nasalis, whereas the dilators are the dilator naris anterior and posterior. Nasal muscles are innervated by temporal, zygomatic, and buccal branches of facial nerve. The elevators shorten nasal length and dilate nostril. Procerus takes origin from the periosteum of the nasal bones and the aponeurosis of the transverse nasalis and inserts into the glabellar skin. Levator labii superioris alaeque nasi muscle originates from medial infraorbital margin and inserts at muscle and skin of nasolabial fold, nasal alae, and upper lip. The levator labii superioris alaeque nasi muscle causes flaring of the nasal ala and nasal tip ptosis when smiling **(Fig. 9)**.

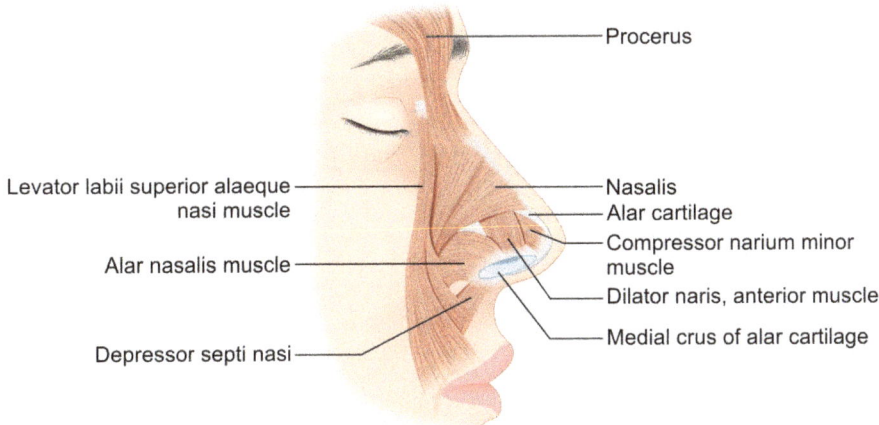

Fig. 9: Muscles of nose.

The depressors lengthen nasal length and dilate nostril. Nasalis is a paired muscle that is situated over the dorsum of the nose. It has two parts: Alar and transverse. The alar part is also known as dilator naris posterior, and the transverse part is called the compressor naris. The main portion of the dilator naris posterior (alar nasalis) originates from the periosteum of the maxilla above the canine tooth and inserts into the alar base. It dilates the nostril as it pulls the ala laterally. All these actions of nasalis normally happen prior to each inspiration, in order to prevent the external nasal valve from collapsing. The depressor septi nasi muscle originates from the periosteum of the maxilla above the canine tooth and inserts into the footplates of the medial crura with attachment to the anterior nasal spine and membranous septum. This muscle lowers the nasal tip during smiling or making a facial expression.

The transverse nasalis muscle takes its origin from the periosteum of the maxilla superolateral to the incisive fossa. Its fibers then run in superomedial direction, expanding into a thin aponeurosis over the bridge of the nose. Via this aponeurosis, the muscle inserts at the dorsum of the nose by blending with its counterpart from the opposite side and the procerus muscle. The transverse nasalis compresses the nasal aperture and wrinkles the nasal skin.

Dilator naris anterior originates from the surface of the lateral crus and inserts into the rim of the nostril.[7]

The muscles are interconnected by an aponeurosis termed the nasal superficial musculoaponeurotic system (SMAS).[8]

Blood Vessels and Lymphatics

Blood vessels and lymphatics are found superficial to the nasal musculature.[9] The layers of the soft-tissue in the nose are epidermis, dermis, subcutaneous tissue, muscle and fascia, areolar tissue and perichondrium or periosteum.

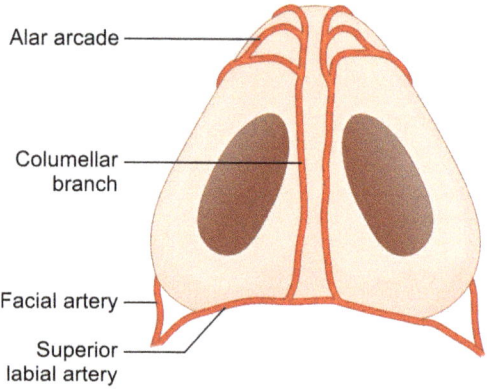

Fig. 10: Blood supply of nose.

During rhinoplasty dissection should be done in the areolar tissue plane (i.e., submusculoaponeurotic) which preserves nasal blood supply and minimizes postoperative edema.

The external nose is supplied by both the internal carotid artery and the external carotid artery via the ophthalmic artery and the facial artery, respectively. The ophthalmic artery mainly supplies blood to the upper part of the nose via the external nasal branch of the anterior ethmoidal artery and the dorsal nasal artery; the facial artery gives rise to the angular and superior labial arteries, which supply the lower part of the nose. The nasal tip receives blood supply from the ophthalmic artery via the dorsal nasal artery superiorly. Facial artery via the lateral nasal artery, and the superior labial artery via the columellar artery supply nasal tip inferiorly **(Fig. 10)**.

Veins follow the arterial pattern. They have direct communication with the cavernous sinus and lack valves.

Even with the good vascularity of the nose, smoking delays postoperative healing.[8]

Lymphatics arise from superficial mucosa. Submandibular nodes collect lymph from the external nose and anterior part of the nasal cavity. Upper deep cervical nodes drain the rest of the nasal cavity, either directly or through the retropharyngeal nodes.

Nerve Supply of the Nose

The sensory supply of the nose is derived from the ophthalmic and maxillary divisions of the trigeminal nerve.

The external nasal branch of anterior ethmoidal nerve innervates the nasal tip. It runs from nasal dorsum to nasal tip after coming out between nasal bone and upper lateral cartilage. Sometimes, patients are seen having temporary sensory discomfort due to nerve injury or edema during early phase after rhinoplasty. The nerve injury is more common after hump reduction or wide

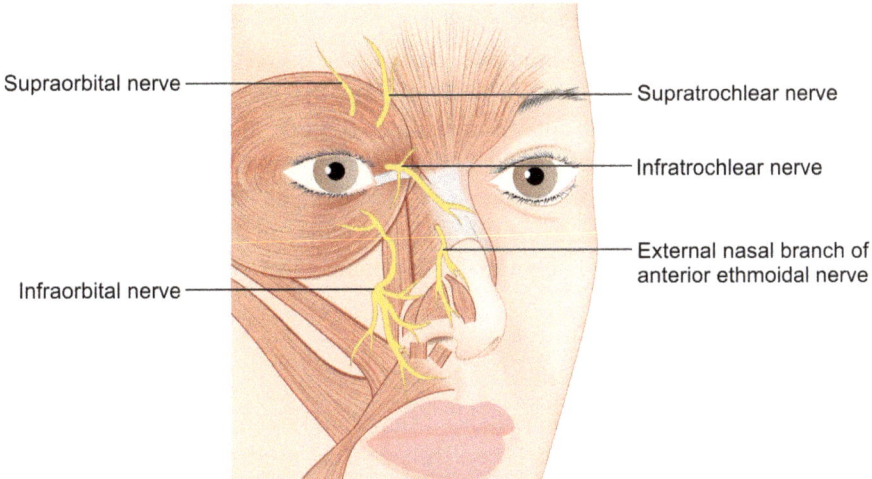

Fig. 11: Nerve supply of nose.

subperiosteal dissection, which usually recovers spontaneously after several months during postoperative period.

Infratrochlear nerve supplies medial eyelids, palpebral conjunctiva, nasion, and bony dorsum.

Infraorbital nerve, a branch of maxillary nerve, innervates the lateral wall of lower nose, columella, and nasal vestibule **(Fig. 11)**.

The internal branch of anterior ethmoidal nerve innervates the anterior portion of lateral nasal wall and septum. Posterior ethmoidal nerve supplies superior half of the nasal cavity. Nasopalatine nerve, a branch from the sphenopalatine ganglion, is the main sensory innervation for the septum. Sphenopalatine nerve conveys sensation from posterior and central regions of the nasal cavity.[8]

Bony Vault

The bony vault is pyramidal in shape. The lateral walls consist of the frontal processes of the maxilla and the nasal bones with union to the nasal process of frontal bone in the midline. A "rocker deformity" occurs when lateral osteotomy is done too far cephalically, onto the nasal process of the frontal bone. When infracture of the bone is done, the superior segment narrows but the caudal segment moves out laterally, causing visible deformity and persistent widening. To avoid this deformity, osteotomies should either be done below the level of the medial canthus, or course medially before arriving at the nasal process of the frontal bone. The bony width of the bony lateral wall of the nose should be approximately 75% of the distance of a normal alar base on frontal view.[10]

Middle Cartilaginous Vault

The middle cartilaginous vault is formed by the upper lateral cartilages that are attached to the dorsal margin of the septum like wings. The cephalic ends extend deep to the nasal bones for a distance of 1 cm. The internal nasal valve is the triangle formed by caudal edge of upper lateral cartilage, septum, and nasal floor. Action of the internal valve is paradoxical, narrows on inspiration and widens on expiration. The optimal angle between the septum and upper lateral cartilage is 15°.[11] The width of the nasal valve can be increased with spreader grafts.

Lower Cartilaginous Vault

The lower cartilaginous vault consists of a pair of lower lateral cartilages. The lower lateral cartilage comprises a thin vertical medial crus resting on its footplate, the curved dome, also known as the middle crus, and the widened lateral crus **(Figs. 12 to 14)**.

The medial crus is subdivided into lower footplate segment and superior columellar segment. The footplates vary in shape, size, and angulation. The superior columella segment forms the narrow waist of the columella and its length determines the nostril length **(Fig. 15)**.

Columella-lobular junction is the junction between the paired vertically oriented medial crura and the divergent angular middle crura. It is the breakpoint in the columella's "double break."

Middle crus begins at the columella-lobular junction and ends at the lateral crura. It has two segments: a lobular segment and a domal segment. The shape of the lobular segment affects the tip shape. The domal segment is situated in

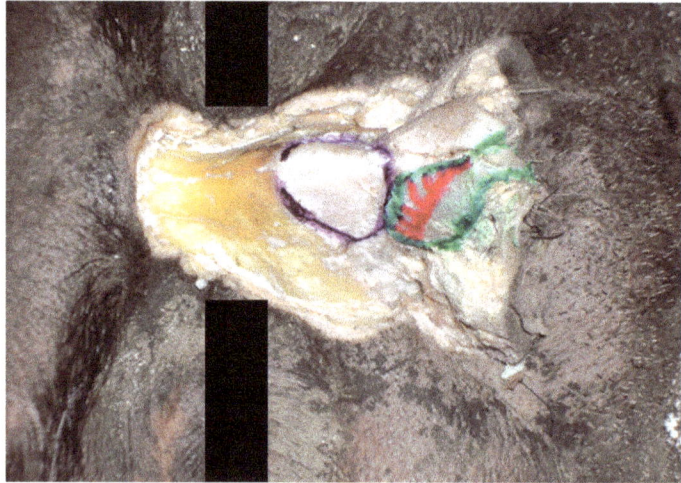

Fig. 12: Upper lateral cartilage (outlined by blue line) and lower lateral cartilage (outlined by green line) in cadaver.

Anatomy and Physiology

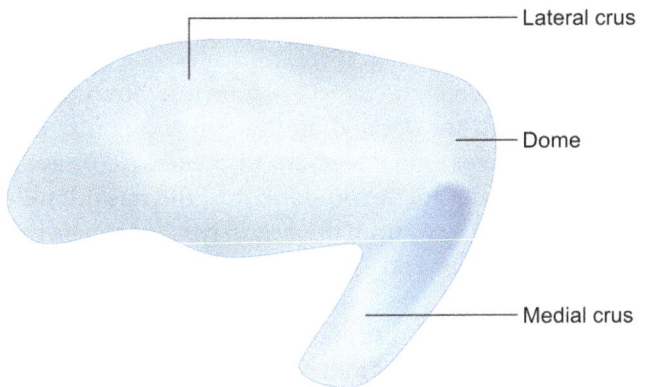

Fig. 13: Lower lateral cartilage.

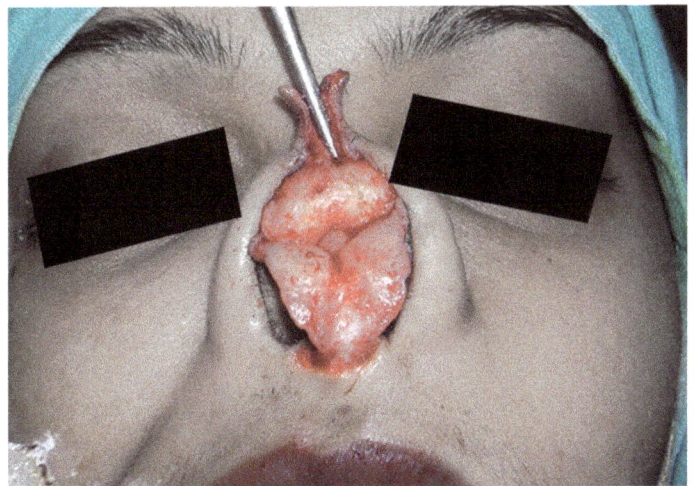

Fig. 14: Lower lateral cartilages and weak triangle after skeletonization.

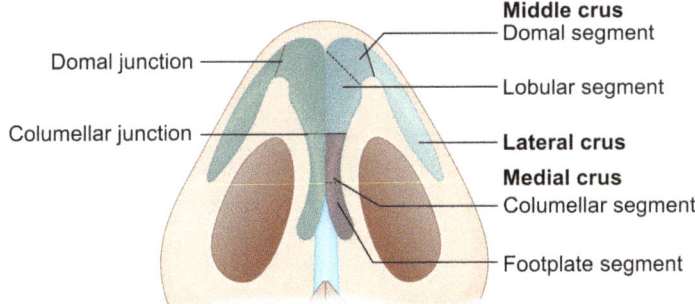

Fig. 15: Tip anatomy.

between medial and lateral genu and forms the domal notch, which in turn determines the soft triangles **(Fig. 16)**.

Domal junction indicates the transition from middle crura to lateral crura. The tip-defining points are situated on the domal junction line. The most aesthetic shape is a convex domal segment adjacent to a concave lateral crura.

The lateral crus is the main component of the nasal lobule. Laterally, the crus goes posteriorly away from the nostril rim and tapers in size.

The external nasal valve consists of the alar rim and the fibrofatty tissue in the nasal ala **(Fig. 17)**. Excessive resection of the lateral crura may cause weak external valve unable to resist the negative pressure of inspiration. At the external valve, inspiration is initiated with the nasalis muscle contracting and pulling up the lateral crus.[11]

On profile view, the columella is visible slightly lower than the alar border. The normal columellar show is 2–4 mm. In excessive columellar show, it is

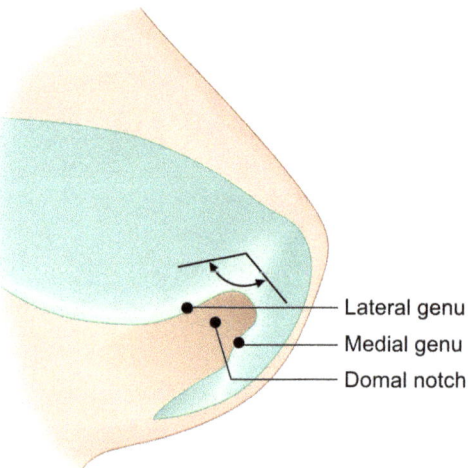

Fig. 16: Domal segment (middle crus) of lower lateral cartilage.

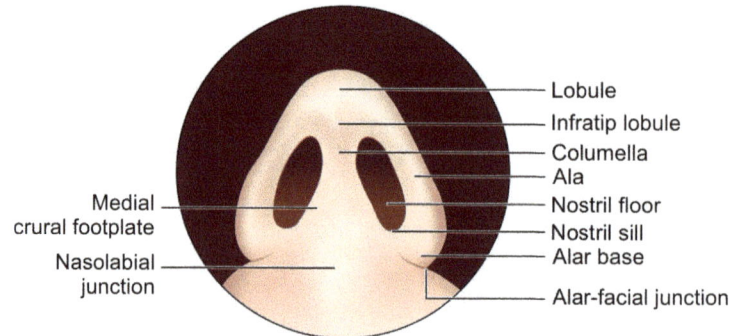

Fig. 17: Diagram of lobule, ala, and columella.

necessary to differentiate between alar retraction and a hanging columella.[12] At the upper ends, both medial crura diverge outward at an angle of 30° forming the width of the tip. The thin skin of columella is adherent to medial crura. Hanging columella is caused by either a weakened medial crural complex after rhinoplasty or by long caudal septum and/or prominent anterior nasal spine. The deformity can be detected by palpation of the medial crura and the caudal septum and then correction is done. The length of the columella should be equal to the height of the upper lip.[13]

The ideal projection of the nasal tip, or the distance of the tip from the face, is measured by using the Goode rule. Tip projection should be 55–60% of the distance between the nasion and tip-defining points.[8]

The nasal tip has two tip-defining points situated in the horizontal plane, which are the points on the domes of the nasal alae.[14]

The volume, width, definition, projection, rotation, and shape of the tip depend on the underlying anatomy and overlying surface aesthetics.

Tip analysis is done before operation and the tip factors such as volume, definition, width, projection, rotation, and position are studied to formulate the operative plan **(Fig. 18)**.

Tip volume depends on the size of the lateral crura. In most of the tip plasties, resection of the cephalic part of the lateral crura is done. This makes the tip smaller, improves definition, and rotates the tip slightly upward. Tip suturing also becomes easier.

Tip definition is the visibility of the dome-defining points from the rest of the alar cartilage. The best tip definition is produced by a convex domal segment with an adjacent concave lateral crura. The skin envelope is also very important.

Width is related to the interdomal distance and is measured on the skin surface between the two tip-defining points.

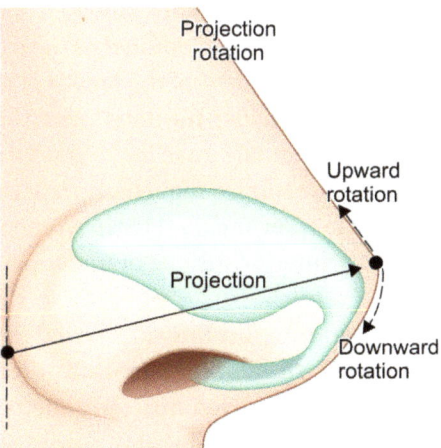

Fig. 18: Projection and rotation of nasal tip.

There are different tip shapes including broad, boxy, pinched, pinocchio, and various other shapes. The boxy tip comprises thick alar cartilages, but weak alar sidewalls which can collapse if not supported with rim grafts.

Nasal tip surgery is the most difficult part of rhinoplasty. One who can perform tip plasty well is said to be a masterhand in rhinoplasty.

The following fibrous connections are important for maintenance of the shape of the nasal tip:
- Fibrous connection between the upper lateral and lower lateral cartilages.
- Connecting the lateral border of the lower lateral cartilages to the pyriform aperture. Three to four accessory cartilages are interspersed in the fibrous tissue.
- The interdomal ligament and anterior septal angle.
- Attachment of the lower end of the medial crus to septal cartilage.
- The ligamentous connection between nasal skin and dorsal septum to the posterior margins of the domes (Sling of Pitanguy).

The nasal tip is mobile and fixed to upper lateral cartilages and the septum by scroll ligaments and the midline Pitanguy's ligament. These ligaments are formed by the thickening of the SMAS in the supratip region and allow upward and downward movement of the nasal tip.[15]

Anderson first proposed the rhinoplasty tripod theory. The structure of the two lower lateral cartilages forms a functional tripod that provides support to the nasal tip. The two lateral crura form two legs of the tripod, and two conjoined medial crura form the third leg. The medial crura are shorter than the lateral crura. The medial crural foundation is supported by the attachments to the septum. Intercartilaginous incisions and removal of the cephalic part of the lateral crura (cephalic trimming) disrupts the interlocking arrangement of the upper and lower lateral cartilages.

The width of the alar base should be approximately the same width as the intercanthal distance. Ideal alar width is defined as the distance between the alar facial grooves which is equal to 70% of the length of the nose.[5]

The female nose is relatively smaller, the dorsum and lobule narrower than that of the male. In profile, the female nose looks good with a slight supratip depression while, in the male dorsum, a slight hump is acceptable. The normal nasolabial angle is 90–105° in men and 95–115° in women.[16]

In an aesthetic face, the anterior surface of the upper and lower lips rest on the nasomental line.[17]

When the chin lies anterior to this line, it is called prognathic and when it lies posterior to this line, it is called retrognathic. A retrognathic chin can give the impression of an overprojected nose and the reverse happens in a prognathic chin. Genioplasty or chin implant procedures are therefore often combined with rhinoplasty.[18]

Nasal Septum

The three major constituents are perpendicular plate of ethmoid, vomer, and septal cartilage. These articulate with other bones which contribute in a minor way to the formation of the septum. These minor components are anterior nasal spines of maxillae, nasal crests of maxillary and palatine bones, rostrum and crest of sphenoid bone, nasal spine of frontal bones and crests of nasal bones **(Fig. 19)**. The perichondrium of the septal cartilage is continuous with the periosteum of the ethmoid bone but the subperichondrial space of septal cartilage is not continuous with the subperiosteal space of premaxilla and vomer **(Fig. 20)**. The mucoperichondrium covering the septal

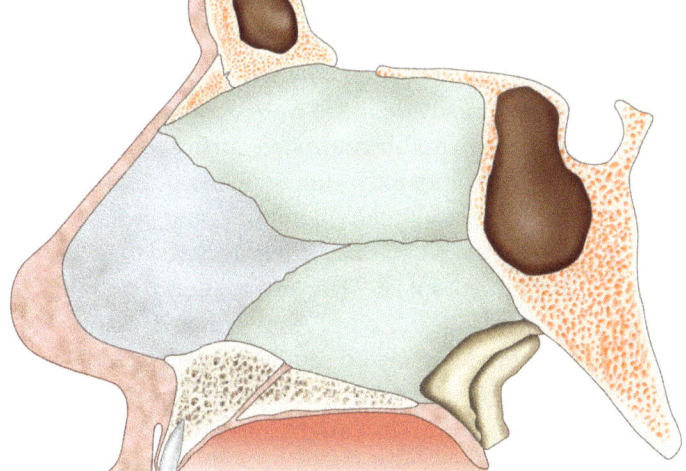

Fig. 19: Septum.

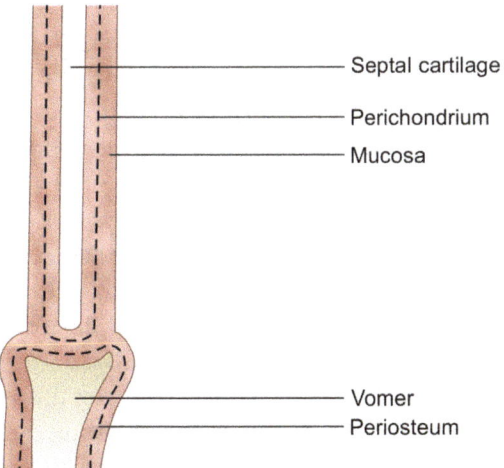

Fig. 20: Distribution of perichondrium and periosteum in nasal septum.

cartilage inserts tightly into the junction of the septal cartilage with crest of the maxilla, where mucoperiosteum enveloping the crest of the maxilla is also inserted firmly. During septoplasty, tears at the mucoperichondrial flaps usually occur at the junction of the septal cartilage with the crest of maxilla. As the resilient connective tissue fibers present at the junction are stronger than the mucoperichondrium itself, there is a chance of tearing the mucoperichondrium rather than the fibers of the junction if one attempts blunt dissection. Though the periosteum of the perpendicular plate of ethmoid and vomer is not continuous, their separation during septoplasty operation is not a problem.

The perpendicular plate of the ethmoid is continuous with the cribriform plate superiorly. Any traumatic manipulation of the superior part of the bony septum may cause a CSF rhinorrhea and/or anosmia, particularly in patients with a history of recent fractures or females with osteoporosis. If the superior bony septum is deviated causing nasal obstruction, it should be partially resected sharply rather than pulled or twisted during septoplasty.

Inferoposteriorly, the vomer forms the bony nasal septum. Inferior to the vomer, the crest of the maxilla is situated anteriorly, and the crest of the palatine bone is situated posteriorly. When this crest is deviated to form septal spur, it must be resected during septoplasty. The anteroinferior margin of the caudal septum is attached to the anterior nasal spine of maxilla. The anterior septal angle is the junction of the dorsal and caudal borders of septal cartilage and the posterior septal angle is the area where the septal cartilage articulates with the nasal spine anteroinferiorly. The flared wings of the upper lateral cartilages are firmly attached to the dorsal part of septal cartilage in their upper four fifths and provide shape and support to the middle third of the nose.

The part of the septum, anterior to the imaginary line (Cottle's line) dropped from the nasal process of frontal bone to the anterior nasal spine, provides principal support to the nose. The septal part posterior to this line provides minimum nasal support and, therefore, can be excised with less concern than septal cartilage anterior to this line **(Fig. 21)**.

Gross deviations of the ethmoid not only cause posterior airway obstruction but also may prevent adequate lateral wall infracture by osteotomy in order to make the nose narrow. If this bony deviation is not corrected, it can be responsible for postoperative nasal obstruction after osteotomies.

The membranous septum is highly mobile and is situated in between the caudal margin of the septal cartilage and the columella. It consists of two layers of vestibular skin with intervening subcutaneous tissue. Transfixion incision is made, either partially or completely, at the junction of the septal cartilage and the membranous septum. Complete transfixion incision causes division of the fibers of the depressor septi muscle and detachment of medial crura footplates from the caudal septum, thereby reducing the vital tip support mechanism

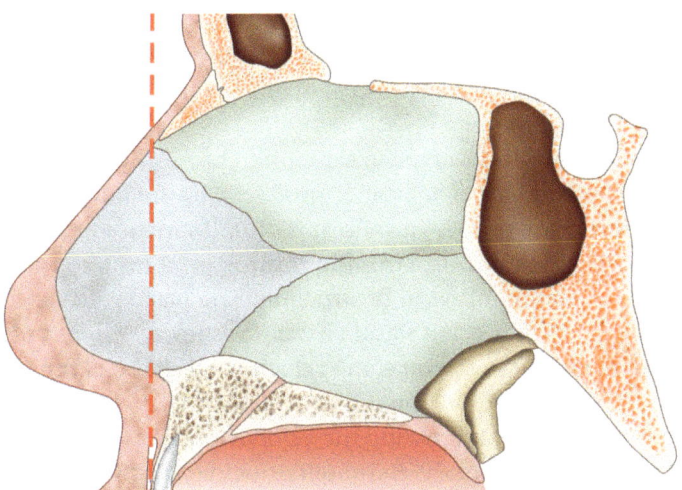

Fig. 21: Cottle's line: Imaginary line dropped from the nasal process of frontal bone to the anterior nasal spine.

leading to deprojection of the tip. To prevent this, partial transfixion incision can be made. In most cases of rhinoplasty, the membranous septum is preserved to prevent unpleasant surgical results.[19]

Function of the septum: It supports the dorsum of the nose and maintains the position of the nasal tip and columella. It separates the nasal cavities and helps in shock absorption for the floor of the frontal sinus.

PHYSIOLOGY OF THE NOSE

A knowledge of physiology of the nose is essential and should be acquired by those who want to be a rhinoplasty surgeon. The nose provides some protection to the lower respiratory passages through its treatment of the inspired air. The air is purified, warmed, and humidified. Vibrissae of the vestibule entrap coarser particles. The cilia of the nasal cavity are bathed in a viscous layer of mucus. Fine particles stick to the mucus and are impelled as a continuous "conveyor belt" into the nasopharynx. The complete sheet of mucus is cleared into the pharynx every 10–20 minutes. The inspiratory air currents are mainly moistened by the transudation of fluid through the respiratory epithelium. It is further moistened by the secretion from the mucosal glands and goblet cells of the respiratory epithelium.

Adults condition more than 14,000 L of air per day, requiring more than 680 g of water, approximately 20% of our daily intake of water. The air currents are affected by a number of factors, including the structure of the cartilaginous framework, the shape and direction of the nasal septum, the degree of nasolabial angle, the size of the nasal turbinates, and the thickness of the nasal mucosa.

In adults, the length of the nasal airway is about 10 cm. Within this air passage, the air is conditioned to approximately 31–37°C in temperature with a 75% relative humidity. About 70 kcal of energy are needed to perform the functions of air conditioning.[20]

The position and shape of the nasal septum have only a partial role for an efficient nasal airway. Nasal resistance produced by the intranasal structures is very important for proper nasal respiration. Inadequate resistance due to overwide airway found in atrophic rhinitis or complete turbinectomy produces the sensation of nasal obstruction. The nasal valve and the nasal valve area produce significant nasal airway resistance. The nasal valve area regulates nasal airflow, resistance, the velocity and shape of the air stream.[15] The airflow from the external nares passes to the internal nasal valve, where the air passage narrows increasing the velocity of flow while narrowing the column of air. According to the Bernoulli principle, as this airflow increases, the lateral pressure decreases. Normal cartilage of the internal nasal valve does not collapse inward with quiet inspiration. If the valve area is abnormally compliant due to weakened upper lateral cartilages, forceful inspiration will lead to internal collapse and further narrowing with a sensation of obstruction. From this valve area, the air passes along the middle meatus, between the inferior turbinate and septum, and along the upper border of the middle turbinate. The airflow occurs in a parabolic curve, and a smaller amount passes through the inferior meatus and along the floor. The anterior end of the inferior turbinate is important in regulating the airflow. Expiratory air currents pass in roughly the same parabolic curve as the inspiratory currents. Frictional resistance at the internal nasal valve allows only part of the expired air to reach the outside directly. Eddies are formed by the remainder, partly under cover of the middle turbinate.

In long nose with drooping tip, the air currents are directed more superiorly under the nasal roof. In saddle nose, instead of the normal parabolic curve, the air currents are directed along the nasal floor.

The nasal cycle varies from person to person. Nasal mucosa undergoes rhythmic cyclical congestion and decongestion, thus controlling the airflow through the nasal passages. The nasal cycle lasts from 2 to 4 hours.

Inspiratory flow usually occurs as laminar airflow. Duration of inspiration is about 2 seconds. Expiratory airflow has more components of turbulent flow. Duration of expiration is about 3 seconds.[21]

The nose is responsible for nearly half of the total airway resistance; a third of the resistance is contributed by the external valve and two thirds by the internal valve. The internal valve regulates respiration by limiting the airflow so that it does not exceed the ability of the nose to process it. During deep inspiration enlargement of the nostril and narrowing of the internal valve occurs, whereas during expiration narrowing of the nostril and enlargement of the internal valve occurs.

REFERENCES

1. McCollough EG. Rhinoplasty: A humbling experience. J Oral Maxillofac Surg. 1989;47:1132-41.
2. Tardy ME, Brown R. Surgical anatomy of the nose. New York: Raven Press; 1990.
3. Toriumi DM, Becker DG. Anatomy. Rhinoplasty Dissection Manual. Philadelphia: Lippincott Williams & Wilkins; 2010.
4. Gunter JP, Rohrich RJ, Adams WP. Dallas Rhinoplasty: Nasal Surgery by the Masters, 2nd edition. St. Louis, USA; Quality Medical Publishing Inc.; 2007.
5. Powell N, Humphreys B. Proportions of the aesthetic face, 1st edition. New York: Thieme Stratton; 1984.
6. Burget GC, Menick FJ. The subunit principle in nasal reconstruction. Plast Reconstr Surg. 1985;76(2):239-47.
7. Kim TK, Jeong JY. Surgical anatomy for Asian rhinoplasty. Arch Craniofac Surg. 2019;20(3):147-57.
8. Chang EW. (2013). Nasal Anatomy. [online] Available from: emedicine.medscape.com/article/835134-overview. [Last accessed May, 2023].
9. Toriumi DM, Mueller RA, Grosch T, Bhattacharya TK, Larrabee WF. Vascular anatomy of the nose and the external rhinoplasty approach. Arch Oto/Head Neck Surgery. 1996;122:24-34.
10. Shah AR. (2010). Anatomy of the nose. Rhinoplasty Information. [online] Available from: https://www.shahfacialplastics.com/blog/rhinoplasty-articles/anatomy-nose-rhinoplasty-information. [Last accessed May, 2023].
11. Shubailat G. Secondary rhinoplasty. Indian J Plast Surg. 2008;41:80-7.
12. Gunter JP, Rohrich RJ, and Friedman RM. Classification and correction of alar-columellar discrepancies in rhinoplasty. Plast Reconstr Surg. 1996;97:643.
13. Simons RL. Nasal tip projection, ptosis, and supratip thickening. Ear Nose Throat J. 1982;61(8):452-5.
14. Daniel RK. Tip Refinement Grafts: The Designer tip. Aesthetic Surg J. 2009;29(6):528-37.
15. Daniel RK, Palhazi P. The Nasal Ligaments and Tip Support in Rhinoplasty: An Anatomical Study. Aesthet Surg J. 2018;38(4):357-68.
16. Bernstein L. Aesthetics in Rhinoplasty. St. Louis. MO: CV Mosby; 1978.
17. Aufricht G. Combined plastic surgery of the nose and chin; resume of twenty-seven years' experience. Am J Surg. 1958;95(2):231-6.
18. Guyuron B, Raszewski RL. A critical comparison of osteoplastic and alloplastic augmentation genioplasty. Aesthetic Plast Surg. 1990;14(3):199-206.
19. Tardy ME. Rhinoplasty: The Art and the Science, 1st edition. Philadelphia, USA: WB. Saunders Co; 1997.
20. McCarthy JG (Ed). Plastic Surgery, Volume 3, The Face, Part 2. Philadelphia; US: Saunders; 2011.
21. Kerr A (Ed). Rhinology. Scott-Brown's Otolaryngology, 6th edition. Oxford: Butterworth-Heinemann; 1997.

CHAPTER 3

Instruments and Preoperative Assessment

INTRODUCTION

Appropriate instruments are necessary to perform a reliable operation. The main goal is to do rhinoplasty with minimal tissue injury, to prevent unpredictable scar formation, and to make sure of good long-term results. Sharp and good-quality instruments should be used to lessen surgical trauma and to enter the correct surgical planes leading to reduced bleeding, less duration of the operation and, ultimately, better outcome.

INSTRUMENTS

The following basic instruments are required for rhinoplasty **(Fig. 1)**:
- Kilner alar retractor to expose alar rim during making marginal incision
- Fomon ball point retractor to retract during external rhinoplasty
- Fomon angular scissors for cutting dorsal part of septum
- Malinac retractor to retract nasal skin
- Aufricht retractor to retract the skin during external rhinoplasty
- Chisel (9 mm) for removal of hump
- Freer mucoperichondrial elevator to elevate mucoperichondrium during septoplasty
- Gillies osteotome (5 mm) for medial osteotomy
- Silver nasal chisel (3 mm) for right lateral osteotomy

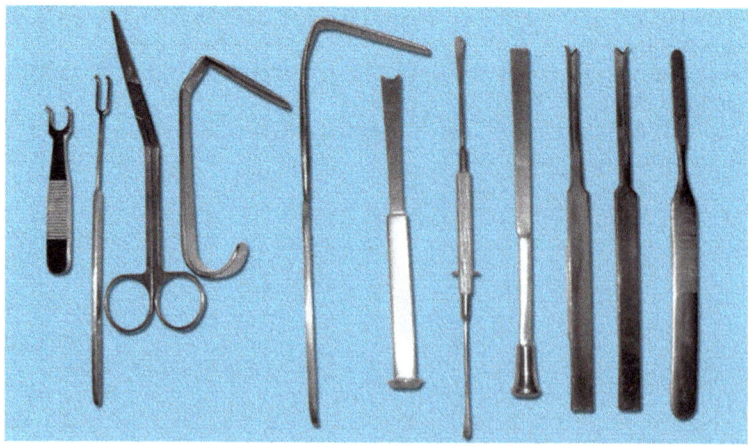

Fig. 1: Instruments used in rhinoplasty.

- Silver nasal chisel (3 mm) for left lateral osteotomy
- Rasp (pull) for rasping small hump and bony irregularities.

Many options are available when choosing a suture needle. Round body needle is ideal for soft tissue and fascia. Needles are also available in conventional cutting or reverse cutting form. A conventional cutting needle has a cutting edge on the inside of the curve and a flat edge on the outside, whereas a reverse cutting needle is the opposite, having a flat surface on the inside with cutting edge to the outside. Reverse cutting needles have minimum risk of cutting through tissue in a direction perpendicular to the wound edge.

PREOPERATIVE ASSESSMENT

The final result of any rhinoplasty operation depends on the individual patient's anatomy and the skill of the surgeon. No two noses are similar. The surgeon must diagnose the limitations inherent in each patient. Patients with minimal deformities usually expect perfection; but patients with major deformities like a severe crooked nose or a large hump may not complain if there is any minor imperfection after the surgery.

Proper selection of cases and their preoperative assessment is very important.

Preoperative assessment depends on a sense of beauty, harmony, and proportion combined with keen observational skills. More mistakes in rhinoplasty result from not seeing than from not knowing. The surgeon, therefore, must train himself accordingly.[1] The result of the operation should be a beautiful nose, harmonic with the rest of the face.[2] Attractive women with beautiful face have less marked jaw, and smaller noses, in comparison with men.[3] In males, the nasal profile should be straight or slightly convex, in women straight or slightly concave.[4]

Facial proportions guide us in planning procedures but should not be taken as absolute. It is to be noted that the ideal measurements vary between ethnicities.[5] An attractive western nose, although may be beautiful as a nose itself, does not harmonize with the Asian face. Anatomic characteristics of the Asian nose along with differences in aesthetic standards demand that they be approached in a different way.

The western concept of the ideal nose is the leptorrhine nose, which comprises a thinner dorsum and more slender nostrils than the other two general nasal types, platyrrhine (broad) and mesorrhine (intermediate). African American noses are thought to be broader and flatter (platyrrhine). Among leptorrhine noses, the Greek subtype (straight profile) is considered as the most desired variant over the Roman (convex) or Armenoid (convex with ptotic tip) subtypes. Latin American patients are mixed-race patients commonly known as mestizo, Hispanic, or Latino people. Most Latin patients consider their noses too big and too broad for their faces. Patients usually like their noses to be more defined, with greater definition but without looking bigger.[6] Every attempt should be made to create a nose that is harmonious with the individual's face and respect the cultural differences in the concept of beauty. In a study done by Mehta N (2017) on Indian noses, North Indians have been found to have the longest and the narrowest nose (leptorrhine). Broadest nose was found among South Indians and people from the Himalayan area had the shortest nose. On average, Indian population had a mesorrhine nose.[7]

Inspection and palpation of nose are done. The skin is examined for thickness and elasticity. In noses with thin skin, less postoperative edema and quick wound healing are observed but rhinoplasty should be done very carefully as postoperative structural irregularities will be visible more prominently in these cases. The elasticity of the skin is less in the elderly. Skin with moderate thickness produces the best result in rhinoplasty. It is difficult to achieve a good definition of the nose in patients with thick nasal skin with plenty of subcutaneous tissue.[8] The nose should be examined for its length and projection, and any deformities of the tip, columella, cartilaginous and bony dorsum, and radix. Examination of columellar width and length is done. In case of too short medial crura, a longitudinal cartilage graft is needed. Correction of overprojection of tip may need reduction of the width and length of medial crura.[9] Projection of the nasal tip is measured by the distance from the junction of the upper lip with subnasale to the tip. The nostril looks like falling water drop, and its width is same as the width of the columella. The long axis of the nostrils is directed anteriorly and medially about 45° to the axis of the columella.[10] Ala is palpated to feel the thickness of the cartilage. Tip support is tested by pressing the tip downward and then releasing it to see the tip recoil.

Deviations of the nose can be assessed by drawing a vertical line from the midpoint between the medial canthi to the upper lip and central incisors, provided there are no marked facial asymmetries **(Fig. 2)**.[11]

First, nasal cavity is examined without nasal speculum to evaluate the internal valve region. Internal nasal valve is situated at a distance of about 1.3 cm posterior to the nostrils.[12] Cottle test is a technique used to assess an internal valve disorder. Here, the cheek is pulled laterally during quiet inspiration to widen the cross-sectional area of the internal nasal valve. If the patient feels an improvement in breathing with this maneuver, the Cottle test is positive. This is an indication for placement of spreader graft to improve the angle of the internal valve. During normal inspiration, nose is inspected for any alar collapse. A false-positive Cottle test may be found in patients with alar collapse. A false-negative Cottle sign may occasionally be observed in patients with scarring in the valve area.[13] With nasal speculum, the nose is examined for deviated nasal septum (DNS), hypertrophy of turbinates, or any nasal pathology. To visualize the deeper part of the nasal cavity, the axis of the headlight should be at the same level as the visual axis. A probe is introduced into one nasal cavity to gently support and lateralize the internal and external

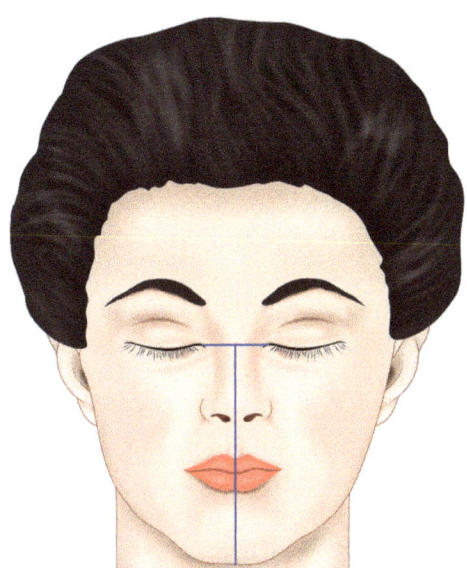

Fig. 2: To appreciate deviation, a vertical line is drawn from the center point between the pupils or medial canthi.

nasal valves. The patient is asked about any improvement in airflow while gently closing the opposite nostril. The location of support that gives maximal improvement in airflow is noted (modified Cottle test).[14]

The posterior septum is seen with a nasal endoscope. The endoscope is also necessary in diagnosing polyps, examining the severity and extent of posterior septal deviations and bony spurs, and identifying septal perforation or mucosal injury.

Rhinomanometry is done for an objective assessment of nasal airway resistance. Active rhinomanometry does flow measurement from the respiratory cycle. The three types of active rhinomanometry are anterior, postnasal, and posterior rhinomanometry. In passive rhinomanometry, airflow from an external source, such as an air pump is used.[15] Anterior rhinomanometry and acoustic rhinomanometry are most commonly used for clinical measurement of nasal airflow. Acoustic rhinomanometry can locate areas of constriction. However, acoustic rhinometry has a limited role in preoperative assessment and postoperative determination of objective outcomes. Unfortunately, efforts to link rhinometry measures with subjective perception of nasal patency have not met with convincing results.[16,17]

The expectations and mental status of the patient should be assessed.

To identify the high-risk patient during consultation is a major problem.[18] If a dissatisfied patient meets a surgeon who is satisfied with his work, the situation becomes very unpleasant.[19] Frequently, emotional disappointment of the patient causes dissatisfaction rather than an improper surgical technique.[20]

The surgeon should identify those patients who may create problems in postoperative period. Usually, these patients have unreasonable expectations, hyperesthetic, obsessive-compulsive, hesitant, depressive, impolite, fickle, flattering, noncooperating, "VIP" or overly talkative.[2] The simplified acronyms SYLVIA (secure, young, listens, verbal, intelligent, attractive) and SIMON (single, immature, male, overly expectant/obsessive, narcissistic) describe some of characteristics of the ideal and the high-risk patient, respectively.[21] Patients having body dysmorphic disorder usually concentrate on one part of the body, most commonly on the nose. Body dysmorphic disorder is a subjective perception of ugliness or physical defect that results in distress, although the appearance is within normal limits.[22] It is a chronic condition and affects both sexes equally. Picavet et al. found that only 2% of those undergoing rhinoplasty for a medical reason had body dysmorphic disorder whereas 43% of those undergoing rhinoplasty for purely cosmetic reasons had body dysmorphic disorder.[23] The outcome of the surgery is usually not satisfying for the patients with underlying psychiatric problem.[24] Psychiatric disorders were seen as a contraindication, even though this opinion was not supported by clear evidence.[25] By contrast, the motivation of the patients with posttraumatic deformities is high and usually results in a positive reaction to rhinoplasty.[26]

Detailed history is taken about the patency of both nostrils, asthma, headache, snoring, if there is any tendency for bleeding, family history of bleeding, hypertension and cardiac problems, allergy, aspirin intake, if prone to keloid formation, nasal injury, previous nasal surgery, sinus diseases and any addictions.[27] After examination of the nose, the surgical possibilities, expectations and limitations are discussed with the patient, taking the help of preoperative photographs. Patients should be informed about the possibility of postoperative pain, swelling of the face, bruising around the eyelids, nasal blockage due to anterior packing and the dressing. The patient should be asked to sign a document of "informed consent."

Time spent in preoperative assessment is never wasted, indeed, it is one key to a good result.[28]

The following investigations are necessary before rhinoplasty operation:
- Examination of blood for blood group, hemoglobin%, total count (TC), differential count (DC), erythrocyte sedimentation rate (ESR), bleeding time (BT), clotting time (CT), sugar, urea, creatinine, hepatitis B virus (HBV) antigens, hepatitis C virus (HCV) antibodies, human immunodeficiency virus (HIV) test
- Computed tomography (CT) scan of PNS in some cases
- X-ray chest—posteroanterior (PA) view
- Electrocardiogram
- Psychological evaluation if needed
- Photographs for external nasal deformity
- Nasal endoscopy.

PHOTOGRAPHY

Photographs are essential for preoperative planning and for comparison with postoperative results **(Figs. 3A to F)**. In most cases, four views are taken:

1. *Frontal view* is taken with the patient looking straight into the camera with horizontal position of the eyebrows. An equal amount of pinna should be seen on both sides.
2. *Lateral view* (on both sides) is taken with the Frankfort plane (the line passing through the superior border of the external auditory canal and the inferior border of the infraorbital rim) remaining horizontal. The nearest eyebrow should be completely visible, whereas the contralateral eyebrow must be invisible.
3. *Basal view* is taken with both the nostrils visible clearly and the tip of the nose in a more or less vertical position. The head is deflected backward so that the nasal tip is projected just between the eyebrows. The upper lip is seen completely whereas the chin and ears are not.
4. *Oblique view* (on both sides) provides extra information about the lateral nasal wall. The body and head are in the same position as for the side view except that the head is now turned 135° instead of 90°. The nasal tip is aligned with the cheek contour. The oblique view is required to determine whether the nasal hump is a midline or a side wall defect. The left oblique view provides information about the right nose and vice

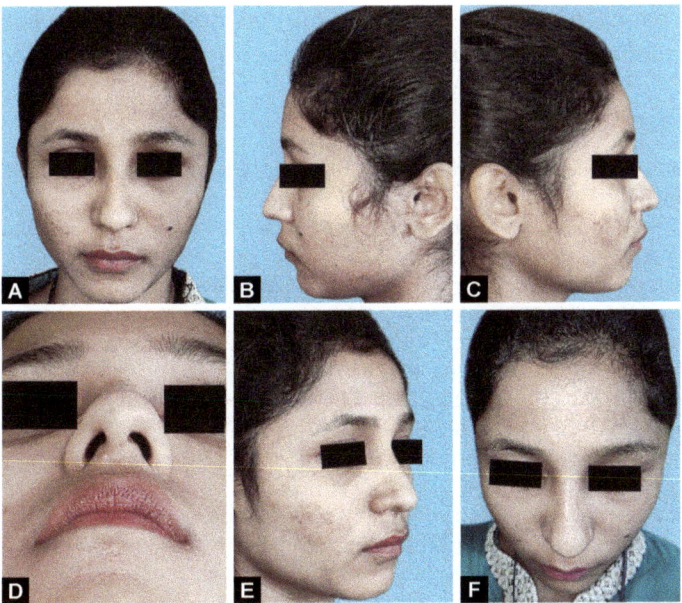

Figs. 3A to F: (A) Frontal view; (B) Left lateral view; (C) Right lateral view; (D) Basal view; (E) Oblique view; and (F) Helicopter view.

versa. In the oblique view, the caudal edge of the lateral crus and the lobule are best studied.

Sometimes, an additional view like topdown or *helicopter view* becomes necessary. In the helicopter view, the nasal tip is located at the central point of the lip. In this view, aesthetic lines and lateral crural convexity are best understood. Dorsal deviations are also seen.

Photography can be taken with any SLR camera in a photography studio. 100-mm macrolens is used to get a better view.

For background, blue color can be used to avoid reflection or absorption of excessive light rays. To prevent shadow formation, 1-m distance should be kept between the background and the patient. 2-m distance is required between the patient and the camera.

Going closer to the patient and zooming out will make a "fisheye" photograph, where the nose and cheeks will be larger and the pinna smaller.

Apaydin F et al. (2009) mentioned that they used a studio with two flashes and a full-frame SLR camera with 105-mm macrolens to take lifesize 1:1 photograph. This is helpful for aesthetic and photometric analysis and for postoperative comparison. These photographs are transferred into Rhinobase, a special program used to store the data of the patient and enabling the surgeon to use an automated facial analysis tool.[29]

Computer morphing of the preoperative photographs has been found to increase communication with the patient and helps in judging expectations of the patient.[30] It is necessary to show different options to the patient to perceive what the patient really wants. However, the patient should be explained that it is only a method of communication and does not imply a guaranteed result.

REFERENCES

1. Fomon G, Bhll J. In: Thomas CC (Ed). Rhinoplasty: New concepts. Charles C. Thomas: Springfield; 1970. p. 111.
2. Tardy ME. Rhinoplasty—The Art and the Science, 1st edition. Philadelphia, USA: WB Saunders Co.; 1997.
3. Perrett DI, May KA, Yoshikawa S. Facial shape and judgements of female attractiveness. Nature. 1994;368(6468):239-42.
4. Tezel E, Durmus FN. A new instrument for achieving a natural nasofrontal angle. J Plast Reconstr Aesthet Surg. 2009;62(12):617-19.
5. Fang F, Clapham PJ, Chung KC. A systematic review of interethnic variability in facial dimensions. Plast Reconstr Surg. 2011;127(2):874-81.
6. Cobo R. Structural rhinoplasty in Latin American patients. Facial Plast Surg. 2013;29:171-83.
7. Mehta N, Srivastava RK. The Indian nose: An anthropometric analysis. Journal of Plastic, Reconstructive & Aesthetic Surgery. 2017;70(10):1472-82.
8. Mathes SJ, Hentz VR. Plastic Surgery, Vol. II- The Head and Neck, Part-I, 2nd edition. Philadelphia, USA: Saunders Elsevier Inc.; 2006.
9. Gunter JP, Rohrich RJ, Adams WP. Dallas Rhinoplasty-Nasal Surgery by the Masters, 2nd edition. St. Louis, USA: Quality Medical Publishing Inc.; 2007.

10. Elsahy N. Plastic and reconstructive surgery of the nose, 1st edition. Philadelphia, USA: WB Saunders Co.; 2000.
11. Shah AR. (2010). Anatomy of the nose. Rhinoplasty Information. [online] Available from: https://www.shahfacialplastics.com/blog/rhinoplasty-articles/anatomy-nose-rhinoplasty-information. [Last accessed May, 2023].
12. Trenite GJN. Rhinoplasty: A Practical Guide to Functional and Aesthetic Surgery, 3rd edition. Netherlands: Kugler Publication, Hague; 2005.
13. Krzeski A. Wyklady z chirurgii nosa, 1st edition. Via Medica Gdansk, Poland; 2005.
14. Constantinides M, Galli SK, Miller PJ. A simple and reliable method of patient evaluation in the surgical treatment of nasal obstruction. Ear, Nose Throat J. 2002;81:734.
15. Kerr A, ed. Rhinology. Scott-Brown's Otolaryngology, 6th edition. Oxford: Butterworth-Heinemann;1997.
16. Reber M, Rahm F, Monnier P. The role of acoustic rhinometry in the pre- and postoperative evaluation of surgery for nasal obstruction. Rhinology. 1998;36(4):184-7.
17. Hardcastle PF, White A, Prescott RJ. Clinical and rhinometric assessment of the nasal airway- do they measure the same entity? Clin Otolaryngol Allied Sci. 1988;13(3):185-91.
18. Slator R, Harris DL. Are rhinoplasty patients potentially mad? Br J Plast Surg. 1992;45:301.
19. Moses S, Mahler D. After aesthetic rhinoplasty: new looks and psychological outlooks on post-surgical satisfaction. Aesthetic Plast Surg. 1984;8:213.
20. Goin MK, Rees TD. A prospective study of patients' psychological reactions to rhinoplasty. Ann Plast Surg. 1991;27:210.
21. Adamson PA, Chen T. The dangerous dozen: avoiding potential problem patients in cosmetic surgery. Facial Plast Surg Clin North Am. 2008;16(2):195-202.
22. Jakubietz M, Jakubietz RJ, Kloss DF, Gruenert JJ. Body dysmorphic disorder: diagnosis and approach. Plast Reconstr Surg. 2007;119(6):1924-30.
23. Picavet VA, Prokopakis EP, Gabriels L, Jorissen M, Hellings PW. High prevalence of body dysmorphic disorder symptoms in patients seeking rhinoplasty. Plast Reconstr Surg. 2011;128(2):509-17.
24. Alavi M, Kalafi Y, Dehbozorgi GR, Javadpour A. Body dysmorphic disorder and other psychiatric morbidity in aesthetic rhinoplasty candidates. J Plast Reconstr Aesthet Surg. 2011;64 (6):738-41.
25. Meerloo J. The fate of one's face. Psychiatric quarterly. 1956;30:31.
26. Dziewulski P, Dujon D, Spyriounis P, Griffiths RW, Shaw JD. A retrospective analysis of the results of 218 consecutive rhinoplasties. Br J Plast Surg. 1995;48(7):451-4.
27. Krzeski A. [Podstawy chirurgii nosa]. In: Polish, 1st Edn. Via Medica, ISBN 83-89861-10-0, Gdansk, Poland; 2004.
28. Taylor JR. Things I wish I had been taught about rhinoplasty. Can J Plast Surg. Winter. 2010;18(4):129.
29. Apaydin F, Akyildiz S, Hecht DA, Toriumi DM. Rhinobase: a comprehensive database, facial analysis, and picture-archiving software for rhinoplasty. Arch Facial Plast Surg. 2009;11(3):209-11.
30. Ozkul T, Ozkul MH. Computer simulation tool for rhinoplasty planning. Comput Biol Med. 2004;34(8):697-718.

Anesthesia

Rhinoplasty can be done under local or general anesthesia. Most patients of rhinoplasty tolerate local anesthesia well. The endotracheal tube during general anesthesia distorts the patient's mouth and the full view of the patient's face cannot be obtained. Local anesthesia (topical along with infiltration) is preferred because of low risks and more or less blood less surgical field.

Oral tranquilizers (diazepam), given the night before and 2 hours before surgery and a discussion about the anesthetic and surgical procedures, are very helpful for the patient's peaceful state of mind. Combination of pentazocine 30 mg or pethidine 50 mg with promethazine 25 mg is given intramuscularly 1/2 hour before the surgery. The aim of premedication is to achieve relief of anxiety, making the patient calm and cooperative.

The patient should lie on the table in a slight reverse Trendelenburg position with the head elevated by about 20°. This helps in venous and lymphatic drainage and causes less bleeding. Before infiltration, sterile cotton pledgets soaked in 4% lignocaine solution mixed with adrenaline are placed inside the nasal cavities for surface anesthesia. One cotton pledget is placed along the middle meatus posteriorly up to the sphenopalatine foramen. Another cotton pledget is placed anterosuperiorly up to the root of the nose for effect on the anterior ethmoidal nerve. The pledgets are removed after 5–10 minutes.

Lignocaine 2% in combination with 1:100,000 or 1:150,000 dilution of adrenaline is the most commonly used injectable agent for infiltration anesthesia in rhinoplasty. The lower concentration is used in older patients or in patients with any cardiovascular problem or peripheral vascular disease. Incision is made after 10–15 minutes. The lignocaine with adrenaline has an effective duration of 1.5–2 hours of anesthesia. However, bupivacaine (0.25%–0.5%), which has a considerably prolonged anesthetic effect, can be used; but in higher concentration (0.5%), it may cause tissue damage. Infiltration should be done slowly at low pressure, using a long thin needle (27 gauge).

The infraorbital nerves are blocked by inserting the needle through the lateral wall of nose toward the infraorbital foramen and about 0.5 mL of the solution is injected.[1] The infraorbital foramen is situated about 6–8 mm inferior to the infraorbital rim, in line with the pupil. The foramen can be reached by a percutaneous or sublabial injection, with the needle introduced superolaterally toward the foramen, the noninjecting hand protecting the eye. Regional anesthesia by nerve block technique facilitates outpatient nasal surgery and avoids the need for general anesthesia.[2]

The needle prick is done at the junction of the floor of the right nostril and columella and is advanced up to the left alar facial junction **(Fig. 1)**. The needle is next rotated and infiltration is done into the columella as the needle is withdrawn **(Fig. 2)**. Without removal, the needle is rotated into the nasal base of the right side and the procedure is repeated **(Fig. 3)**.

The ala is retracted cephalically with thumb to expose the caudal margin of the upper lateral cartilage. The needle is inserted parallel to the long axis of the exposed upper lateral cartilage through the intercartilaginous

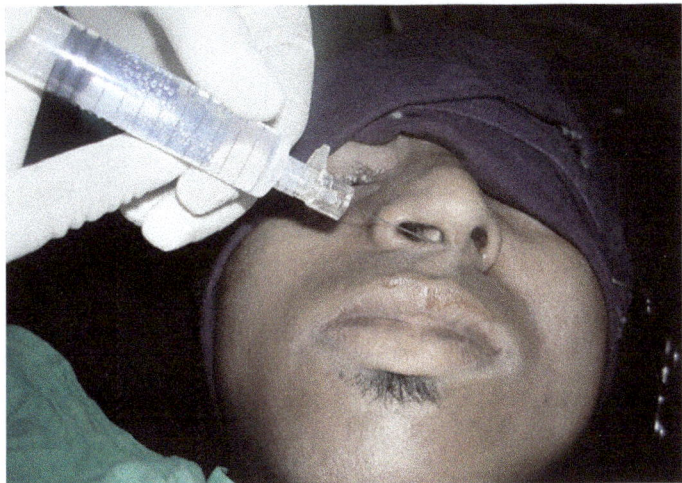

Fig. 1: Needle prick for initiation of infiltration of base and floor of nose.

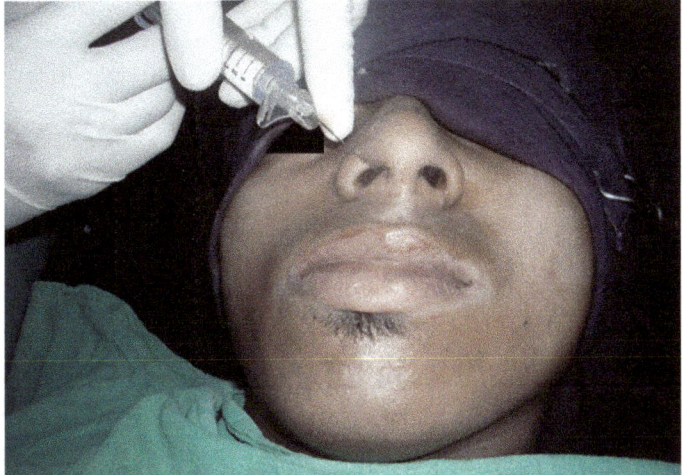

Fig. 2: Needle is rotated and infiltration is done into the columella as the needle is withdrawn.

incision area **(Fig. 4)**. Any pain sensation of the needle prick may be masked by simultaneous blunt pinching of the skin elsewhere on the nose or face. This phenomenon is called "lateral inhibition" **(Fig. 5)**. The needle is pushed along the lateral wall and dorsum of nose and infiltration is done just superficial to the perichondrium of the upper lateral cartilages and the periosteum of the nasal bones. With rotation and advancing the needle, fresh areas can be infiltrated over the dorsum. The infiltration is repeated on the opposite side of the nose. Infiltration in the immediate supraperichondrial and supraperiosteal planes

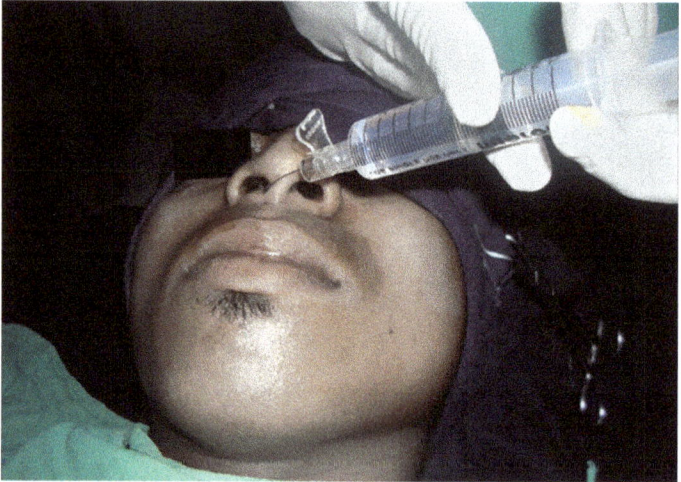

Fig. 3: Needle is rotated into the nasal base of the right side for contralateral infiltration.

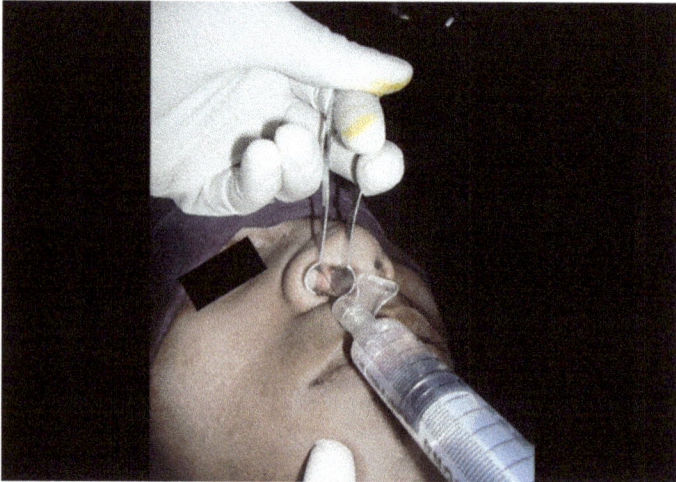

Fig. 4: Intercartilaginous penetration of the needle into proper plane over nasal dorsum.

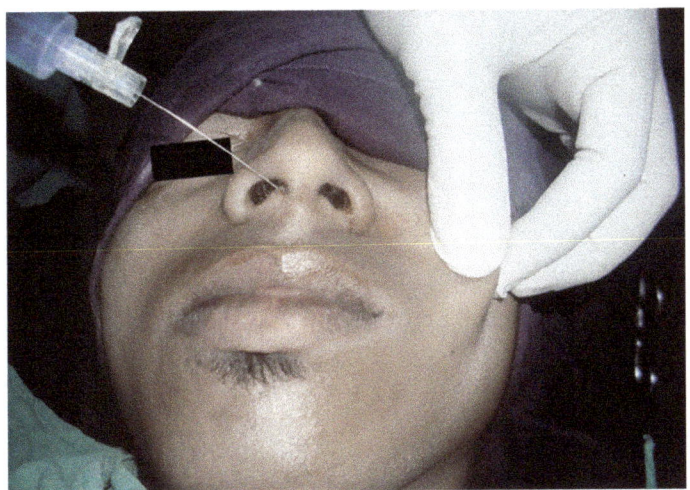

Fig. 5: A firm but gentle pinching of the cheek simultaneous with intranasal needle prick—"lateral inhibition."

over the upper and lower lateral cartilages and nasal bones causes an almost bloodless field for rhinoplasty. If the infiltration is done in the subcutaneous tissue or epithelium instead of the surgical planes, larger quantities of local anesthetic are required to get the same effect, and there may be distortion of the nose.[3]

In the soft tissue around the domes of the lower lateral cartilages, 0.3 mL of local anesthetic is injected. Multiple injections of 0.1 mL of local anesthetic are done at the incision area. The infratrochlear nerve is blocked by placing the solution between medial canthus and the dorsum, and the external nasal nerve is blocked by placing the solution at the level of lower border of nasal bones on each side.

If osteotomies are to be done, then the needle is introduced over the site of the incision for lateral osteotomy and inserted up to the radix close to the maxilla **(Fig. 6)**. The needle is then slowly withdrawn, injecting approximately 1 mL of anesthetic solution. The same procedure is done on the opposite side. Infiltration of the local anesthetic on either side of the ascending process causes less bleeding during lateral osteotomy. In case of correction of alar flaring, 0.25 mL of anesthetic is injected directly into the alar lobules. Infiltration is also done beneath the lateral crus between cartilage and underlying vestibular skin when required **(Fig. 7)**.

For septoplasty, 0.5–1.0 mL of the solution is injected at multiple sites in the subperichondrial and subperiosteal planes. The injection will cause hydrodissection leading to easier elevation of the septal flap. This is very useful for dissecting over fractures in the cartilage, bone, or along the crest of the maxilla.

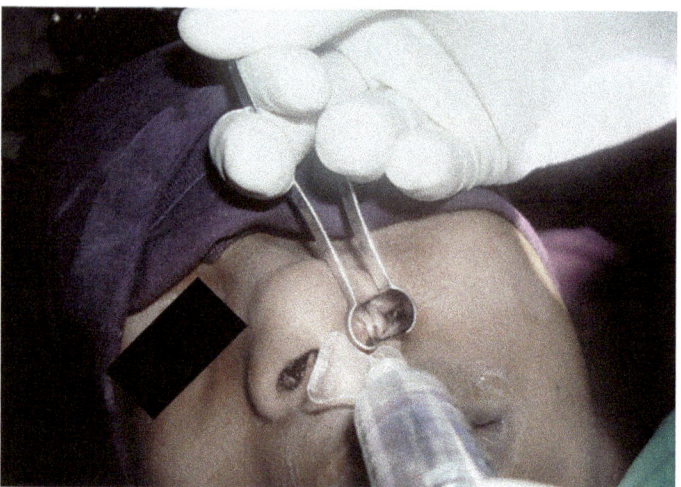

Fig. 6: Infiltration at the site of entry of osteotome for lateral osteotomy.

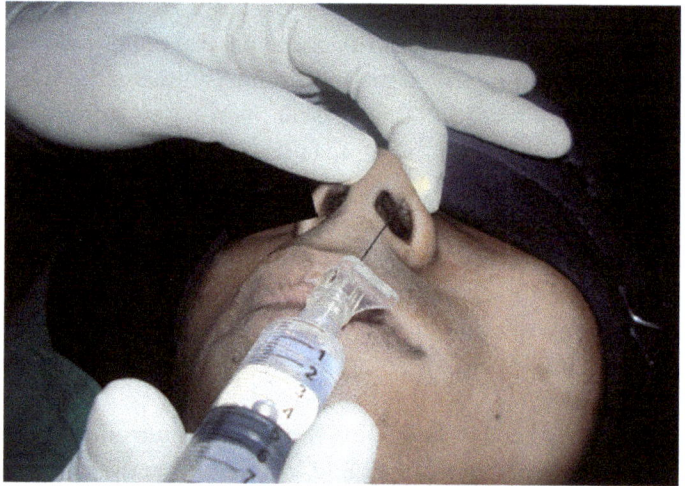

Fig. 7: Infiltration beneath lateral crus between cartilage and underlying vestibular skin.

To lessen bleeding from the sphenopalatine blood vessels, an injection is made on the posterosuperior part of the septum bilaterally.

Vibrissae are cut with scissors and the vestibules are again cleaned with Povidone iodine solution.

General anesthesia is used in children, apprehensive patients, and when rib cartilage is harvested as graft for augmentation. The endotracheal tube should be introduced in such a way as to avoid distortion of the lip. So, it is recommended to use an oral Ring-Adair-Elwyn (RAE) endotracheal tube fixed to the middle of the lower lip.[4]

The anesthesia in rhinoplasty should provide a clear surgical field, absence of patient movement, smooth emergence from anesthesia, a quick return of consciousness and protective airway reflexes and no postoperative nausea and vomiting.[5]

A clear surgical field is maintained by use of moderately controlled hypotension by the anesthesiologist and infiltrating 2% lignocaine with 1:100,000 adrenaline in the subcutaneous planes by the surgeon. Adrenaline in local anesthetic may cause an increase in end-tidal carbon dioxide ($EtCO_2$) or QT lengthening or arrhythmia in electrocardiography (ECG) and warns the surgeon to stop injecting solution.

Prevention of straining, bucking, and coughing by the patient during emergence from anesthesia is important for avoiding the formation of hematoma.[6] A rapid return of consciousness and protective airway reflexes is essential, as managing the patient's airway with mask ventilation after rhinoplasty is very difficult.

Conscious sedation of the patients with obstructive sleep apnea (OSA), and those with obesity, should be done with extreme care.[7] Mask ventilation and tracheal intubation may also be difficult in OSA patients.[8]

Maintenance of moderately controlled hypotension (systolic blood pressure <100 mm Hg; mean arterial pressure 60–70 mm Hg) is helpful for optimal surgical conditions. There is a fear of postoperative nausea and vomiting in general anesthesia, which should be controlled by antiemetic drugs.[9]

REFERENCES

1. Beeson WH. The nasal septum. Otolaryngol Oin North Atli. 1997;20:743-67.
2. Molliex S, Navez M, Baylot D, Prades JM, Elkhoury Z, Auboyer C. Regional anaesthesia for outpatient nasal surgery. Br J Anaesth. 1996;76(1):151-3.
3. Tardy ME. Rhinoplasty: The Art and the Science, 1st edition. Philadelphia: WB Saunders Co.; 1997.
4. Nolst Trenite GJ. Rhinoplasty: a practical guide to functional and aesthetic surgery of the nose. The Hague, Netherlands: Kugler Publications; 2005.
5. Nekhendzy V, Ramaiah VK. Prevention of perioperative and anesthesia-related complications in facial cosmetic surgery. Facial Plast Surg Clin N Am. 2013;21:559-77.
6. Caloss R, Lard MD. Anesthesia for office-based facial cosmetic surgery. Atlas Oral Maxillofac Surg Clin North Am. 2004;12:163-77.
7. Hillman DR, Platt PR, Eastwood PR. Anesthesia, sleep, and upper airway collapsibility. Anesthesiol Clin. 2010;28:443-55.
8. Kheterpal S, Han R, Tremper KK et al. Incidence and predictors of difficult and impossible mask ventilation. Anesthesiology. 2006;105:885-91.
9. Kasperbauer JL, Facer GW, Kem EB. Reconstructive surgery of the nasal septum. In: Papal ID, Nachlas NE (Eds). Facial plastic and reconstructive surgery. Philadelphia: Mosby Year Book; 1992. pp. 337-43.

Basic Technique

INTRODUCTION

Rhinoplasty is a difficult operation because of the variations in the patient's nasal anatomy and aesthetic expectations.

PRINCIPLES

- The surgeon should correct the main deformities, otherwise the patient will not be happy.
- Operation will be smoother if the preoperative planning is done in more detail.
- An operative procedure having maximum gain and minimum risk should be done.
- Operative sequence should be written step by step and should be visible in the operating room.

OPERATIVE STEPS

In rhinoplasty, the operative steps can be planned in the following order:[1]
- Incision
- Mobilization of soft tissue
- Removal of hump
- Septoplasty
- Preliminary contouring of the lower lateral cartilages
- Osteotomies
- Shortening the nose
- Final contouring of all parts including tip plasty
- Reconstruction of internal valve
- Sutures and dressing.

This sequence of steps can change according to the discretion of the surgeon. Rigid adherence to these steps is not required. The surgeon can modify the surgical plan according to the response of the tissues. Elevation of flaps in septoplasty is done before osteotomies but final correction of septum is done later. In most of the rhinoplasties, it is technically easier and more predictable to reconstruct the projection of the nasal tip first, followed by alignment of the osseocartilaginous dorsum to harmonize with the tip position. Osteotomies for nasal narrowing should be the last step in the surgical sequence of rhinoplasty, immediately before the application of the splint, to reduce operative swelling and oozing.[2]

The patient lies in supine position with head end elevated about 20°.

Rhinoplasty is an operation with risks, primarily because of the limited predictability of the final result, which is due to the dynamics of the healing process. A perfect result during immediate postoperative period may be totally different 1 year later. During the healing process, many different types of tissues are involved, namely cartilage, bone, skin, mucosa, fascia, perichondrium, periosteum, fat, muscles, nerves, and vessels. The individual reactions of these tissues, especially the cartilage, are not always under the control of the surgeon. The patient sometimes blames the surgeon for the result while the surgeon tends to call it a complication. Some "complications" are in fact a mistake in preoperative analysis or surgical planning, surgical technique, or in postoperative care.

Various studies report complication rates in the range of 8–15%. Complications may occur even after satisfactory surgeries. All surgeons experience complications.

In 70% of the patients for revision rhinoplasty, nasal obstruction is the main complaint,[3,4] because of residual deviations of septum, vestibular stenosis, narrowing of the internal nasal valve, or alar collapse. The loss of mucosal sensitivity caused by surgical scars can give the impression of a blocked nose. This is called "empty nose syndrome" in which the patient complains of nasal obstruction in the absence of an obstructive cause.[5]

REFERENCES

1. Sheen JH. Aesthetic rhinoplasty. St. Louis. MO: CV Mosby; 1978.
2. Tardy ME. Rhinoplasty-The Art and the Science, 1st edition. Philadelphia, USA: WB Saunders Co; 1997.
3. Bracaglia R, Fortunato R, Gentileschi S. Secondary rhinoplasty. Aesthetic Plast Surg. 2005;29(4):230-9.
4. Foda HM. Rhinoplasty for the multiply revised nose. Am J Otolaryngol. 2005;26(1): 28-34.
5. Wang Y, Liu T, Qu Y, Dong Z, Yang Z. Empty nose syndrome (in Chinese). Zhonghua Er Bi Yan Hou Ke Za Zhi. 2001;36:203-5.

CHAPTER 6

Incisions and Approaches

INCISIONS

- *Killian incision:* A vertical incision is made in the septal mucoperichondrium, 1.5 cm behind the margin of the caudal septal cartilage. This is a very useful incision for harvesting graft and correction of deviations of septum by submucosal resection (SMR).
- *Hemitransfixion incision:* A vertical incision is made over vestibular skin approximately 2 mm posterior and parallel to the caudal border of septal cartilage, preserving the integrity of the membranous septum. This incision is commonly made for septoplasty operation.
- *Transfixion incision:* A vertical incision is made through the membranous septum just in front of the caudal border of the septal cartilage. All parts of the septum become accessible by this incision, and in combination with intercartilaginous incisions, excellent exposure of the valve area and the nasal dorsum is obtained.
- *Intercartilaginous incision:* The incision is made on the caudal border of upper lateral cartilage and is extended toward the anterior septal angle. During incision, the ala is retracted with the help of Kilner retractor and pressure is given over the upper lateral cartilage by middle finger of left hand to expose the caudal border of the upper lateral cartilage **(Fig. 1)**.

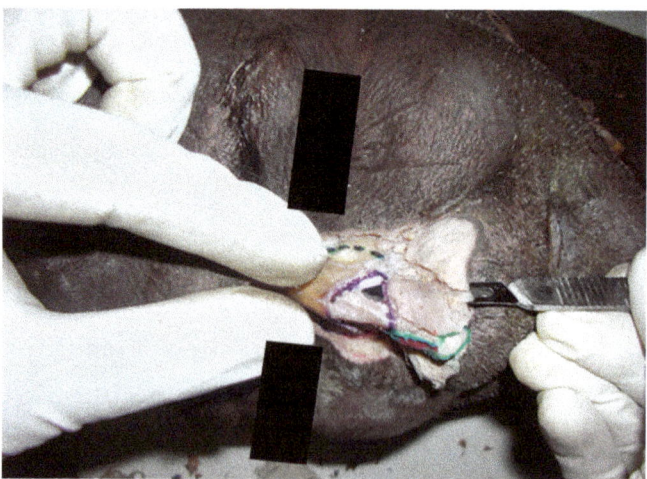

Fig. 1: Cadaver dissection showing intercartilaginous incision between upper and lower lateral cartilages by number 15 blade.

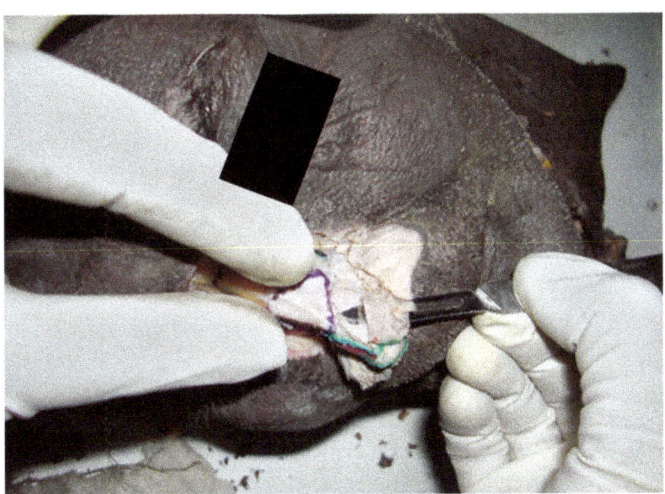

Fig. 2: Cadaver dissection showing intracartilaginous or cartilage-splitting incision through the lateral crus of lower lateral cartilage.

- *Intracartilaginous or cartilage-splitting incision:* Here the internal nasal valve area is avoided, and the incision is made below the level of intercartilaginous incision. The cartilage above the incision, i.e., the cephalic part of lateral crus can be excised and thus cephalic trimming is done easily **(Fig. 2)**. Using Kilner retractor and the middle finger of left hand the lower lateral cartilage is exposed. The caudal and cephalic borders of the lateral crus are located. Vestibular skin is incised 6–8 mm cephalic to the caudal border of the lateral crus. The vestibular skin is dissected free with scissors in a posterior direction to just beyond the cephalic edge of the lateral crus. Then incision is made on lateral crural cartilage and the remaining soft tissue is removed from cephalic part by dissecting superficially to it and the cephalic portion is excised.
- *Marginal incision:* Beginning laterally, the incision is made over vestibular skin caudal to the caudal border of the lateral crus of the lower lateral cartilage. It extends medially around the soft triangle toward the columella up to the flaring of medial crura. The marginal incision must not pass through the soft triangle. During incision, the caudal margin of the lateral crus is made prominent by pressing the lobule from outside with the middle finger of left hand and retracting the margin of ala by Kilner retractor **(Fig. 3)**.
- *Rethi Goodman incision:* This incision is used during external rhinoplasty **(Fig. 4)**. Bilateral marginal incisions are made. The columellar portion of the marginal incision is made 2–3 mm behind the lateral margin of the columella as it will help in subsequent suturing of the columellar strut. Then inverted V-shaped transcolumellar incision is made near the

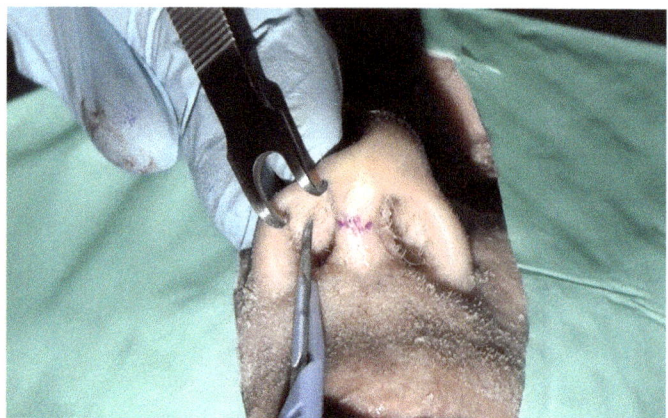

Fig. 3: Marginal incision in cadaver.

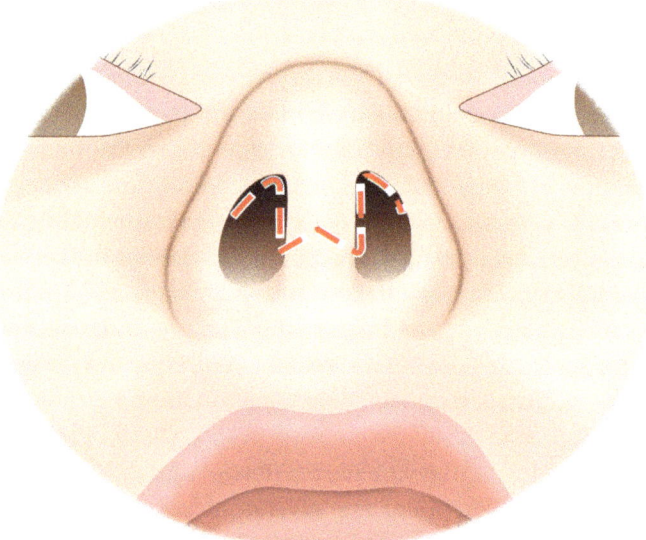

Fig. 4: Bilateral marginal and inverted V-shaped transcolumellar incision for external rhinoplasty.

start of bifurcation of medial crura and connected with the two marginal incisions. There are various modifications of the transcolumellar incision. The inverted V-shaped incision can be made with transverse wings. A small 3-mm equilateral inverted-V incision is made by number 11 blade, whose apex is at the narrowest part of the columella. The transverse wings are made by number 15 blade, across and behind the columellar pillars. The transcolumellar incision is made in the upper two-thirds, usually at its narrowest point, to ensure the medial crural footplates provide enough

support to prevent a depressed scar. The vertical columellar portions of the marginal incisions are made about 2 mm inside the vestibule and joined by careful dissection of the columellar skin with sharp scissors. These blades of the scissors can then be used as a support upon which the transcolumellar incision is made. If the columella is very short in relation to the desired tip projection, a V-Y lengthening procedure can be done after making a V incision at the base of the columella.[1]
- *Mid columellar incision:* A vertical incision is made between two medial crura over the columella and a dorsal midline pocket is made for placing the dorsal graft for augmentation. This is an easy technique but postoperative columellar scar may occur.
- *Rim incision:* An incision is made along the rim of the nostril. The incision is avoided as it may cause alar notching.

SURGICAL APPROACHES

There are various surgical approaches for exposure of the lower two-thirds of the nose. Rhinoplasty should be done by the surgical approach that provides the best exposure; minimal tissue distortion, edema, and scarring; and least disruption of tip-supporting mechanism[2,3] **(Fig. 5)**.

The approaches of the lower two-thirds of the nose are endonasal or external. The approaches are:
- *Endonasal:*
  - Transcartilaginous (cartilage splitting and intracartilaginous)
  - Intercartilaginous
  - Delivery approach
- External (open)

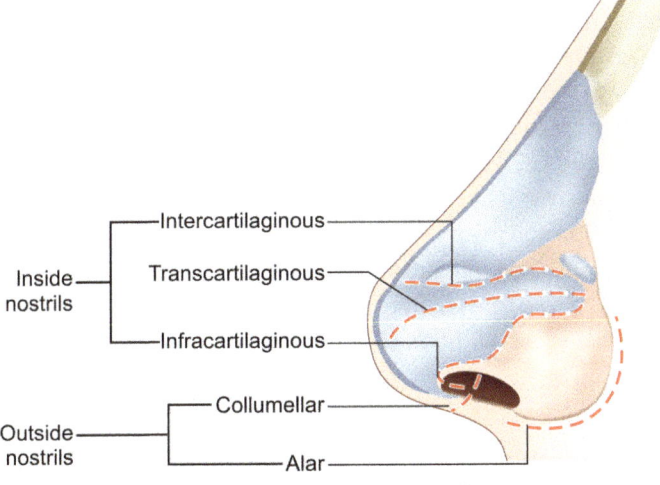

Fig. 5: Skin incisions for rhinoplasty.

Endonasal

The endonasal approach is usually preferred for patients needing mild hump reduction, conservative tip modification, uncomplicated revision rhinoplasty, and other conditions where conservative changes are required. Advantages of endonasal approach are less dissection and less edema and its disadvantage is less exposure.

Cartilage-splitting Approach

The approach is done via intracartilaginous incision. Here the vestibular skin and lateral crus of lower lateral cartilage are incised 6–8 mm cephalic to the caudal border of the lateral crus. The incision avoids the nasal valve area. The cephalic part of lateral crus which is present above the incision can be excised (cephalic trimming). The dorsum of the nose can be approached through this incision with no chance to damage the soft triangle area. This approach is useful for uncomplicated tip plasty and it preserves the natural shape of the tip.

Delivery Approach

It is also called internal approach or closed technique. Many surgeons prefer delivery approach over external approach as there is less postoperative tip edema and no chance of transcolumellar scar. Adequate exposure is obtained for various tip modifications.

Bilateral intercartilaginous incisions are made with a number 15 blade. It will help in retrograde dissection between the skin and lateral crura by curved Fomon scissors. Marginal incisions are made on both sides caudal to the caudal border of lower lateral cartilage. The marginal incision should avoid the soft triangle area. Through the marginal incision, undermining and dissection between the skin and lateral crura can be done. The lateral crus, dome, and upper part of the medial crus are completely freed from the overlying skin. Through the intercartilaginous incision, a long plain dissecting forceps is introduced and the forceps brings out the nose between the caudal margin of the lower lateral cartilage and overlying skin and the alar cartilage is delivered like a bucket handle. The fibrofatty tissue over the lateral crus is removed with the help of fine scissors and toothed dissecting forceps under direct vision. The excessive fibrofatty tissue between two domes and upper ends of medial crura is removed. Cephalic part of the lateral crus is excised after stripping the cartilage from the underlying vestibular skin (cephalic trimming) **(Fig. 6)**. Injury to the vestibular skin is avoided to prevent subsequent stenosis.

External

In external approach, there is better exposure but more postoperative tissue edema.[4] The external approach is indicated for correction of deformities and

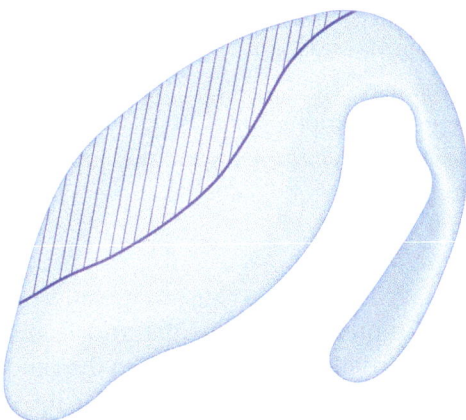

Fig. 6: Cephalic trimming.

asymmetries of the nasal tip, dorsum, and septum, which may be difficult to perform in endonasal technique.[5] Here, bilateral marginal incisions are made, continuing along the caudal border of the lower lateral cartilage to a level just anterior to the flare of the medial crural footplates. At this level, a transcolumellar incision connects the marginal incisions. The transcolumellar incision is either an inverted "V" or a stepped incision to minimize scar formation.[6] When suture realignment of the transcolumellar incision is performed precisely, the healed incision site is often invisible and seldom results in an objectionable scar. A septoplasty can be done either by a separate hemitransfixion incision or via the external approach.

In the external approach, intercartilaginous incisions are not used. So, the valve area is not disturbed and the important major tip support mechanism of the scroll area is preserved. However, mobilization of the skin-soft tissue envelope from the lower cartilaginous vault and the division of the medial intercrural fibrous tissue may lead to loss of minor tip support mechanism, and therefore mild tip ptosis may occur in some cases. There may be mild difficulty assessing the supratip area and the desired tip projection, due to lack of traction of the soft tissue prior to closure of the transcolumellar incision.

In the external approach, easier and more accurate placement and suture fixation of spreader grafts and spreader flaps can be done. The spreader grafts are placed longitudinally between the upper lateral cartilages and septum extramucosally.[7]

One of the advantages of the external approach is better surgical exposure leading to a more precise anatomic diagnosis. The external approach also allows accurate tissue manipulation, grafting, and suturing. Disadvantages are the transcolumellar incision, excessive dissection resulting in loss of support, and prolonged tip edema due to transection of lymphatics of columella. Tip edema may take as long as 6 months to subside. External approach may cause hypoesthesia of the tip and prolongs the surgical procedure itself.[8]

Indications of the external approach:
- It can be done in all rhinoplasties.
- Difficult tip rhinoplasty
- Complicated septal deviations
- Revision rhinoplasty with complex structural grafting
- For teaching purposes
- Cleft lip nasal deformity
- Repair of septal perforation.

The complete transfixion incision causes separation of the caudal septum from the membranous septum and the medial crura leading to interruption of the attachment of the medial crural footplates to the caudal septum, a major tip support mechanism. However, in overprojecting tip, it helps the surgeon by facilitating retropositioning of the tip. If no nasal shortening is required, complete transfixion incision should be avoided.

When limited access to the nasal tip and nose is required, a limited partial transfixion incision is preferred, preserving the major tip support mechanism while providing adequate exposure. The partial incision is carried from just beyond the anterior septal angle to any extent just short of the medial crural attachment to the caudal septum.[9]

REFERENCES

1. Gorney M. Reconstruction of the post cleft nasal deformity. In: Rees TD (Ed). Rhinoplasty 'Problems and Controversies', 9th edition. St Louis: Mosby; 1988. p. 410.
2. Daniel RK. Aesthetic plastic surgery: rhinoplasty. Boston MA: Little, Brown & Co.; 1993.
3. Sheen JH, Sheen AP. Aesthetic Rhinoplasty, 2nd edition. St Louis: Mosby; 1987.
4. Guida RA. Surgical approaches to the nasal skeleton. Operative techniques in otolaryngology head and neck surgery. 1999;10(3):228-31.
5. Anderson JR, Reis WR. Rhinoplasty: emphasizing the external approach. New York: Thieme; 1986.
6. Johnson CM, Toriumi DM. Open structure rhinoplasty. Philadelphia: Saunders; 1990.
7. Tardy ME. Cartilage autografts reconstruction of the nose. In: Tardy ME (Ed). Rhinoplasty: the Art and the Science, Volume II. Philadelphia: WB Saunders; 1987. pp. 648-724.
8. Bafaqeeh SA, al-Qattan MM. Alterations in nasal sensibility following open rhinoplasty. Br J Plast Surg. 1998;51(7):508-10.
9. Tardy ME. Rhinoplasty: the Art and the Science, 1st edition. ISBN 0-7216-8755-5. Philadelphia: WB Saunders Co; 1997.

Mobilization of Soft Tissues (Skeletonization)

INTRODUCTION

The skin of the upper third of the nose is thicker than the middle-third region. The inferior third also has thick skin like the upper third, where it contains large sebaceous glands. In the lower third, the skin is fixed to the underlying structures. Average skin thickness was reported to be more at the nasofrontal groove (1.25 mm) than at the rhinion (0.6 mm).[1]

The nasal muscles are situated beneath the skin in four groups: (1) The elevators, (2) the depressors, (3) the compressor, and (4) the dilators. The procerus is present over the nasion between the aponeurosis of the transversus nasalis muscle and the frontalis. It is attached to the nasal bones and to the upper lateral cartilages, at the midline of the dorsum.

The depressor septi nasi goes from the orbicularis oris to the columellar skin and is attached to the feet of the medial crura of lower lateral cartilages.

Depressor septi nasi muscles can be cut to widen the nasolabial angle, to lengthen the upper lip, or to rotate the nasal tip. Resection of hypertrophic procerus muscle can be done to deepen the frontonasal angle.[2]

The muscles are connected together by an aponeurosis named the nasal superficial musculoaponeurotic system (SMAS).[3]

Blood vessels and lymphatics are present superficial to the layer of nasal muscles.[4] The nasal SMAS contains all the nasal vessels, and from this layer, perforating branches arise from the arteries to form the subdermal plexus and reach the skin. The SMAS can also be considered a protective layer in between the nasal framework and the skin. The layers of the soft-tissue envelope of the nose are epidermis, dermis, subcutaneous tissue, muscle and fascia, areolar tissue, and perichondrium or periosteum. During surgery, dissection should be done in the areolar tissue plane (i.e., submusculoaponeurotic) which maintains vascular supply and reduces postoperative edema.

The purpose of separation of soft tissues from the skeleton is to expose the skeletal structure and to allow the tissues to redrape over the newly made framework. Undermining of soft tissues is done either with curved blunt ended scissors or with the help of number 15 blade. Number 15 blade is preferred as it causes less damage to the surrounding tissues during dissection. During undermining, the knife is used with gentle sweeping movements and the fingers of the left hand should follow the course of the knife blade to prevent damage of the skin. The dissection is carried over the upper lateral cartilage, extending over the dorsum.[5] The soft tissue over the lower lateral cartilages is

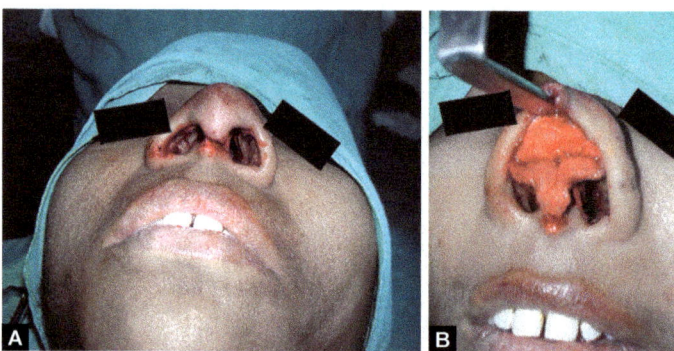

Figs. 1A and B: (A) Rethi Goodman incision; and (B) Mobilization of soft tissues during external rhinoplasty.

freed in a retrograde manner with the help of Fomon scissors passed through the intercartilaginous incision.

The soft tissue of the bony vault should be dissected in a subperiosteal plane after making an incision 2–3 mm above the lower edge of the nasal bones. With Cottle periosteal elevator, the periosteum and skin are elevated as a single layer from the nasal bones. During elevation of periosteum, the lateral limit of the dissection is kept to a minimum and is not carried too laterally over the area of proposed lateral osteotomy sites. The elevation should be symmetrical on both the sides **(Figs. 1A and B)**. The subperiosteal dissection can be extended along the most lateral aspect of the bony vault to allow for powered lateral osteotomies such as with a Piezo device. The edge of the nasal bones is palpated before making the incision over the periosteum, to prevent separation of the upper lateral cartilages from the nasal bones. If the separation occurs, it can be corrected by a camouflaging onlay graft or cartilage spreader grafts.[6]

Mobilization of the soft tissue in the proper surgical plane causes minimal bleeding. During freeing the cartilaginous vault, false passage may occur into the SMAS. To avoid this, dissection should be started in the midline between or just dorsal to the domes during external rhinoplasty. The excess subcutaneous tissue at the supratip area can be trimmed if required, but this should be done very conservatively to prevent damage to the blood supply of the overlying skin. Prolonged supratip edema and pollybeak deformity due to dissection in the wrong plane damaging the transverse nasal muscle are the potential complications of the external approach.

If augmentation is done by placement of grafts, the overlying soft tissue should have adequate viability. If blanching of the skin over the graft occurs, reducing the size of the graft will prevent necrosis of the skin.

In cases of revision rhinoplasty, the normal tissue planes are absent. So, there is more risk, compared with primary rhinoplasty, of damage to the skin-soft tissue envelope. Restoration of skin-soft tissue envelope is difficult if it is damaged. The damaged skin causes an aesthetically bad appearance.[7]

In atrophic rhinitis of long duration, the thick puckered skin is usually fixed to the underlying structures and mobilization of skin-soft tissue envelope is difficult. If rhinoplasty is done in patients with atrophic rhinitis, extra care and patience are needed to avoid buttonhole formation during elevation of the skin.

REFERENCES

1. Lessard M, Daniel RK. Surgical anatomy of septorhinoplasty. Arch Otolaryngol Head Neck Surg. 1985;111(1):25-9.
2. Meyer R. Residual bony deformity. Nasofrontal angle. In: Meyer R (Ed). Secondary Rhinoplasty: Including Reconstruction of the Nose, 2nd edition. New York: Springer; 2002. p. 68.
3. Chang EW. (2015). Nasal anatomy. [online] Available from: emedicine.medscape.com/article/835134-overview. [Last accessed April, 2023].
4. Toriumi DM, Mueller RA, Grosch T, Bhattacharya TK, Larrabee WF. Vascular anatomy of the nose and the external rhinoplasty approach. Arch Oto Head Neck Surgery. 1996;122:24-34.
5. Sheen JH. Aesthetic Rhinoplasty. St. Louis, MO: CV Mosby; 1978.
6. Tardy ME. Rhinoplasty: the Art and the Science, 1st edition. Philadelphia: WB Saunders Co; 1997.
7. Rettinger G, Zenkel M. Skin and soft tissue complications. Facial Plastic Surgery. 1997;13:51-9.

CHAPTER 8

Nasal Spine

INTRODUCTION

The anterior nasal spine is a pointed midline bony projection of the premaxilla. The nasal septum is fixed to the nasal spine and the crest of maxilla by fibrous attachment. The positions of the lower parts of the medial crura depend on the shape and size of the anterior nasal spine. The nasal spine has the footplates of the medial crura on each side of it and thereby, the shape of the footplates and columella is determined by them. During assessment of deviation of the caudal part of nose, the nasal spine should be examined to make sure that it is in midline and straight. Although useful information can be obtained by palpation, direct inspection is very important to understand a malpositioning of the nasal spine affecting the footplates. During external rhinoplasty, after mobilization of the skin-soft tissue envelope, separation of the medial crura and direct inspection of the nasal spine can be done **(Fig. 1)**.

A tilted nasal spine is repositioned to correct the deviated caudal nose. The malpositioned nasal spine can be placed midline with an incomplete fracture at its base, done with a chisel. The straight septum keeps the spine in the central position. Nasal splints placed at the end of the operation also support the caudal nose and nasal spine.

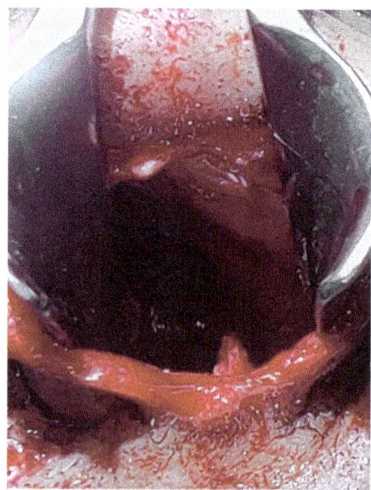

Fig. 1: Anterior nasal spine seen after separation of the medial crura during external rhinoplasty.

The decision for the modification of the anterior nasal spine should be made preoperatively. The nasal spine is usually the first bony part to be reduced after skeletonization. Proper resection of the nasal spine improves the appearance of the face by adding length to the lip and by deepening the nasolabial angle.[1] The soft curve over the subnasion should be retained and the vertical line of the upper lip should be parallel to the facial plane.

A prominent anterior nasal spine may cause excessive columellar show, overprojection of the nose, and tethering of the upper lip. The nasal spine is sometimes removed to make the nose short or to decrease the projection of the nose. After removal of a large anterior nasal spine, the upper lip becomes straight, and it meets the bottom of the nose at a more distinct angle.

Rees mentioned that there should be a very conservative surgical approach to the caudal septum and anterior nasal spine.[2] Over-resection of the nasal spine can lead to columellar retraction, foreshortening of the nose, and sharp retrusive angle of the subnasion and the plane of the lip moves posteriorly, giving the lip an unattractive retrusive look.

In patients with unilateral cleft lip, nasal spine is deviated toward the opposite side. Replacing the nasal spine from the noncleft side to the central position is done by a greenstick fracture at the base of the spine with an osteotome and fixation by sutures to prevent redeviation of the septum and nasal spine.[3]

REFERENCES

1. Sheen JH. Aesthetic rhinoplasty. St. Louis, MO: CV Mosby; 1978.
2. Rees T. Aesthetic plastic surgery. Philadelphia, USA: WB Saunders Company; 1994. p. 245.
3. Nolst Trenite GJ. Rhinoplasty: a practical guide to functional and aesthetic surgery of the nose. The Hague, Netherlands: Kugler Publications; 2005.

CHAPTER 9

Removal of Hump

The purpose of nasal hump removal is to improve the beauty of the nose based on aesthetic, cultural, and evolutionary influences. Most surgeons prefer to perform the tip plasty procedure before doing the dorsal hump reduction.[1]

Humps are of three types:
1. Bony
2. Bony and cartilaginous
3. Cartilaginous

Bony and cartilaginous hump is most commonly seen.

Pseudohump is the prominent osteocartilaginous area caused by sagging of the cartilaginous vault. In most cases, the cause is trauma, septal abscess or submucosal resection (SMR) operation.

The hump should be removed above an imaginary line drawn between the depth of nasofrontal angle and tip projection. The amount of the hump to be removed is marked with gentian violet on the side of the nose **(Fig. 1)**. In the humped nose, the bony contribution is usually considerably less than that of the cartilaginous contribution. So, much less bony convexity is to be removed than normally expected.

Most tall patients usually accept minor degrees of bony hump convexity above an otherwise straight profile.

Hump reduction can be done by endonasal approach but the incidence of postoperative profile irregularities has been reduced when it is done through

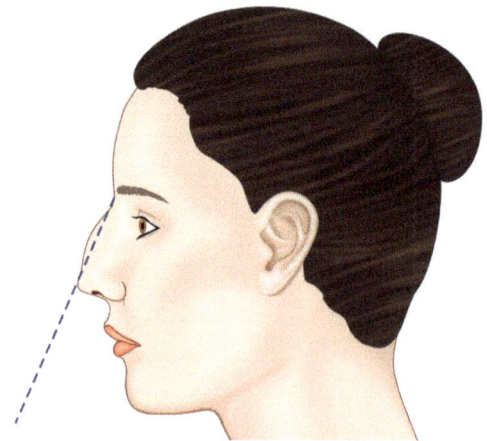

Fig. 1: Resection of hump is done above the line.

the open approach. Generally, if the patient has an isolated dorsal hump, an endonasal approach is done. However, if major modifications to the nose are necessary, the open approach is preferred.[2,3]

A bony hump is either reduced with a rasp or resected. A very small hump can be rasped with a sharp downcutting rasp or removed with an osteotome or chisel. Using a saw, the minimum amount of dorsum reduced is 4.5 mm. So, a saw cannot be used during removal of small amount of bone. Small and medium humps (i.e., 3 mm or less) can usually be reduced with rasping **(Figs. 2 and 3)**. Rasping should be done first along the left and right dorsal aesthetic lines, and then centrally using controlled, short rasp excursions.[4] Rasping causes trauma to surrounding soft tissues, and, therefore, should be done with the minimum number of short, firm strokes. The rasp should be fine enough and held obliquely to provide maximum effective cutting motions and to avoid the possibility of the potential separation of the upper lateral cartilage

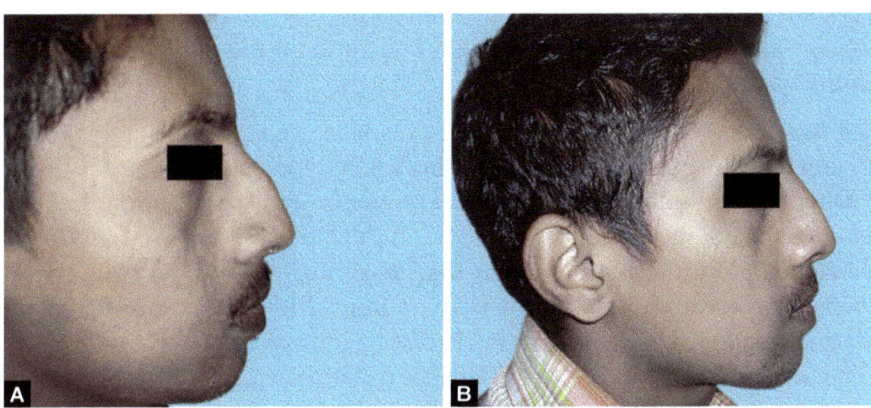

Figs. 2A and B: (A) Preoperative; (B) Postoperative views of nasal hump corrected by rasping.

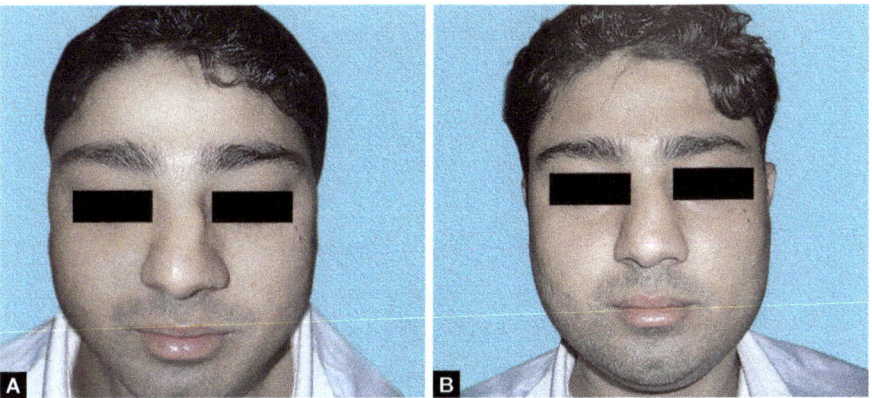

Figs. 3A and B: (A) Preoperative; (B) Postoperative views of bony hump with deviated nasal septum (DNS). Septoplasty and rasping were done. Slight postoperative edema is present.

from the undersurface of the nasal bone. Avulsion of the osteocartilaginous junction can be avoided by gently rasping with as little pull on the area. After rasping, the bone dust is removed by suction tip. The dorsum is palpated with a finger moistened with hydrogen peroxide to see any bony irregularities.

To prevent damage to the periosteum over the bony dorsum, the periosteum is elevated before rasping or hump reduction. The elevation of periosteum is done carefully to prevent accidental dislocation of the articulation of the caudal nasal bones to the underlying cephalic margins of the upper lateral cartilages, which results in step deformity as the upper lateral cartilage is partially avulsed and falls medially.

This deformity (inverted V-deformity) can be corrected by cartilage spreader grafts or camouflaging with onlay grafts. Severe upper lateral cartilage avulsion may result in medialization of the internal nasal valve with nasal obstruction.

Two methods are available for reducing the cartilaginous hump: a transverse en bloc reduction using a knife and an incremental technique using scissors.

En bloc hump reduction: A number 11 blade is used to resect cartilaginous hump because of its long straight cutting edge. To prevent perforation, the tip of the blade is broken off. Symmetrical resection of the cartilaginous hump is done by maintaining a 90° angle between the knife and the septum. During lowering the cartilaginous dorsum, the "m" configuration of the vault should be maintained by preserving mucosal continuity whenever possible. After the cartilage is incised, the osteotome is placed right at the bony-cartilaginous junction, and the assistant gently taps the osteotome to cut the bony part and the hump is removed in one piece **(Figs. 4 and 5)**.

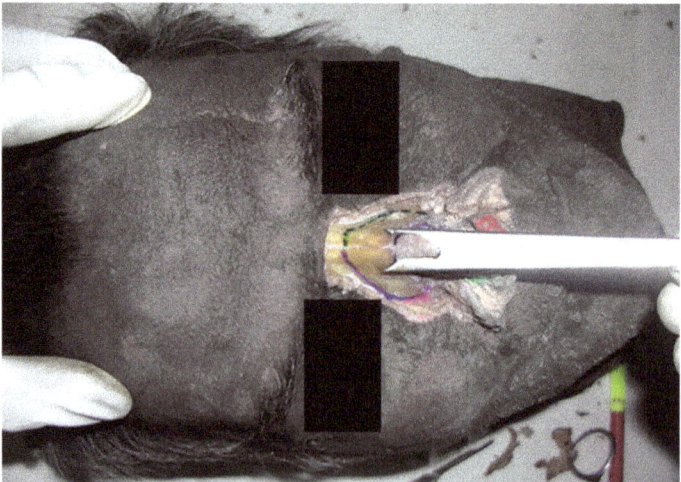

Fig. 4: Cadaver dissection showing en bloc hump removal.

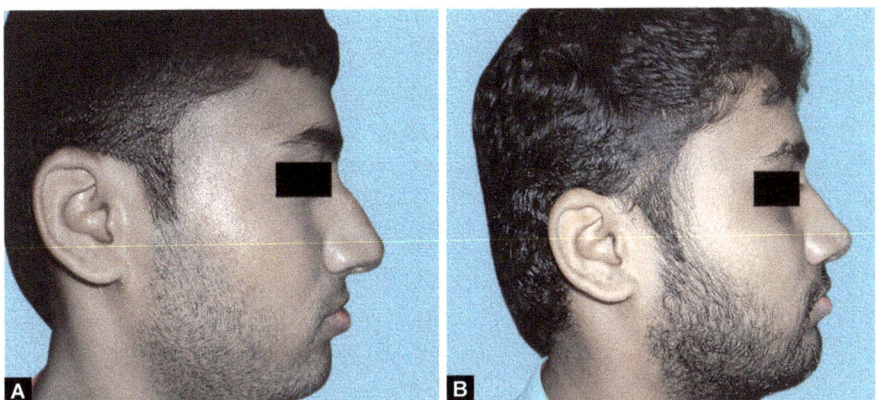

Figs. 5A and B: (A) Preoperative; and (B) Postoperative views of nasal hump removal.

For bony hump removal, Mcindoes or Gillies osteotome of 8–10 mm size can be used. After hump is incised completely, it is grasped with a straight artery forceps and then it is first pushed up and then pulled out. After hump removal, the dorsum should be examined by inspection and palpation. The fingertip moistened with normal saline, gently palpates both the left and right dorsal aesthetic lines, and then centrally to detect any bony irregularities, which can be made smooth with a rasp.[5]

The amount of hump reduction is measured in such a manner that the removal stops short of the desired final result. At least 10% of the hump should be left for final precise reduction by scalpel for the cartilaginous portion and rasping for the bony portion.

In some centers, powered rasp is used. It has a speed of approximately 15,000 rpm, and it moves back and forth approximately 2 mm. So, it is a very precise instrument.

There is a difference in skin thickness over the dorsum of the nose. At the tip and root of the nose, the skin is thicker. But at the bone-cartilage junction, the skin is very thin. So, during hump removal, a little bit less amount should be excised at the area where the skin is thin. If accidentally, more than required amount of the hump is removed, a part of it should be reinserted to prevent saddle-nose deformity.[6] To avoid collapse of the cartilaginous part of the nose, spreader grafts may be placed in between the upper lateral cartilages and the septum.[7] Spreader grafts maintain the width, strength, and straightness of the nose **(Fig. 6)**.

Before taking a decision about reduction of the nasal dorsum, one should consider projection at the radix, the rhinion, and the tip. The degree of hump reduction must be balanced with radix augmentation and modification of tip projection.

Extramucosal tunnels are made to separate the mucosa from the undersurface of the dorsum allowing the dorsal hump to be reduced without

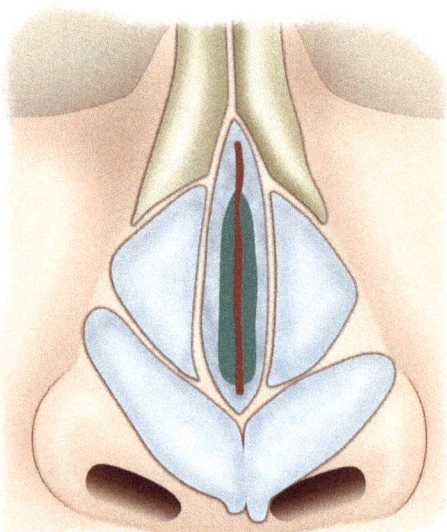

Fig. 6: Spreader grafts.

damaging the underlying mucosa. After exposure of the septum, local anesthesia is injected under the dorsum for hydrodissection and mucosa is dissected with the elevator. The mucosa is also elevated from the undersurface of the upper lateral cartilages when a large hump is to be reduced.

Incremental hump reduction: Many surgeons prefer component or incremental hump reduction. Dorsal hump reduction is done incrementally using rasps or chisel for the bony hump and scissors for the cartilaginous hump. Bony hump reduction is preferred before the cartilaginous hump as it reveals the amount of the necessary cartilaginous hump removal. In most cases, the bony hump is quite thin (<1 mm) and rasping is effective and conservative. Osteotomy has a risk of too much excision. Powered burrs and rasps may be used during bone reduction for better control. When the bony dorsum comes down to the level of the profile line drawn on the skin before operation, then cartilaginous hump is removed.

The cartilaginous hump is divided into three parts (septum and two upper lateral cartilages) by scissors or a number 15 number blade inserted extramucosally. The dorsal part of septal cartilage is excised incrementally with the scissors followed by conservative excision of the upper lateral cartilages **(Fig. 7)**. By excision of the dorsal part of septal cartilage, reduction of the profile height is done, while excision of the dorsal border of upper lateral cartilages narrows dorsal width.[8] Usually, upper lateral cartilage removal is 33–50% of the dorsal septal cartilage excision. Then, dorsal aesthetic lines are examined and minor corrections, if required, are done.

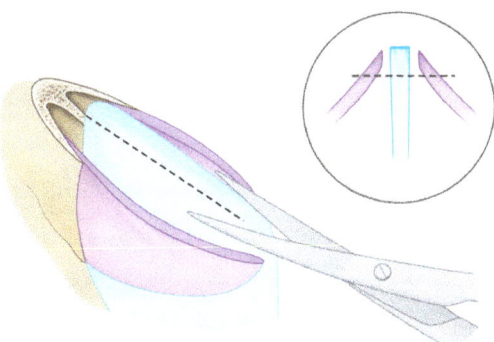

Fig. 7: Incremental hump reduction.

The dorsal margins of the upper laterals are sutured together in the midline after hump resection over spreader grafts **(Figs. 8 and 9)**.

Extramucosal tunnels are needed in cartilaginous hump reduction of >1 mm and spreader grafts are required in hump reduction of >2 mm.

Spreader grafts: Spreader grafts are strut-shaped cartilage grafts, usually taken from septal cartilage. A typical dimension is 24 × 8 × 2 mm; however, the size can vary considerably. The grafts are inserted into submucoperichondrial pockets adjacent to the dorsal part of the septum, in between the upper lateral cartilages and septum.

Resection of the dorsal hump converts the superior portion of the septum into a narrow "I" from a broad "T", leading to collapse of the upper lateral cartilages inward. Spreader grafts reform the broad "T" of the septum and thereby avoid a collapsed inverted-V deformity and widen the internal nasal valve angle. The grafts are secured in place with two 25 needles piercing all the five layers consisting of the upper lateral cartilage, the spreader graft, the septum, spreader graft, and opposite upper lateral cartilage. The caudal part is sutured first with 5-0 PDS usually in three layers, i.e., the spreader grafts and the septum, whereas the cephalic suture unites all five layers.

After a high bony hump removal, longer spreader grafts are required to place the grafts into the bony open roof to achieve normal dorsal width. In case of overly rotated tip, longer spreader grafts are placed extending caudally to enclose a columellar strut which makes the tip derotated. If the spreader graft extends beyond the anterior septal angle, it is called extended spreader graft.

Spreader flaps: The dorsal margins of the upper lateral cartilages can be folded medially into the nose and sutured to the septum. These are called spreader flaps or "autospreaders." The spreader flaps maintain middle-third width and are an alternative to spreader grafts.[9] If a small hump is removed, there may be insufficient upper lateral to use as a flap and in such cases spreader grafts are used.

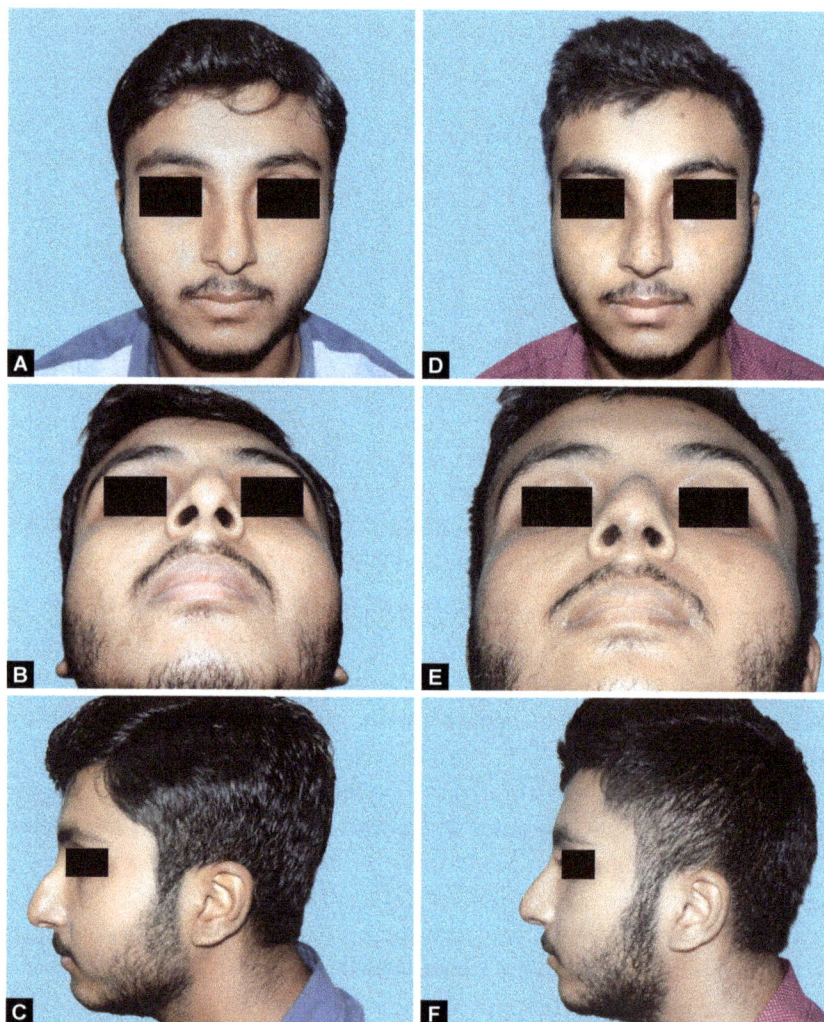

Figs. 8A to F: (A to C) Preoperative; and (D to F) Postoperative views of a crooked nose with deviated nasal septum (DNS) and hump. Septoplasty, intranasal medial and lateral osteotomies and percutaneous transverse osteotomies were done. Bony hump was rasped, cartilaginous hump was removed by incremental technique and spreader grafts were placed. Tip plasty was done by domal equalization suture. To rotate the tip upward, a triangular piece of caudal septal cartilage (with the base of the triangle toward the dorsum) was excised.

If the middle-third width is good, as in removal of very small hump in long nasal bones, spreader grafts are not needed and the upper lateral cartilages are sutured back onto the septum.

Sheen (1978) described radix augmentation as a "balancing procedure" to minimize hump reduction. Either a complete (5 × 5 cm) or partial sheet of deep temporal fascia is used for radix augmentation.

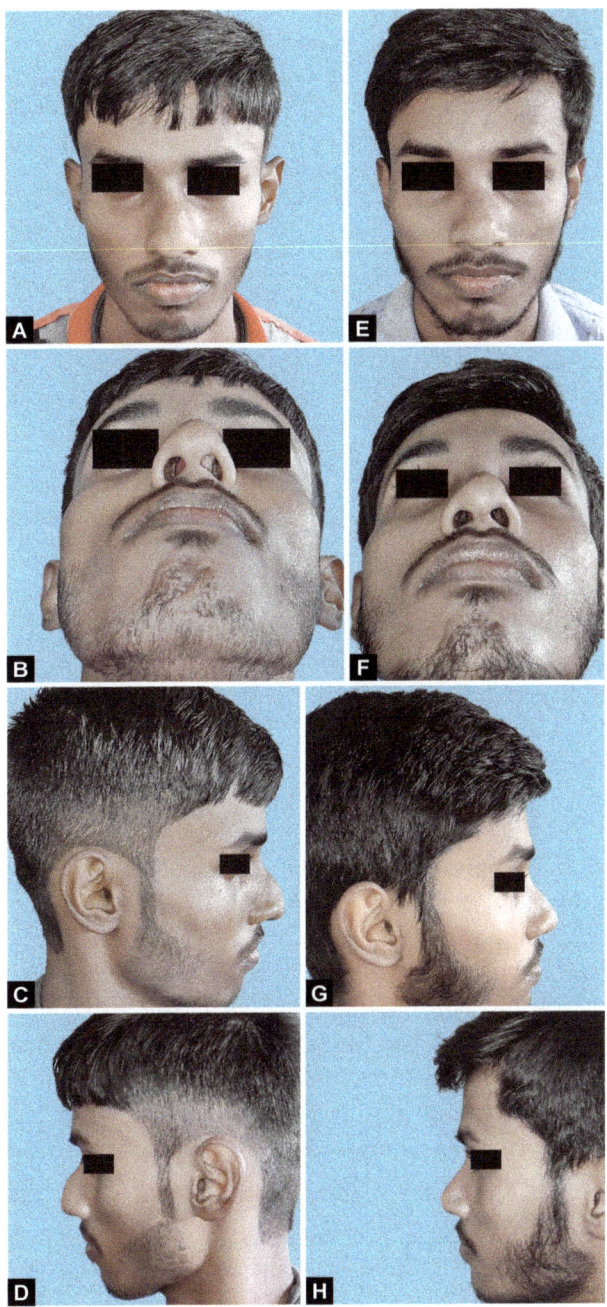

Figs. 9A to H: (A to D) Preoperative; and (E to H) Postoperative views of nasal hump, crooked nose with gross deviated nasal septum (DNS). Septoplasty, hump removal, placement of spreader grafts, and cephalic trimming were done by external approach. Bony hump was rasped, cartilaginous hump was removed by incremental technique. Tip plasty was done by domal equalization suture. Caudal deviation of septum was corrected by "tongue-in-groove technique."

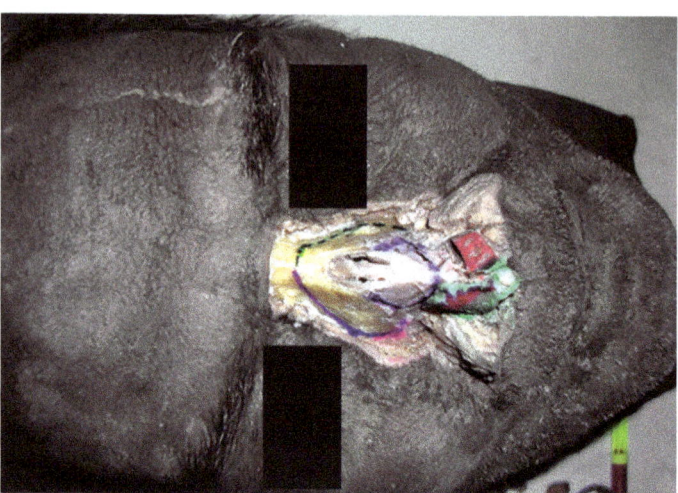

Fig. 10: Cadaver dissection showing "open-roof" deformity following hump removal.

"Open-roof" deformity: Removal of a hump usually causes a defect on the bony dorsum called "open roof" **(Fig. 10)**. This deformity should be corrected to avoid bony irregularities, a flat nasal dorsum, and to prevent an ingrowth of endonasal trigeminal nerve fibers beneath the skin of the dorsum. This deformity with hyperesthesia of the nasal dorsum is called "open-roof syndrome."[10]

Lateral osteotomies are done to close the open or wide roof resulting from hump removal. Combined transverse percutaneous osteotomy with a 2-mm osteotome from just above the medial canthus and intranasal low-to-low lateral osteotomy can also be done. The roof is then closed by digital pressure. Another cause of open-roof deformity is excessive nasal packing, which can splay the nasal bones in lateral direction. In the small nose with a large hump, overzealous lowering of the osseocartilaginous vault with lateral osteotomies may significantly compromise nasal airway by further reducing the cross-sectional diameter of the nasal cavities.[11] After removal of hump in small nasal bones, a dorsal cartilage graft may be required to hide an open-roof deformity.[12] Osteotomies performed on a narrow nose may result in overly narrowed nasal bones. Intermediate osteotomy can be performed in some cases to correct severely asymmetric bony vaults.[13]

Rocker deformity: The osteotomies should not be made too far cephalically beyond the intercanthal line, to avoid a rocker deformity, where the superior parts of the nasal bones are lateralized when the inferior parts of the nasal bones are pushed inward.[14]

"Polly-beak deformity" may occur due to inadequate resection of the cartilaginous hump, or excessive resection of the bony part, resulting in low dorsum, a relatively high septal angle and lack of tip support.

Inverted-V deformity: Too much resection of the upper lateral cartilage as compared with the septum results in the inverted-V deformity.[15] There is a loss of continuity between the nasal bones and the upper lateral cartilages, creating a visible triangular shadowing of the midvault on frontal view. This can also give a "pinched appearance" to the cartilaginous dorsum and cause narrowing of the nasal valve. Spreader grafts can be placed to correct this.[16]

REFERENCES

1. Adamson PA, Litner JA, Dahiya R. The M-Arch model: a new concept of nasal tip dynamics. Arch Facial Plast Surg. 2006;8(1):16-25.
2. Gunter JP. Gunter's approach. In: Gunter JP, Rohrich RJ, Adams WP, Jr. (Eds). Dallas rhinoplasty: nasal surgery by the Masters. St. Louis, Mo: Quality Medical Publishing; 2002. pp. 1049-75.
3. Gunter JP, Rohrich RJ. The external approach for secondary rhinoplasty. Plast Reconstr Surg. 1987;80:161.
4. Rohrich RJ, Muzaffar AR, Janis JE. Component dorsal hump reduction: the importance of maintaining dorsal aesthetic lines in rhinoplasty. Plast Reconstr Surg. 2004;114:1298-308.
5. Rohrich RJ, Hollier LH. Rhinoplasty-dorsal reduction and spreader grafts. In: Gunter JP, Rohrich RJ (Eds). 16th Annual Dallas Rhinoplasty Symposium. Dallas: University of Texas Southwestern Medical Center; 1999. p.153.
6. Skoog T. A method of hump reduction in rhinoplasty. Arch Otolaryngol. 1966;83:283-7.
7. Vuyk HD. Cartilage spreader grafting for lateral augmentation for the middle third of the nose. Face. 1993;3:159-70.
8. Daniel R. Radix and dorsum. In: Daniel R (Ed). Mastering rhinoplasty. Berlin: Springer-Verlag; 2010.pp.67-100.
9. Gruber RP, Park E, Newman J, Berkowitz L, Oneal R. The spreader flap in primary rhinoplasty. Plast Reconstr Surg. 2007;119:1903-10.
10. Huizing EH, de Groot JAM (Eds). Functional reconstructive nasal surgery. Stuttgart, New York: Thieme; 2003.
11. Tardy ME. Rhinoplasty: the Art and the Science, 1st edition. Philadelphia, USA: WB Saunders Co.; 1997.
12. Sheen JH. Aesthetic Rhinoplasty. St. Louis. MO: CV Mosby; 1978.
13. Lee HM, Kang HJ, Choi JH, Chae SW, Lee SH, Hwang SJ. Rationale for osteotome selection in rhinoplasty. J Laryngol Otol. 2002;116(12):1005-8.
14. Nolst Trenite GJ. Surgery of the osseocartilaginous vault. Rhinoplasty. Kugler Publications, The Hague: The Netherlands; 1998.
15. Sheen JH. Aesthetic Rhinoplasty, 2nd edition. St. Louis, Mo: Mosby; 1987.
16. Toriumi DM. Management of the middle nasal vault in rhinoplasty. Operative techniques in plastic and reconstructive surgery. 1995;2(1):16-30.

CHAPTER 10

Septoplasty

INTRODUCTION

Symptomatic deviated septum was found in 26% of patients with nasal obstruction in a study done on randomly chosen adults.[1] Trauma is a major cause of septal deviation. It may be a recent trauma or a childhood trauma. In childhood, even insignificant nasal trauma can produce unilateral microfractures affecting the growth of the septal cartilage. Trauma usually causes asymmetric damage to the septal cartilage. After some time, there will be overgrowth of the dominant side of the septal cartilage in comparison to the other side leading to a deviation with the convex side showing the dominant growth pattern.

Mladina classified the septal deviations into seven types:
- *Type 1:* Unilateral vertical crest in the valve area that does not reach the valve itself
- *Type 2:* Unilateral vertical crest in the valve area touching the nasal valve
- *Type 3:* Unilateral vertical crest located posteriorly in the nasal cavity
- *Type 4:* S-shaped deviation
- *Type 5:* Almost horizontal septal spur
- *Type 6:* Massive unilateral bony spur
- *Type 7:* Combination of these types.[2]

Freer (1902) and Killian (1904) introduced the submucous resection (SMR) operation for treatment of deviated septum. SMR is the foundation of modern septoplasty techniques.[3,4] In SMR, the dorsocaudal L-strut of at least 1 cm width is preserved while the rest of the nasal septum is removed. However, the straightened cartilage and bone pieces may be reinserted between the mucoperichondrial flaps to prevent complications.

In 1947, Cottle described the hemitransfixion incision and the procedure of conservative septal surgery.[5] In septoplasty, the area of deviation is corrected or resected leaving behind as much cartilage and bone as possible.

Septoplasty can be done at any age above 6 years.

The success of functional rhinoplasty depends on proper postoperative function of the septum, turbinates, and nasal valve area. During inspection of the nose in basal view, the caudal septum may be seen projecting into one of the nostrils and can reveal alar collapse during nasal breathing. Internal valve disorder can be diagnosed by Cottle test. Rhinomanometry is commonly used to assess nasal obstruction. Among various methods of rhinomanometry,

TABLE 1: Nasal Obstruction Symptom Evaluation (NOSE) questionnaire.

	No problem	Mild	Moderate	Bad	Severe
1. Nasal congestion	0	1	2	3	4
2. Nasal blockage or obstruction	0	1	2	3	4
3. Difficulties in nasal breathing	0	1	2	3	4
4. Disturbance in sleeping	0	1	2	3	4
5. Difficulties in nasal breathing during exercise or exertion	0	1	2	3	4

Total score (× 5): 0–100

anterior active rhinomanometry is most commonly done. Measurement of intranasal volume, and the size and location of minimal cross-sectional area are done by acoustic rhinomanometry. But the use of rhinomanometry is limited and subjective symptoms reported by the patients and the validated Nasal Obstruction Symptom Evaluation (NOSE) questionnaire are used as subjective assessments of nasal airway **(Table 1)**. The NOSE survey is a brief questionnaire consisting of five self-rated items, each scored from 0 to 4. The NOSE score represents the sum of the responses to the five individual items and multiplying the sum by 5. The final score ranges from 0 to 100.

INDICATIONS

- Nasal obstruction due to septal deviation.
- *Epistaxis:* Septoplasty is done to gain access to a posterior bleeding vessel for cauterization or packing. Septal deviation may also cause mucosal drying and crusting leading to intermittent epistaxis.
- *Sinusitis due to septal deviation:* Septoplasty may be combined with functional endoscopic sinus surgery (FESS).
- *Chronic dacryocystitis with septal deviation:* Endoscopic dacryocystorhinostomy (DCR) is combined with septoplasty.
- *Nasal bone fracture with dislocation or fracture of septum:* Reduction of nasal bone fracture is combined with septoplasty.
- In rhinoplasty, septoplasty is done to harvest septal cartilage graft and as a part of septorhinoplasty.
- *Hypophysectomy*: By transseptal-transsphenoidal approach.

For septoplasty, hemitransfixion incision is made at the caudal edge of the septal cartilage preserving the integrity of the membranous septum. Then, an anterior tunnel is made between the septal cartilage and the mucoperichondrium. Theoretically, unilateral elevation may leave a better blood supply to the septal cartilage, but elevation of the mucoperichondrium in both sides provides better exposure in severe septal deviations. The blood vessels of the septum run between the perichondrium and the mucosa.

Elevation of the mucoperichondrial flap from the septal cartilage is done at the avascular subperichondrial plane during septoplasty. Unilateral anterior tunnel is usually made in concave side of the septum. Inferior tunnels are made by elevating mucoperiosteum separately on both the sides over the premaxillary and maxillary crests **(Fig. 1)**. The anterior and inferior tunnels are joined without causing any injury or perforation of the flaps **(Fig. 2)**. The inferior part of the septum is detached from the anterior nasal spine, premaxilla, and the maxillary crest and a strip of cartilage is excised along the inferior border. Next, the posterior part of the septal cartilage is detached from the bony septum by a firm pressure with the septal elevator. The septum can now be moved aside like a swinging door and gives access to the bony septum. The mucoperiosteal flaps are elevated from the ethmoid and vomer on both sides and the deviated part of the bony septum is either excised or fractured.

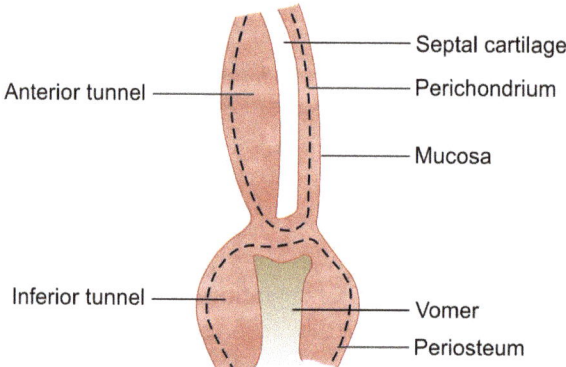

Fig. 1: Anterior tunnel and bilateral inferior tunnels during septoplasty.

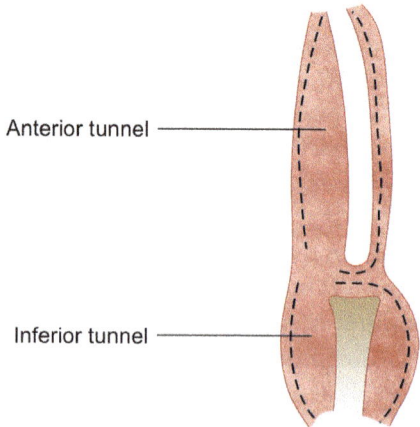

Fig. 2: Anterior and inferior tunnels made continuous in right side.

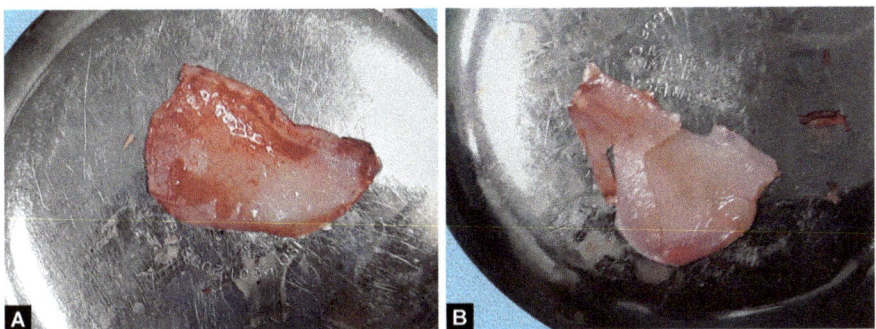

Figs. 3A and B: Deviated excised cartilage (A) can be made straight by incisions (B) and replaced between the mucoperichondrial flaps and sutured with the remnant cartilage.

The bony septum is sharply "bitten off" with a small Takahashi forceps. If the bony septum is twisted out, there is a chance of damage of the cribriform plate leading to cerebrospinal fluid (CSF) leak.

The bony spur along the floor is removed by a gouge but the anterior nasal spine is preserved. When the upper lateral cartilages prevent the straightening of the external deviation, these must be separated from the septum and spreader grafts are placed. The deviated septal cartilage can be weakened on its concave side by cross-hatching with partial-thickness incisions to relieve intracartilaginous tension.[6] Vertical scoring is done to correct vertical bending and horizontal scoring is done to correct horizontal bending of the cartilage. Parts of the excised cartilage may be replaced between the mucoperichondrial flaps, to avoid their direct adherence **(Figs. 3A and B)**.

A weakened deviated septum can be supported by bilateral stenting sandwich grafts. These grafts are placed in the submucoperichondrial plane on both sides of the deviation. Septal cartilage or perpendicular plate of ethmoid may be used as grafts. If ethmoid bone is used, small holes are made over it by a 3-mm drill bur. A 4-0 PDS suture is used to fix the stenting grafts.

For caudal deviation of septum, multiple vertical half-thickness cuts are done on the concave side. Excision of excess cartilage is done from the caudal end of the septal cartilage. Suture fixation is done with Vicryl suture taken from the concave side. Splinting by a small piece of septal cartilage or ethmoid bone may be done from the convex side. Vertical wedge resection on the convex side may also be done. The caudal end of the septum is fixed with the anterior nasal spine.

Swinging Door Technique

Metzenbaum (1929) advocated the use of the swinging door technique **(Fig. 4)**.[7] A dislocated caudal septum can be corrected by the swinging door technique, with or without splints. Here, incision is made at the site of angulation. A small

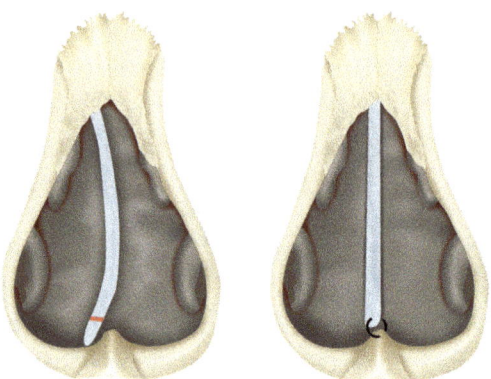

Fig. 4: Swinging door technique.

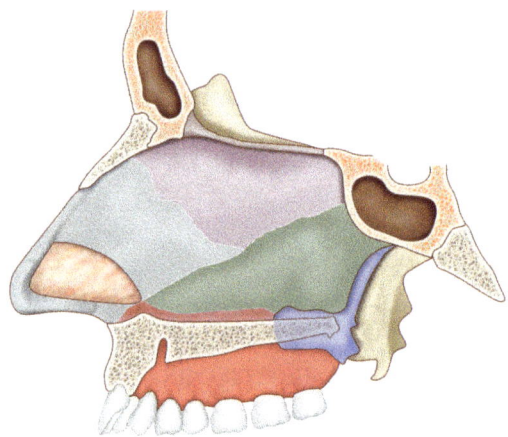

Fig. 5: Septal extension graft.

strip of cartilage can be excised at the site of angulation to achieve mobility. The caudal septum is fixed with the nasal spine by a suture taken either through the soft tissue over the spine area or through a drill hole made in the spine. Sometimes, the septum is "flipped" to the contralateral side of the nasal spine, and sutured to the periosteum. To accommodate the caudal septum in its new position, a pocket is made between the medial crura. In severe cases, caudal batten grafts or caudal septal extension grafts can be used to straighten the caudal septum **(Fig. 5)**. The batten graft is secured to the caudal septum by 4–0 PDS.[8]

Lastly, transfixation suture is done after making a new pocket in the columella.

During septoplasty, tears at the mucoperichondrial flaps usually occur at the junction of the septal cartilage with the crest of maxilla. As the resilient connective tissue fibers present at the junction are stronger than the mucoperichondrium itself; there is a chance of tearing the mucoperichondrium rather than the fibers of the junction if one attempts blunt dissection.[9] The nasal cavity should be packed lightly for 1 or 2 days.

Siegel et al. (2000) and Samad et al. (1992) observed that success rate for septoplasty operation is approximately 70%.[10,11]

Septoplasty can also be done by external approach or by endoscope in selected cases.

SEPTOPLASTY BY EXTERNAL APPROACH

The external approach for septoplasty is a technique to correct severe septal deviations, caudal deformities, and mid-dorsal abnormalities when an endonasal approach may be inadequate. In external approach, nasal valve is corrected and dorsal onlay graft is placed if needed. Unobstructed access is obtained to the nasal spine and caudal part of the septum **(Figs. 6 and 7)**.

Spreader grafts are cartilage struts usually used to reconstruct the dorsal nasal roof, and restore the internal valves. The grafts are taken from the septal cartilage, but in case of shortage, conchal cartilage and costal cartilage can be used. They should be 20–25 mm in length, 3–4 mm in height, and 2–3 mm in thickness.[12] During septoplasty in crooked nose, the deviated dorsal segment can be corrected by splinting it with two spreader grafts from both sides by external approach. The concave side can be cross-hatched to break the cartilage memory. Splinting spreader grafts are sutured by 4-0 PDS to keep the dorsal segment straight **(Fig. 8)**.

In revision septoplasty, when the caudal segment is inadequate, a caudal septal extension graft should be used. The graft is sutured to the anterior nasal spine and to the caudal septum **(Figs. 9 and 10)**.[13]

L-strut graft is used when both the dorsal and caudal segments are deviated. Before placing the graft, cross-hatching of the segments is done. The graft is

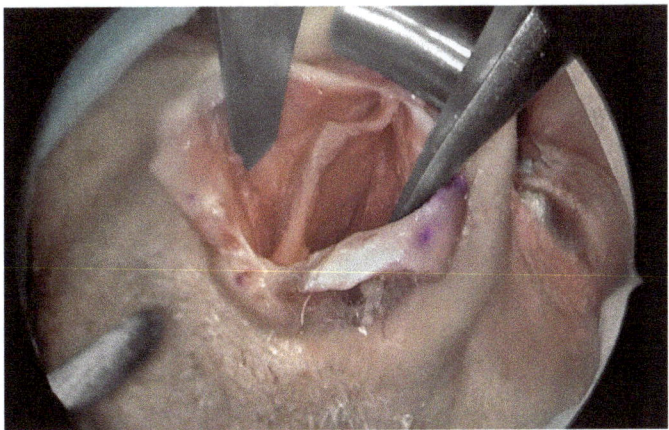

Fig. 6: Elevation of perichondrium in septoplasty by external approach in cadaver.

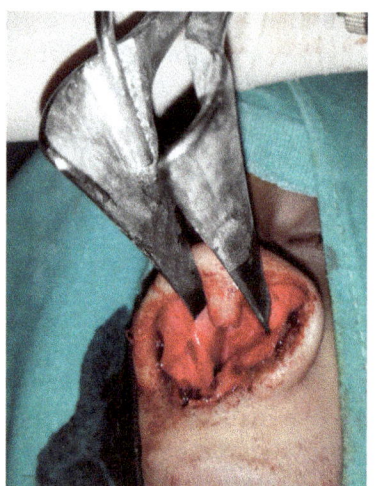

Fig. 7: Septoplasty by external approach.

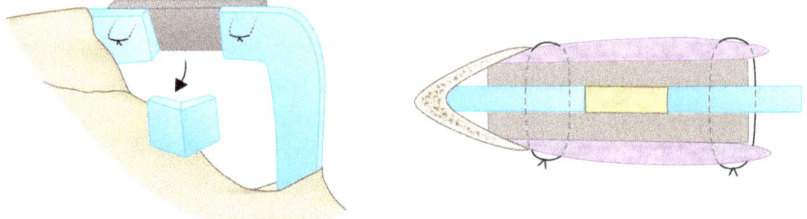

Fig. 8: Dorsal septal deviation corrected by excision and spreader grafts.

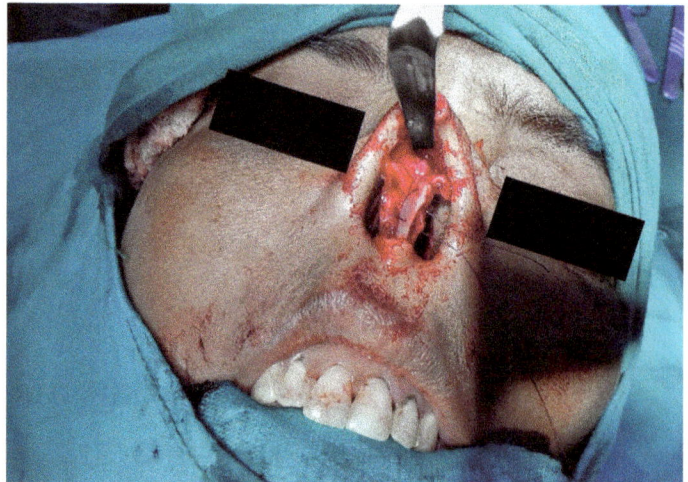

Fig. 9: Septal extension graft sutured with caudal septum.

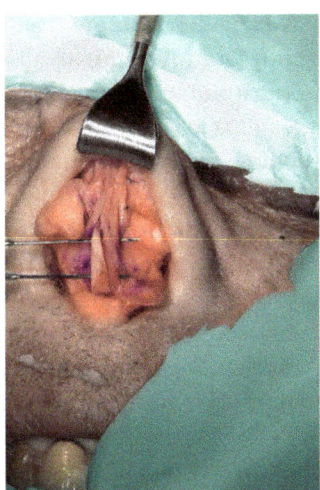

Fig. 10: Suturing of septal extension graft in cadaver.

fixed to a piece of cartilage at the key area and to the anterior nasal spine by multiple sutures.[14] In revision cases, the sixth costal cartilage is used to make a one-piece L-strut.[15] If a big L-strut cannot be obtained, two different pieces of cartilage can be used to replace dorsal and caudal segments. The two pieces are sutured on each other to form an L-strut.[16] If septal cartilage is not obtained in sufficient quantity, conchal cartilage or slices made from eighth rib can be taken as graft.[17]

Tongue-in-groove Technique

The "tongue-in-groove technique," when used in combination with septoplasty helps in correction of caudal septal deviations. Patients having a long caudal septum causing hanging columella are ideal for this technique.[18] Dissection is done to separate two medial crura. The medial crura are moved backward on the midline caudal septum in a "tongue-in-groove" manner and sutured to caudal septum with 5-0 PDS. Thus, procedures like trimming of caudal septum and placement of columellar strut are not required.[19]

ENDOSCOPIC SEPTOPLASTY

Endoscopic septoplasty is a conservative technique where the elevation of the nasal septal flap can be limited minimizing trauma. Furthermore, diagnosing and treating abnormalities of the lateral wall of the nose can be done at the same sitting in the endoscopic approach.

The first endoscopic septoplasty techniques were described by Stammberger (1990) and Lanza (1991).[20,21]

Endoscopic septoplasty provides better exposure, especially in posterior septal deviations. Endoscopy improves the accuracy of the dissection and elevation of mucoperichondrium can be done only in the deviated area of the septum. This technique helps in reducing tears in the mucosa and limited septoplasty is done.[22] Teaching and documentation can also be done in an endoscopic approach.

Endoscope can be placed easily in the mucoperichondrial tunnels. So minimal elevation of flap is needed to get maximum exposure. Incision can be made posteriorly just anterior to the deviated part, resulting in less mucosal elevation anteriorly in the nose and reduced postoperative edema. During endoscopic septoplasty, the bleeding points are identified and the incidence of hemorrhage is reduced. Endoscopy allows better assessment of the critical areas of obstruction such as nasal valve region during surgery. The ability to reduce mucosal elevation is an advantage in revision septoplasty, where the flaps are frequently adherent.[23]

Elevation of mucoperichondrial flap is done with a Cottle's elevator. A suction Freer elevator may be used instead of Cottle's elevator. Elevation of mucoperichodrial flap is done in both sides until the full exposure of septal deformity has been obtained. The deviated part of the septum is then excised with endoscopic scissors.

During FESS, isolated removal of spur is indicated when the septal spur causes obstruction to movement of endoscope and other instruments. Many patients have septal deviation that impedes adequate access to the middle meatus or to the axillary region of the middle turbinate. In those cases, endoscopic septoplasty is done to improve access to the middle meatus and to the frontal recess.

However, endoscopic septoplasty has certain limitations which include the need for frequent cleaning of the tip of the endoscope, loss of binocular vision, and inability to use both hands. In gross septal deviations, wider exposure is needed so, conventional septoplasty with hemitransfixion incision is a better approach. The role of endoscopic septoplasty in complex deviations with external nasal deformities and in caudal septal deviations is limited.

Hwang et al. (1999) described endoscopic septoplasty in 111 patients with promising results.[24]

Kamami (1997) had good results following septoplasties with carbon dioxide laser on 120 patients with limited anterior septal spurs.[25]

EXTRACORPOREAL SEPTOPLASTY

King and Ashley (1952) suggested extracorporeal septoplasty in marked septal deviations involving dorsal and caudal parts of cartilaginous septum as, these are difficult to correct by the conventional technique.[26] In extracorporeal septoplasty, the whole septum is taken out and reconstruction of a new straight septal plate, followed by replantation of this new septum is done.

Then reconstruction of the cartilaginous dorsum is done. Gubisch (1995) first published a big series on this subject.[27]

The surgery can be done by either a closed or open approach. In most of the cases, open approach is done, especially when septal deviation is associated with external nasal deformity. Elevation of mucoperichondrial flaps is done. The upper lateral cartilages are separated from the dorsal border of the septum after extramucosal dissection. After hump removal, the bony septum is vertically fractured as far as possible posteriorly by pressure with a 5-mm chisel. If dorsal hump removal has not been done, a paramedian osteotomy is needed to detach the bony septum from the dorsum. The whole cartilaginous and bony septum is then removed in a single piece after separation of cartilaginous septum from nasal spine and crest of maxilla. The septum is then made straight on the back table by partial-thickness releasing incisions on the concave side and suturing the detached parts of the septum by 4-0 PDS. The ideal reconstructed septal plate should be as large as possible, with stable dorsal and caudal parts. Sometimes, a sharp drill is used to smoothen the cartilage and bone. A piece of perpendicular plate of ethmoid can be sutured onto the cartilaginous septum to make it straight. Occasionally, when there is no tear in mucoperichondrium, a PDS foil is sutured to stabilize the cartilage pieces. In saddle deformity and postoperative cases with little residual cartilaginous septum, the bony septal pieces can be used to reconstruct a stable and straight dorsocaudal L-strut. Multiple holes are drilled on the bony pieces for fixation postoperatively when tissue grows through the holes. The neoseptum is then replanted between the mucoperichondrial and mucoperiosteal flaps. Bilateral spreader grafts are sutured on dorsal part of the septum.[28] If required, conchal cartilage or rib cartilage graft is harvested. The neoseptum with spreader graft is kept within the mucoperichondrial flaps and fixed at the caudal end of the nasal bones, upper lateral cartilages and anterior nasal spine. Fixation is done by drilling holes through the nasal bones and the nasal spine and suturing the neoseptum by PDS. Columellar strut, rim grafts and tip grafts are placed if required. To avoid dorsal irregularities, diced cartilages or folded fascia are placed over dorsum. A quilting suture is done at the caudal septum to stabilize the replanted septum, and to prevent hematoma formation.[29]

Following complications may occur in extracorporeal septoplasty: Septal deviation, upper lip stiffness, saddle nose, dorsal irregularity, septal perforation, and synechia.[30]

Modified extracorporeal septoplasty is based on partial resection of the cartilaginous septum, with preservation of a superocaudal L-strut. This technique has been effective at long-term follow-up in cases of moderate or severe septal deviation. With this technique, structural support is achieved without destabilizing the keystone area.[31]

SEPTOPLASTY IN CHILDREN

Septoplasty is not commonly done in children because of the notion that the septal cartilage is essential for the primary growth of the midfacial structures. But it is a fact that the septum, maxilla, and premaxilla develop independently of one another and septoplasty can be done in small children with gross septal deformity successfully **(Figs. 11A to D)**. Septal deviations usually worsen with the growth of the nose leading to infections of upper respiratory tract and middle ear cavity. Deviations of the caudal part of the septum are commonly found to cause symptoms. Dental problems, malocclusion, facial deformities, and pulmonary hypertension or cor pulmonale may develop when septoplasty is not performed during childhood.[32]

Septoplasty can be done in children successfully without affecting the development of the nose and midfacial region.[33]

However, dissection and removal of septal cartilage and bone should be conservative and minimal, and surgery should be restricted to the deviated part of the septum.[34]

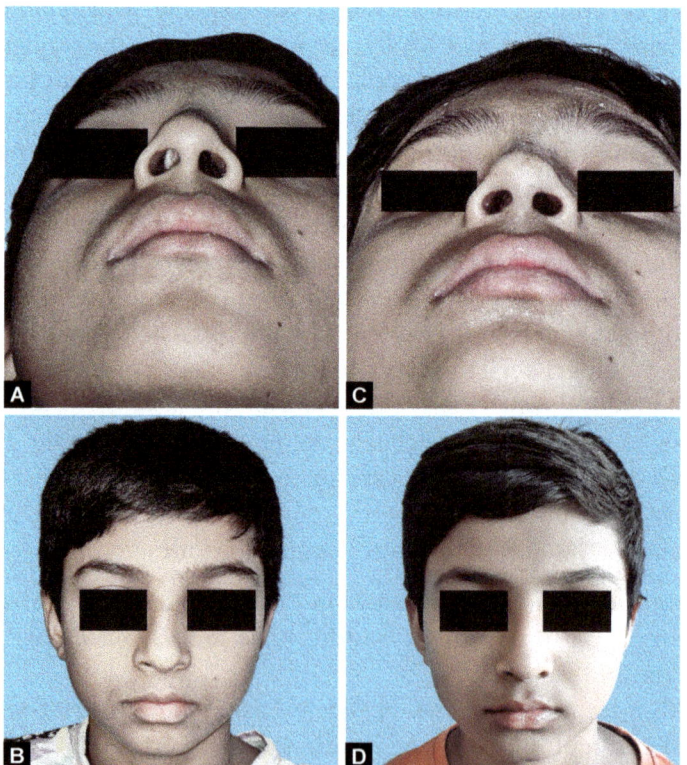

Figs. 11A to D: (A and B) Preoperative; and (C and D) Postoperative views of caudal dislocation of septum with crooked nose in a 10-year-old child, corrected by septoplasty, percutaneous transverse and lateral osteotomies.

Lawrence (2012) mentioned that, in most cases, septoplasty can be done in 6-year-old children.

In western people, maximum growth of the nose is seen between ages 8 and 12 years in girls and at 13 years in boys. Gradual ossification occurs at the septal cartilage. The perpendicular plate of the ethmoid expands from an area near the anterior skull base in the anteroinferior direction.[34] In adults, about 60% of the septum is made of bony components.

Pediatric septoplasty surgeries have been regularly done since the 1970s.[35]

Indications for pediatric septoplasty are the following[36]:
- Severe septal deviation due to nasal trauma
- Cleft lip and nose
- Sleep apnea with complete nasal obstruction
- Severe deviated nasal septum (DNS) causing significant nasal blockage.

During septoplasty in children, special precautions should be taken to preserve the mucoperichondrium, the growth areas (e.g., caudal part of the septum), the anterior nasal spine, and the sutural junctions with the vomer and perpendicular plate. The septum in children is formed mainly by septal cartilage; the contribution of the vomer and perpendicular plate of ethmoid is less. During operation, septal cartilage should not be separated from the perpendicular plate, especially at the dorsal part because this area is important for the length and height of the nasal dorsum and septum. Mobilization of nasal bones by osteotomies along with septoplasty should be avoided to prevent postoperative instability. If there is caudal dislocation of septum, then it should be sutured into the columellar pocket created between the medial crura. When upper lateral cartilages are detached from the dorsal border of septum bilaterally, they should be restored to prevent deformity of the cartilaginous nasal dorsum.[37]

During septoplasty, the pieces of removed septal cartilage are made straight and replaced in between the mucoperichondrial flaps because even after operative trauma, the septal cartilage has some regenerative capacity.[38]

Mucoperichondrium should not be torn during septoplasty as it is essential for cartilage regeneration and survival of transplanted cartilage.

It is to be noted that some cases of septoplasty in children may require a revision surgery in adult age.

Septal dislocation in newborns may be due to birth trauma or due to abnormal intrauterine pressure over nose during pregnancy. Septal dislocation in a newborn baby can be diagnosed by observing the asymmetry of the nostrils, the deviated tip, and the deformed columella. Anterior rhinoscopy can be done with a small nasal speculum. Tip support should be tested by pressing the tip downwards (compression test).

Reduction of the dislocated septum is done within 48 hours after birth under local anesthesia using a small forceps by an upward and rotatory

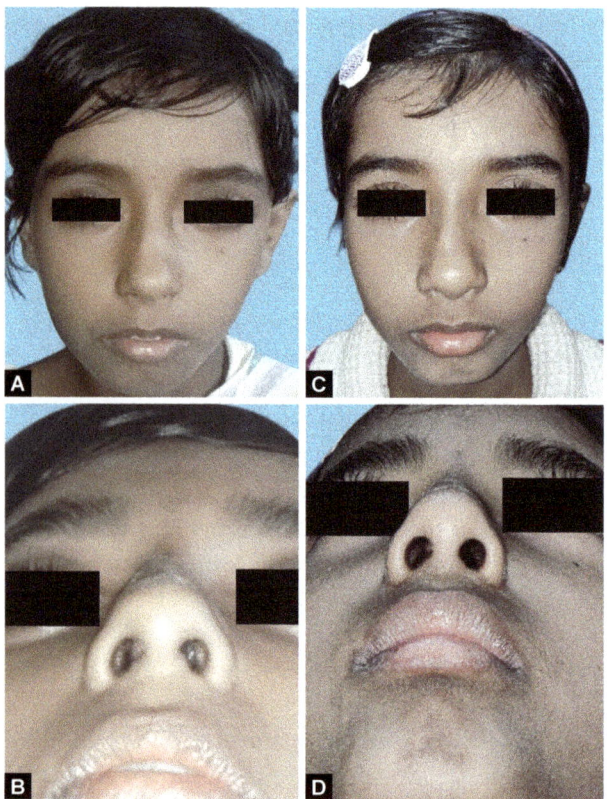

Figs. 12A to D: (A and B) Preoperative; (C and D) Postoperative views of crooked nose with DNS to right in a 10-year-old child, corrected by septoplasty, percutaneous transverse and intranasal lateral osteotomies.

movement toward the vomerine groove. A delayed correction becomes difficult because of fibrosis.

To diagnose deviated nasal septum in neonates, Gray's struts can be used. The septum is considered normal if the struts pass inside the nasal cavities up to the 4-cm mark. DNS is diagnosed when the strut gets stuck before the 4-cm mark on that particular side.[39]

Septorhinoplasty can be done in children in selected candidates for greater functional and anatomic results. The surgery should be conservative and hump removal or other aesthetic procedures should not be done. Septum should not be separated from the upper lateral cartilages. Endonasal lateral osteotomies and percutaneous paramedian and transverse osteotomies can be done if indicated **(Figs. 11 to 13)**.

In children, both external and endonasal approaches can be done. Removal of the deviated vomer and premaxilla does not disturb the normal nasal growth. Placement of grafts for dorsal augmentation and spreader grafts should be avoided.

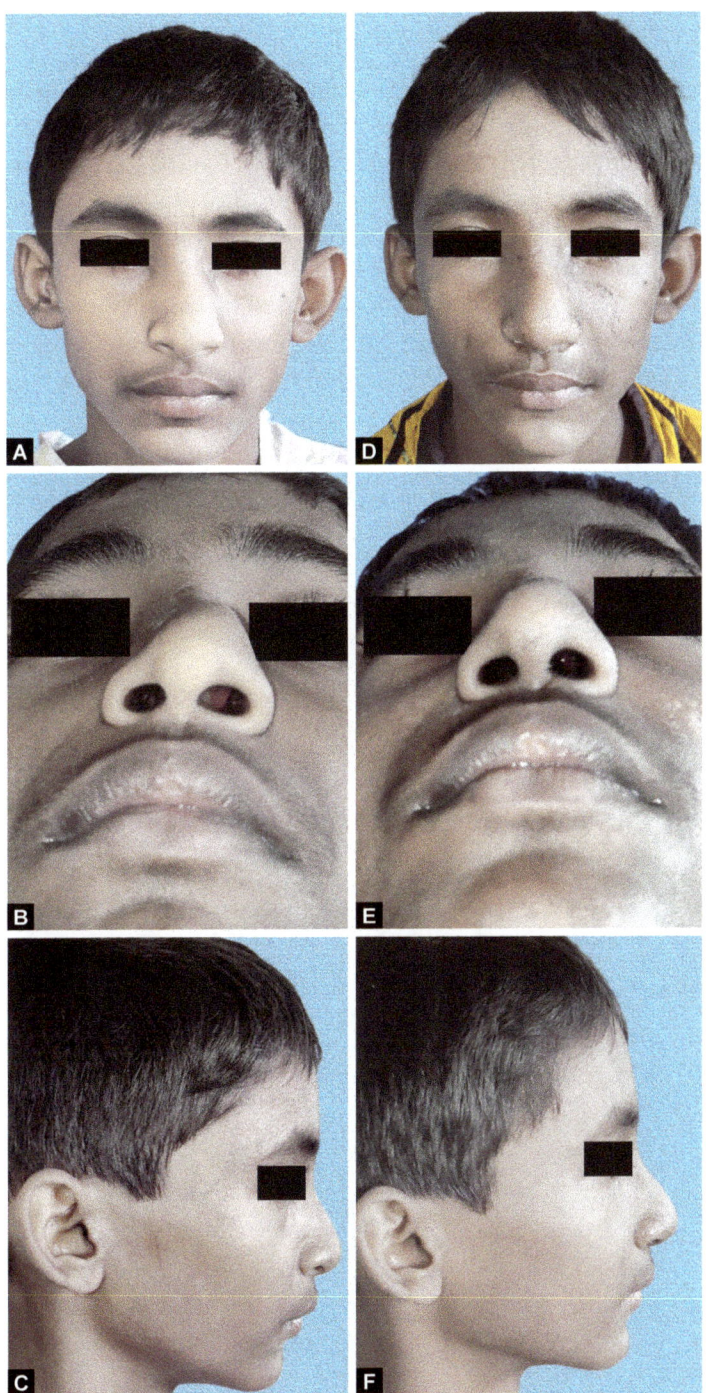

Figs. 13A to F: (A to C) Preoperative; and (D to F) Early postoperative views of crooked nose with DNS to left in a 10-year-old child, corrected by septoplasty, percutaneous transverse and intranasal lateral osteotomies.

CAUDAL DEVIATION OF SEPTUM

Caudal deviation involves that part of the septum which supports the nasal tip and makes the medial boundary of the nasal valve area **(Figs. 14A to C)**. It causes both functional and esthetic problems. Caudal deviation may cause nasal obstruction, epistaxis, recurrent rhinosinusitis, and twisting of the lower third of the nose. Caudal septal deficiency may cause tip ptosis and under projection of tip.[40] Nasal obstruction caused by minimum caudal deviations is much greater than the one caused by large posterior deviations.

The etiology of caudal deviation may be congenital, traumatic, or iatrogenic. Caudal deviation may be mild, moderate, or severe. There is no single method to correct all the cases.[41]

Various types of caudal deviations are anterior subluxation, C- or S-shaped deviations, and combination of horizontal and/or vertical angulations and deviations.

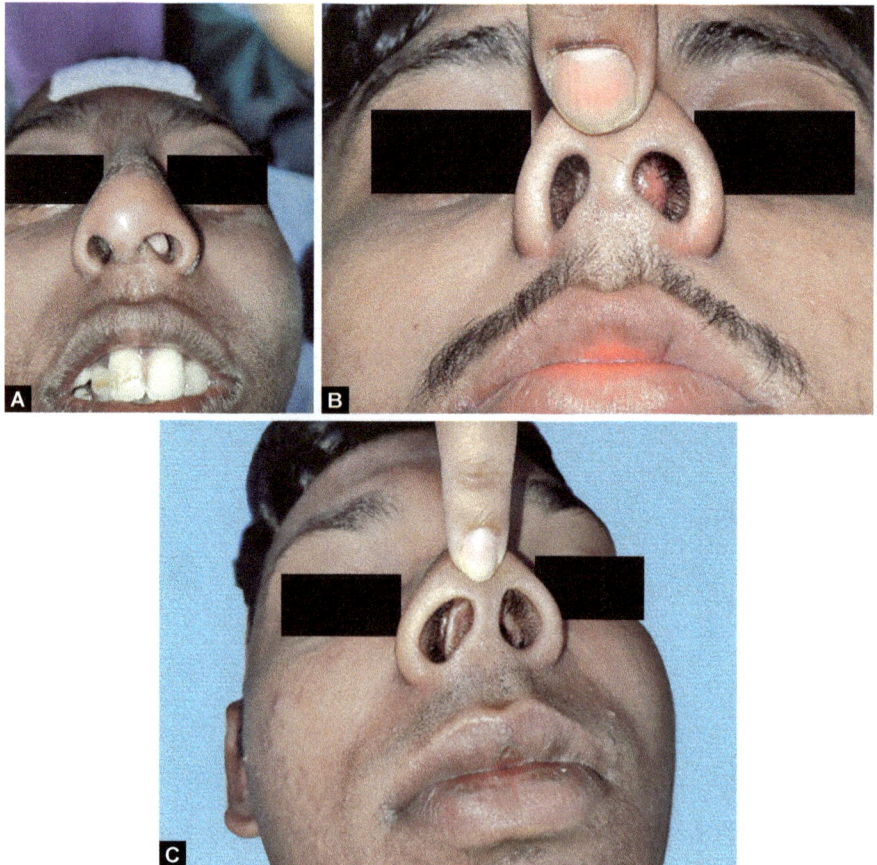

Figs. 14A to C: (A and B) Caudal deviation of septum; and (C) Caudal dislocation of septum.

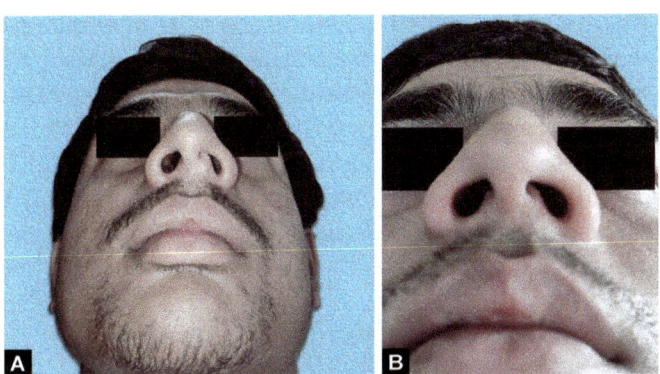

Figs. 15A and B: (A) Preoperative; and (B) Postoperative views of caudal deviation of septum corrected by swinging door technique.

Correction of caudal septal deviation is a difficult procedure. Even after correction the caudal septum may return to its preoperative state because of cartilage memory. There are different methods of corrections like scoring, vertical wedge resection, swinging door technique, placement of spreader grafts or batten grafts, tongue-in-groove technique, columellar strut, septal extension graft, cutting and suture technique, extracorporeal septoplasty, modified extracorporeal septoplasty, and "marionette septoplasty" **(Figs. 15A and B)**.[42]

Scoring is a common method of correction. Vertical or horizontal scoring can be done over concave side of septal cartilage to weaken the cartilage and break the memory in order to prevent recurrence of deviation. But scoring at dorso-caudal strut region weakens the caudal septum and may lead to saddle nose deformities.[43] *Resection of vertical wedge* of cartilage is done on the convex part of septal deformity. This is done in mild and moderate deviations. However, final straightening of the septum is affected by the secondary healing process and there may be recurrence of deviations.

Septal repositioning can be done by the *swinging door method* which was first described by Metzenbaum in 1929.[7] A vertical wedge of cartilage is removed on the convex side of the septum. The caudal septum is then repositioned in a swinging door fashion and sutured with the periosteum over anterior nasal spine or secured after making a burr hole at the nasal spine with 5-0 PDS **(Figs. 16A and B)**.

Translocation of the caudal septum can be done by repositioning the septum to the other side of the anterior nasal spine and sutured with 5-0 PDS. When excess length of the septal cartilage is the cause of the deviation, a caudal strip of septal cartilage is removed and the caudal septum is sutured with the nasal spine.[40]

In severe caudal septal deformity, swinging door technique may not be effective. In these cases, unilateral bony or cartilage batten grafting will be effective.[44] *Batten graft* should be strong and thin and is taken from septal cartilage, rib cartilage, vomer, or perpendicular plate of ethmoid. Scoring or wedge resection of deviated caudal cartilage is done and the batten graft is sutured with the concave side of the septal cartilage using 4-0 PDS to support it and prevent recurrence of deviation **(Fig. 17)**. Holes are made on the bony batten graft by an 18-gauge needle to facilitate suturing **(Fig. 18)**. As the ethmoid bone is a membranous bone, chance of resorption is minimum. Unilateral or bilateral *spreader grafts* can also be used to correct caudal septal deviation.

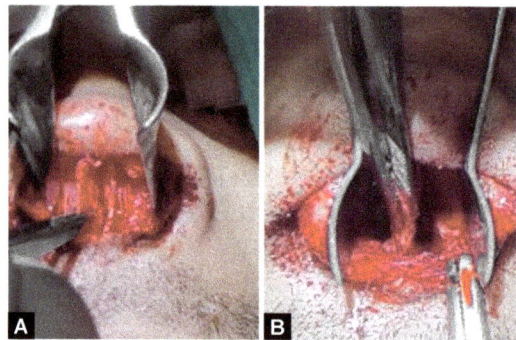

Figs. 16A and B: Swinging door technique: (A) Incision is made at the site of angulation; (B) Caudal septum is fixed with the nasal spine.

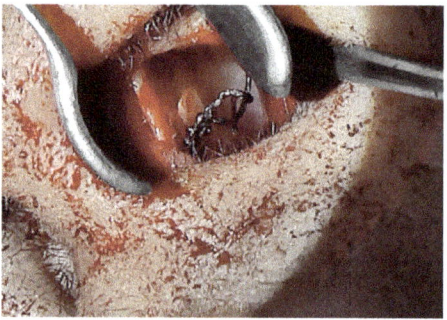

Fig. 17: Bony batten graft has been sutured with the concave side of the septal cartilage.

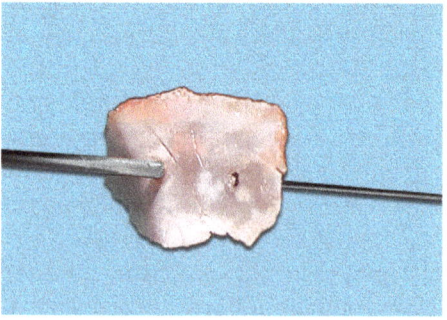

Fig. 18: Holes are made on the ethmoid bone by an 18-gauze needle.

Kridel et al. performed *tongue-in-groove technique* for correcting caudal deviation with excess columellar show. Dissection is done to separate two medial crura. The medial crura are moved backward on the midline caudal septum in a "tongue-in-groove" manner and sutured to caudal septum with 5-0 PDS. Thus, procedures such as trimming of caudal septum and placement of columellar strut are not required **(Fig. 19)**.[19]

In *"cutting and suture technique,"* the deviated parts of cartilaginous and bony septum are excised, leaving 1.5 cm of L-strut. To correct caudal septal deviation, the caudal strut is cut at the most convex part, and the cut ends are overlapped and sutured together with 5-0 PDS. This technique is done by endonasal approach in C-shaped caudal deviation without dislocation of the septum from the anterior nasal spine. There should not be any external nasal deformity. A septal batten graft can be placed on the concave side for additional support **(Figs. 20A to C)**.[45]

In caudal septal deficiency, *septal extension graft or columellar strut* can be used. Septal extension graft is sutured with caudal septal cartilage and can be stabilized in a pocket between the medial crura and sutured with 5-0 PDS as in tongue-in-groove technique. Caudal septal extension graft may lead to deviated nasal tip if it is sutured to the caudal septum in overlapping fashion. To prevent deviated nasal tip, the caudal septal graft can be placed end to end with existing caudal septum and anchoring it to extended spreader grafts and the anterior nasal spine.

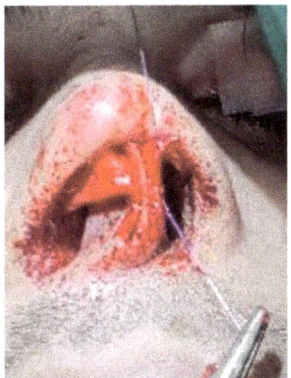

Fig. 19: Tongue-in-groove technique: medial crura are sutured to caudal septum.

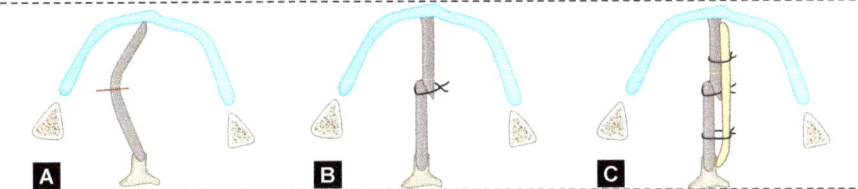

Figs. 20A to C: Cutting and suture technique for caudal deviation of septum: (A) Incision at most convex part; (B) Cut ends are overlapped and sutured; (C) Placement of batten graft.

Columellar strut provides stability, projection, and shape of the columella. It prevents drooping of the tip. The columellar strut is usually 20 mm long, 2.5 mm wide, and 1.5 mm thick, but the actual shape can vary depending upon the need. The graft is usually taken from the vomerine septal cartilage because of its thickness and rigidity. A vertical suture of 5-0 PDS is placed through the columella which holds the strut between the medial crura.

Subtotal extracorporeal septoplasty done by closed approach is called *"marionette septoplasty"*. Here, a small dorsal strut of cartilage is retained near the K-area to facilitate suturing with the L strut, created from the harvested septum.[46]

REFERENCES

1. Vainio-Mattila J. Correlations of nasal symptoms and signs in random sampling study. Acta Otolaryngol Suppl. 1974;318:1-48.
2. Mladina R. The role of maxillar morphology in the development of pathological septal deformities. Rhinology. 1987;25(3):199-205.
3. Freer OT. The correction of deflections of the nasal septum with a minimum of traumatism. JAMA. 1902;16:362-75.
4. Killian G. Die Sumucose Fensterresektion der Nasenscheiwand. Arch Laryngologie Rhinologie. 1904;16:362-94.
5. Cottle MH. Newer concepts of septum surgery: present status. Eye Ear Nose Throat Monthly. 1948;27:403-29.
6. Cottle MH, Loring RM, Fischer GC, Gaynon IE. The maxilla-premaxilla approach to extensive nasal septum surgery. Arch Otolaryngol. 1958;68(3):301-13.
7. Metzenbaum M. Replacement of the lower end of the dislocated septal cartilage versus submucous resection of the dislocated end of the septal cartilage. Arch Otolaryngol HNS. 1929;9:282-311.
8. Toriumi DM. Structural approach to primary rhinoplasty. Aesthet Surg J. 2002;22:72-84.
9. Wentges RTR. Septo-rhinoplasty: applied anatomy and physiology. J Laryngol Otol. 1980;94:467-73.
10. Siegel NS, Gliklich RE, Taghizadeh F, Chang Y. Outcomes of septoplasty. Otolaryngol Head Neck Surg. 2000;122(2):228-32.
11. Samad I, Stevens HE, Maloney A. The efficacy of nasal septal surgery. J Otolaryngol. 1992;21(2):88-91.
12. Sheen JH. Spreader graft: a method of reconstructing the roof of the middle nasal vault following rhinoplasty. Plast Reconstr Surg. 1984;73:230-9.
13. Foda HM. The caudal septum replacement graft. Arch Facial Plast Surg. 2008;10:152-7.
14. Toriumi DM. Subtotal reconstruction of the nasal septum: a preliminary report. Laryngoscope. 1994;104:906-13.
15. Rettinger G. Reconstruction of the pronounced saddle nose. Laryngorhinootologie. 1997;76:672-5.
16. Dyer WK 2nd, Yune ME. Structural grafting in rhinoplasty. Facial Plast Surg. 1997;13:269-77.
17. Tastan E. Presented at the 33th Annual Meeting of the European Academy of Facial Plastic Surgery, Antalya-Turkey, 1-4 September, 2010.
18. Toriumi DM. New concepts in nasal tip contouring. Arch Facial Plast Surg. 2006;8:156-85.
19. Kridel RW, Scott BA, Foda HM. The tongue-in-groove technique in septorhinoplasty. A 10-year experience. Arch Facial Plast Surg. 1999;1(4):246-56.
20. Stammberger H, Posawetz W. Functional endoscopic sinus surgery. Concept, indications and results of the Messerklinger technique. Eur Arch Otorhinolaryngol. 1990;247(2):63-76.

21. Lanza DC. Nasal endoscopy and its applications. Essent Otolaryngol Head Neck Surg. 1991;373-87.
22. Giles WC, Gross CW, Abram AC, et al. Endoscopic septoplasty. Laryngoscope. 1994;104:1507-9.
23. Gupta N. Endoscopic septoplasty. IJOHNS. 2005;57(3):240-3.
24. Hwang PH, McLaughlin RB, Lanza DC, Kennedy DW. Endoscopic septoplasty: indications, technique, and results. Otolaryngol Head Neck Surg. 1999;120(5):678-82.
25. Kamami YV. Laser-assisted outpatient septoplasty results on 120 patients. J Clin Laser Med Surg. 1997;15(3):123-9.
26. King ED, Ashley FL. The correction of the internally and externally deviated nose. Plast Reconstr Surg. 1952;10:116-20.
27. Gubisch W. The extracorporeal septum plasty: a technique to correct difficult nasal deformities. Plast Reconstr Surg. 1995;95(4):672-82.
28. Gubisch W. Extracorporeal septoplasty for the markedly deviated septum. Arch Facial Plast Surg. 2005;7(4):218-26.
29. Gubisch W. Extracorporeal septoplasty for the markedly deviated septum. Archives of Facial Plastic Surgery. 2005;7(4).
30. Gubisch W. Twenty-five years experience with extracorporeal septoplasty. Facial Plast Surg. 2006;22(4):230-9.
31. Persichetti P, Toto V, Segreto F et al. Modified extracorporeal septoplasty: functional results at 6-year follow-up. Ann Plast Surg. 2016;76(5):504-8.
32. Siegel MI. The role of cartilaginous nasal septum in midfacial growth. Plast Reconstr Surg. 1980;65:93-4.
33. Huizing EH. Septum surgery in children; indications, surgical technique and long-term results. Rhinology. 1979;17:91-100.
34. Cemal C, Nuray BM, Seckin U, Lopatin A, Şahin E, Passali D, et al. Septoplasty in children. Am J Rhinol Allergy. 2016,30(2):42-7.
35. Lawrence R. Pediatric septoplasty: a review of the literature. Int J Pediatr Otorhinolaryngol. 2012;76:1078-81.
36. Christophel JJ, Gross CW. Pediatric septoplasty. Otolaryngol Clin North Am. 2009;42:287-94.
37. Verwoerd CD, Verwoerd-Verhoef HL. Rhinosurgery in children: developmental and surgical aspects of the growing nose. Laryngorhinootologie. 2010;89(Suppl 1):S46-S71.
38. Behrbohm H, Tardy ME. Essentials of septorhinoplasty. Philosophy-Approaches-Techniques. New York: Thieme, Stuttgart; 2004.
39. Harugop AS, Mudhol RS, Hajare PS, Nargund AI, Metgudmath VV, Chakrabarti S. Prevalence of Nasal Septal Deviation in New-borns and Its Precipitating Factors: a Cross-Sectional Study. Indian J Otolaryngol Head Neck Surg. 2012;64(3):248-51.
40. Waleed MA, Ibrahim HA, Mohammed AJ, Badi FA. Caudal Septal Deviation: Pertinent Literature Review. J Surg Res. 2021;4:742-48.
41. Haack J, Papel ID. Caudal septal deviation. Otolaryngol Clin North Am. 2009;42:427-36.
42. Ceyhun A. Caudal septal division and batten graft application: a technique to correct caudal septal deviations. Turk Arch Otorhinolaryngol. 2020;58(3):181-5.
43. Heo SJ, Kim JS. Crosshatching incision technique in septoplasty: experimental outcomes under actual surgical settings. Auris Nasus Larynx. 2016;43:518-23.
44. Chung YS, Seol JH, Choi JM, Shin DH, Kim YW, Cho JH, et al. How to resolve the caudal septal deviation? Clinical outcomes after septoplasty with bony batten grafting. Laryngoscope. 2014;124:1771-6.
45. Jang YJ, Yeo NK, Wang JH. Cutting and suture technique of the caudal septal cartilage for the management of caudal septal deviation. Arch Otolaryngol Head Neck Surg. 2009;135(12):1256-60.
46. Kayabasoglu G, Nacar A, Yilmaz MS, Altundag A, Guven M. A novel method for reconstruction of severe caudal nasal septal deviation: Marionette septoplasty. Ear Nose Throat J. 2015;94(6):E34-40.

CHAPTER 11

Osteotomies

INTRODUCTION

To close the open roof, osteotomies are done. Osteotomies should be avoided in narrow noses and in elderly patients with fragile bones. Here the open roof can be corrected by placing dorsal grafts.

LATERAL OSTEOTOMY

A 3-mm guarded osteotome is the ideal instrument for lateral osteotomy. Wide osteotomes cause more mucosal injuries. Bone thickness does not exceed 3 mm at any point on the osteotomy lines.[1] Lateral osteotomies are done to close the open roof following hump removal, to correct the crooked bony vault and to narrow the broad nose.[2,3] The upper limit of lateral osteotomy should be superficial to medial canthus to prevent injury to the medial canthal ligament. Lateral osteotomies are commonly done in a high-low-high direction. Here osteotomy is initiated at a high position on the pyriform aperture leaving a triangle of bone at the base of the pyriform aperture (Webster triangle).[4] Thus, narrowing of the width of the nasal passage at the base is avoided. The osteotomy is then done low along the mid-dorsum to narrow that part and then again in a high direction to avoid overnarrowing at the nasal root. In cases of wide nasal root and wide nasal base, low-to-low lateral osteotomy can be done (**Figs. 1 and 2**). If a high-to-high osteotomy is done, a step deformity will result.

In intranasal lateral osteotomy, a stab incision about 1/2 cm in length is made at the base of the pyriform aperture just in front of the attachment of inferior turbinate and the incision extends to the bone. The periosteum is elevated with Mcindoe elevator just enough to place the chisel or osteotome. The right hand holds the Silver nasal chisel firmly, the left index finger

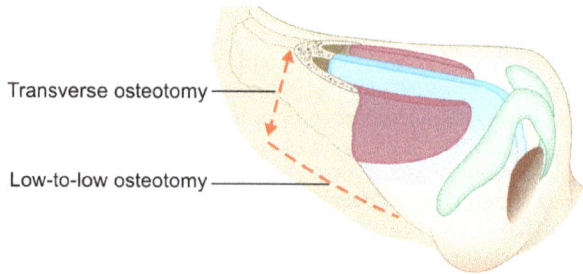

Fig. 1: Lateral and transverse osteotomies.

Osteotomies

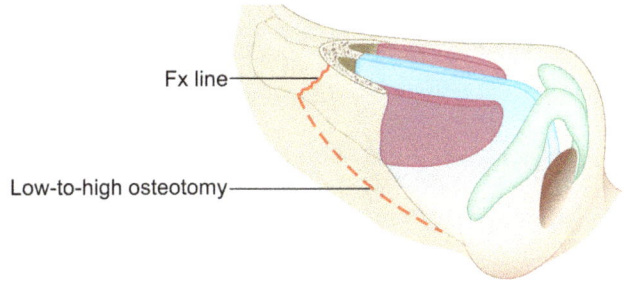

Fig. 2: Lateral osteotomy. (Fx: fracture)

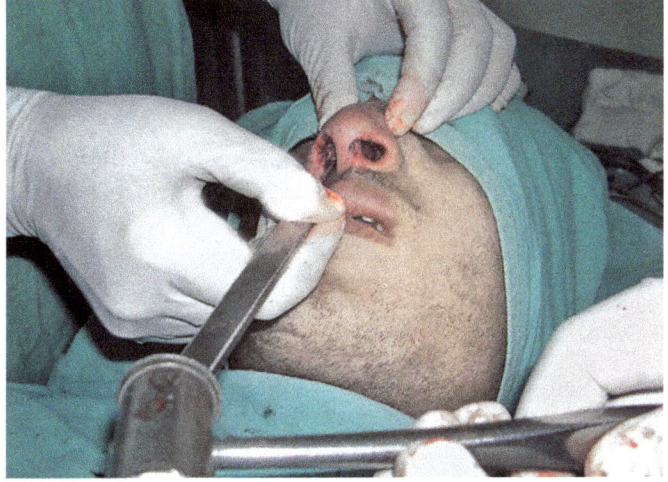

Fig. 3: Intranasal lateral osteotomy by Silver nasal chisel in right side.

palpates the guard of the chisel as it advances, and the assistant strikes the chisel with a hammer in sequence of two taps like "one-two", followed by a pause and to repeat the same sequence. The assistant stops hammering when the tapping tone changes. A gentle upward elevation of the handle of the chisel by a few degrees, or medial rotation of the chisel, completes the osteotomy **(Figs. 3 and 4)**.

Lateral osteotomy can also be done by introducing Joseph saw against the frontal process of maxilla along the nasofacial groove at right angle to the surface of bone. But osteotomy by saw takes more time and produces bone dust.

Percutaneous lateral osteotomy can be done by using 2-mm osteotome introduced through a stab incision in the skin externally over the pyriform aperture. Postage stamp type cuts are made along the line of lateral osteotomy. Another stab incision is made in between the medial canthus and dorsum of nose and transverse osteotomy is done through the incision. The same procedure is also done on the other side, and the bony lateral walls are infractured by digital pressure **(Fig. 5)**.

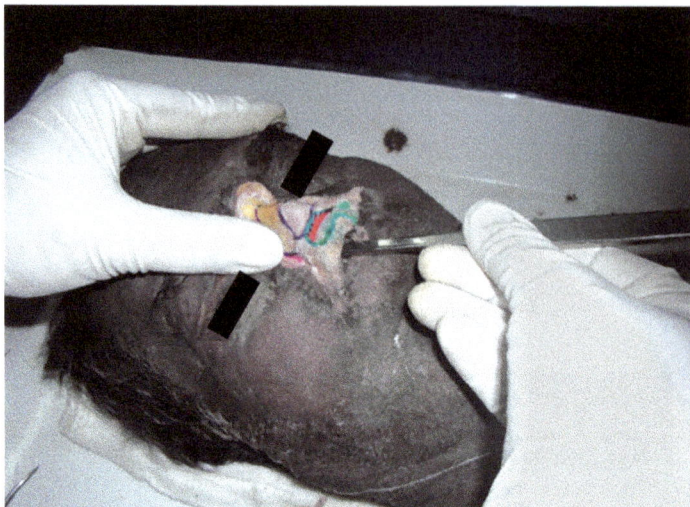

Fig. 4: Cadaver dissection showing lateral osteotomy by Silver nasal chisel palpating the guard of the instrument with thumb of the left hand in internal continuous method.

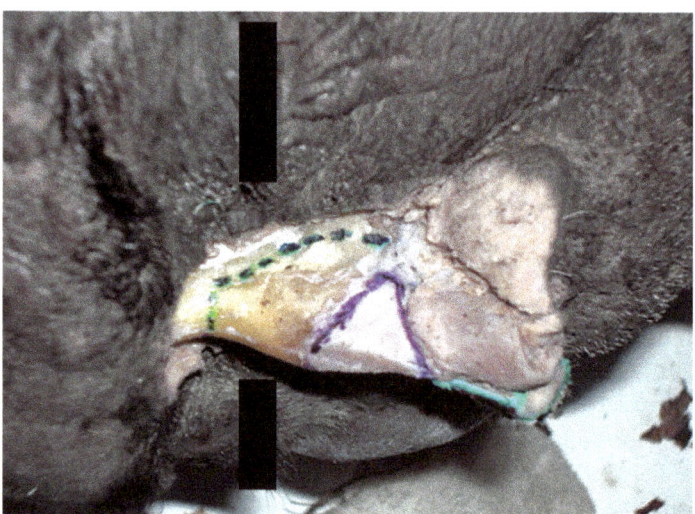

Fig. 5: Cadaver dissection showing stamp type cuts (green) done by 2-mm osteotome in percutaneous lateral and transverse osteotomies.

In sublabial lateral osteotomy, the chisel is introduced sublabially through a small incision in the mucosa over the canine fossa. The periosteum is elevated only till the edge of pyriform aperture and then the chisel is placed at the edge.

To perform curved lateral osteotomy or oblique osteotomy after reaching near the infraorbital border, the chisel is rotated and osteotomy cut is made medially toward the dorsum and the bony wall is infractured. If oblique osteotomy is done, transverse osteotomy is not required **(Fig. 6)**.

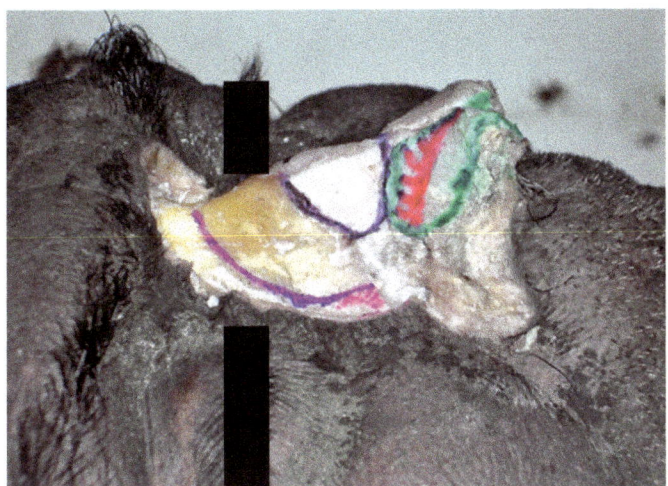

Fig. 6: Cadaver dissection showing curved lateral osteotomy by internal continuous method.

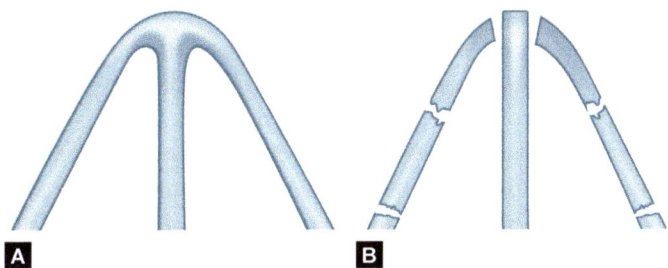

Figs. 7A and B: (A) Wide bony pyramid in axial plane; (B) Medial, intermediate, and lateral osteotomy cuts.

Unilateral lateral osteotomy can be done to narrow a convex lateral wall, when a convex lateral wall gives the impression of ipsilateral deviation of the nose.

INTERMEDIATE OSTEOTOMY

Intermediate osteotomy is done to shorten a markedly convex lateral wall. Intermediate osteotomy is done prior to the lateral osteotomy to prevent fragmentation of the lateral wall **(Figs. 7A and B)**. Indications for the "double osteotomies" are unequal lengths of the lateral bony walls, marked convexity of one bony nasal wall with concavity of the opposite wall, and to straighten a badly traumatized nose. The periosteal attachment should be maintained during double osteotomies or comminution techniques, as the periosteal attachment to the nasal bone fragments prevents displacement and maintains support of the mobilized bony fragments.[5]

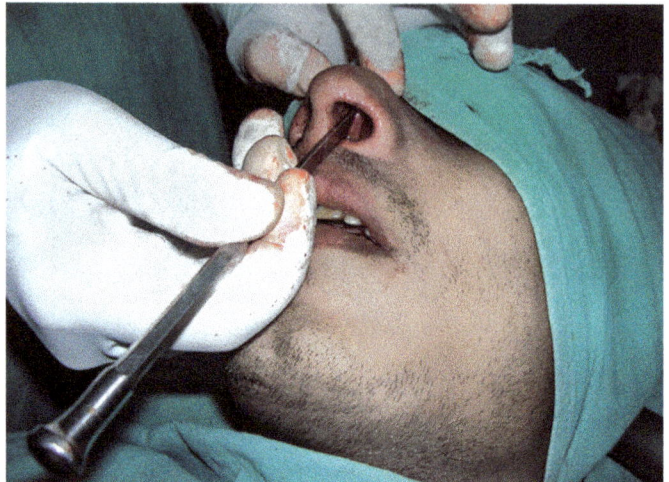

Fig. 8: Medial osteotomy by Gillies osteotome through intercartilaginous incision.

MEDIAL OSTEOTOMY

Medial osteotomies are not required if an open roof results after hump removal. Medial osteotomies are done prior to lateral osteotomies. This helps in making a complete break. Incomplete osteotomies result in bony irregularities and postoperative recurrence of the deformity. A 4-mm wide Gillies osteotome is inserted between the lower end of nasal bone and bony septum and directed 15° lateral from the midline (medial or paramedian osteotomy). The dorsal skin is lifted with the fingers of the left hand to prevent any injury to the skin. The assistant strikes the osteotome with hammer in sequence of two taps like "one-two". The bony cuts are directed upward and laterally **(Fig. 8)**.

TRANSVERSE OSTEOTOMY

When the medial osteotomy cut is completed, the osteotome is rotated laterally to make a fracture at the frontonasal suture which is indicated by an audible click sound. This fracture is called transverse osteotomy. Transverse osteotomy can also be done separately by a 2-mm wide osteotome externally by percutaneous method. The lateral bony walls are now moved in by digital pressure when the upper lateral cartilages also move medially along with the bones. Inward shift of the lateral nasal wall may be difficult in high septal deviations and in incomplete osteotomies.

Medial osteotomy done via an intercartilaginous incision may cause detachment of the upper lateral cartilage from the septum. This detachment can be avoided if the osteotome is placed via a separate small incision above the intercartilaginous incision, just at the junction of the upper lateral cartilages with the nasal bones **(Fig. 9)**.

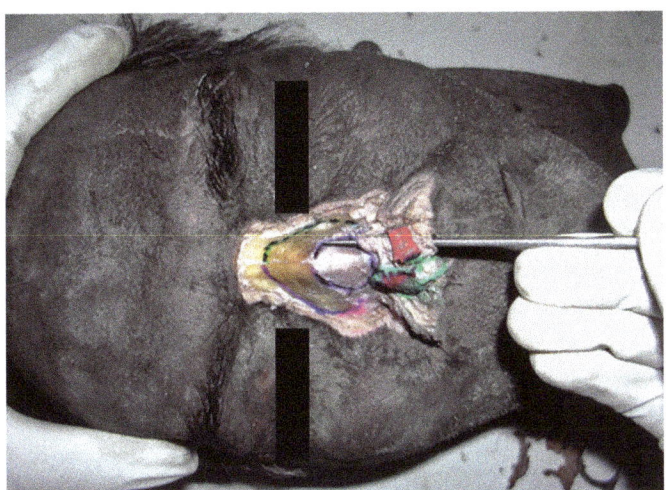

Fig. 9: Cadaver dissection showing medial osteotomy by placing the osteotome at the junction of upper lateral cartilage and nasal bone through intercartilaginous incision.

MICRO-OSTEOTOMY

A 2-mm osteotome is used for micro-osteotomies, which are indicated for correction of asymmetries or irregularities intrinsic to the bones or to correct bony prominences which sometimes occur after lateral osteotomies.

ROCKER DEFORMITY

Osteotomies should stop at the hard nasofrontal bone. A "rocker deformity" may occur when the osteotomies extend too far cephalically into the nasal process of the frontal bone. In a rocker deformity, during inward fracture of the bone after osteotomies, this extra cephalic portion may be displaced laterally.[6] As a general rule to avoid this deformity, osteotomies should not go beyond the level of the medial canthus. Osteotomies can be directed medially before reaching the nasal process of the frontal bone.

Harshbarger and Sullivan mentioned that straight medial osteotomies can cause "rocker deformities" in most of the cases in cadaver. But no "rocker deformities" are seen when medial osteotomies are done in 15° angle.[7]

Lateral osteotomy done by sublabial approach can damage the head of the inferior turbinate, resulting in nasal obstruction.[8] If incomplete osteotomies are done, it will correct the deformity initially, but the deviation will recur within 6 weeks due to the contraction of the fibrous tissue. In a case of incomplete osteotomy, if the osteotome is introduced again, it will produce severe postoperative bruising and swelling, and sometimes black eyes.

If performed at the end of the rhinoplasty, an osteotomy results in less bleeding and less postoperative edema.[9]

Though the internal continuous method is used by many rhinoplasty surgeons, the external perforated osteotomy causes fracture with better control and less intranasal injury and can minimize the associated morbidities such as hemorrhage, edema, and ecchymosis.[10]

In perforated osteotomy, there are small periosteal bridges along the osteotomy line allowing the nasal bones to move inward without displacing the nasal bone at the level of the osteotomy.[11,12] The skin incisions do not lead to any visible scars.[13]

Post osteotomy, nasal obstruction may occur due to narrowing at the nasal valve area. Severe valve stenosis related to infracture after osteotomy may not respond to any simple technique. Revision osteotomy with outfracture is needed in these patients.[14]

The nasolacrimal duct system may rarely be damaged during osteotomy, commonly the nasolacrimal sac, under the medial canthal ligament, and the ostium of the duct in the inferior meatus.[15]

Alireza G et al. (2013) described lateral osteotomy in cadavers performed by a 2-mm diamond burr introduced via an intraoral approach to make the lateral nasal wall thin. The infracture was done by controlled finger pressure. The osteotomy was more accurate and with less complications in comparison with the use of the osteotome.[16]

ROOT OSTEOTOMY

If the bony part of the septum is grossly deviated and pushes the nasal bone laterally, it should be corrected. This is done by making root osteotomy at the bony septum region for several millimeters and fracturing it. With gentle digital manipulation, the bony septum can be mobilized easily into a central position. Percutaneous root osteotomy is done near the intercanthal level by 2-mm osteotome for correction of deviated noses. The study done by Yong JJ et al. (2007) showed the outcome was excellent in 84% of cases and there were no complications such as visible scarring or depression at the osteotomy site.[17]

Osteotomy becomes an easier procedure with less bleeding if power tools are used.[18] The main disadvantage of the osteotome is that it may slip forward suddenly out of control when struck by the mallet. The disadvantage of power tools is cost, and sometimes wider dissection becomes necessary to get adequate exposure.

REFERENCES

1. Kuran I, Ozcan H, Usta A, Bas L. Comparison of four different types of osteotomes for lateral osteotomy: A cadaver study. Aesthetic Plast Surg. 1996;20(4):323-6.
2. Byrd HS, Salomon J, Wood J. Correction of the crooked nose. Plast Reconstr Surg. 1998;102:2148.
3. Meyer R. Crooked nose. In: Gruber RP, Peck GC (eds). Rhinoplasty: State of the Art. St. Louis: Mosby; 1993.

4. Becker DG, McLaughlin RB, Loevner LA, Mang A. Clinical and radiographic rationale for Osteotome selection. Plast Reconstr Surg. 2000;105:1806.
5. Tardy ME. Rhinoplasty: The art and the science 1st edition. Philadelphia, USA: WB Saunders Co.; 1997.
6. Toriumi DM, Becker DG. Anatomy. Rhinoplasty Dissection Manual. Philadelphia: Lippincott Williams & Wilkins; 2010.
7. Harshbarger RJ, Sullivan PK. The optimal medial osteotomy: a study of nasal bone thickness and fracture patterns. Plast Reconstr Surg. 2001;108:2114.
8. Walter C. Septo-rhinoplasty: the correction of the bony parts of the nose. J Laryngol Otol. 1980;94:475-84.
9. Thomas JR, Griner N. The relationship of lateral osteotomies in rhinoplasty to the lacrimal drainage system. Otolaryngol Head Neck Surg. 1986;94(3):362-7.
10. Rohrich RJ, Minoli JJ, Adams WP, Hollier LH. The lateral nasal osteotomy in rhinoplasty: An anatomic endoscopic comparison of the external versus the internal approach. Plast Reconstr Surg. 1997;99(5):1309-12.
11. Tardy ME, Denneny JC. Micro-osteotomies in rhinoplasty. Facial Plast Surg. 1984;1:137.
12. Ford CN, Battaglia DG, Gentry LR. Preservation of periosteal attachment in lateral osteotomy. Ann Plast Surg. 1984;13:107.
13. Gryskiewicz JM. Visible scars from percutaneous osteotomies. Plast Reconstr Surg. 2005;116(6):1771-5.
14. Pontell J, Slavit DH, Kern EB. The role of outfracture in correcting post-rhinoplasty nasal obstruction. Ear Nose Throat J. 1998;77(2):106-8,111-2.
15. Raut VV, Yung MW, Logan BM. Endoscopic dacryocystorhinostomy: anatomical approach. Rev Laryngol Otol Rhinol (Bord). 2000;121(1):53-5.
16. Ghassemi A, Ayoub A, Modabber A, Bohluli B, Prescher A. Lateral nasal osteotomy: a comparative study between the use of osteotome and a diamond surgical burr- a cadaver study. Head Face Med. 2013;19(9):41.
17. Yong JJ, Jong HW, Sinha V, Lee B. Percutaneous root osteotomy for correction of the deviated nose. Am J Rhino Aller. 2007;21(4):515-9.
18. Avsar YI. The oscillating micro-saw: a safe and pliable instrument for transverse osteotomy in rhinoplasty. Aesth Surg J. 2012;32:700-8.

CHAPTER 12

Shortening the Nose and Narrowing of Middle Third of Nose

A patient, short in height, usually likes a shorter nose; whereas in a tall patient, the nose can be reconstructed to remain high and in proportionate length to face and height.[1]

Shortening of the nose can be done by shortening the lateral walls and the septum. Shortening of the lateral wall is done by excising the caudal part of the upper lateral and the cephalic part of the lower lateral cartilages. A rectangular strip of cartilage is excised from the caudal septum with a knife to shorten the septum. This will also lengthen the upper lip without changing the nasolabial angle. Nasolabial angle can be increased by removing a triangular piece of cartilage (with the base of the triangle at dorsum) from the caudal part of the septum **(Fig. 1)**. After excision of cartilage, an excessive part of the membranous septum is removed. Too much shortening of the septum may cause retracted or hidden columella and a drooping tip. Drooping tip can be improved by supporting the columella with the placement of a cartilage strut. Excessive shortening of the lateral wall will cause hanging columella.

Overshortened nose can be corrected by spreader graft, columellar graft, septal extension graft, tip grafts, dorsal grafts, and interposition grafts (between upper and lower lateral cartilages).[2]

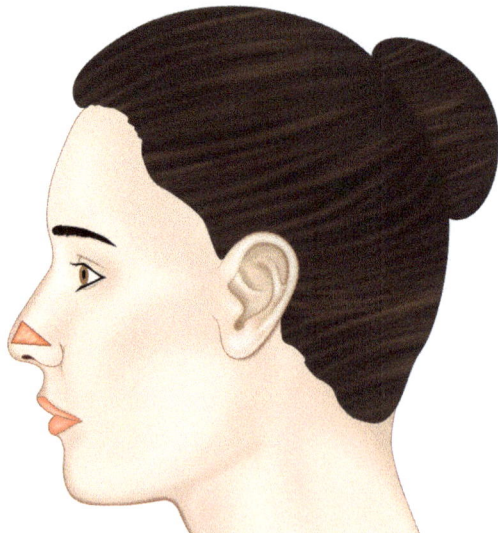

Fig. 1: To open nasolabial angle, a triangular piece of septal cartilage is removed.

Plumping grafts can make a long nose look shorter by an optical illusion. A plumping graft is positioned at the nasolabial angle to augment the area. It also helps to shorten the appearance of the upper lip.

Following osteotomies, medial rotation of the bony cartilaginous complex causes narrowing of the middle third of the nose.

Excision of the subcutaneous tissue overlying the anterolateral walls of the nose also causes thinning of the middle third of the nose.

If the upper lateral cartilages are broad, thick, or convex, the cartilages may be divided submucosally from the septum and excision of a portion of medial borders is done. Vertical shave excision of an excessively thick septal cartilage provides additional narrowing of the cartilaginous dorsum. Excision of the prominent scroll also causes narrowing of the supratip region.[1]

REFERENCES

1. Tardy ME. Rhinoplasty: the art and the science, 1st edition. Philadelphia, USA: WB Saunders Co; 1997.
2. Naficy S, Baker SR. Lengthening the short nose. Arch Otolaryngol Head Neck Surg. 1998;124:809-13.

Tip Plasty

INTRODUCTION

Surgery of the nasal tip to attain a satisfactory result is the most difficult part of rhinoplasty. Fomon's statement in the early part of the 20th century, "He who masters the tip, masters rhinoplasty", remains valid today.[1] The nasal tip is bounded transversely between the tip-defining points and longitudinally from the supratip to the columella breakpoint ("Tip diamond") **(Fig. 1)**. The nasal lobule consists of domes and lateral crura of the lower lateral cartilages. It extends from the junction of the upper lateral cartilages with the lateral crura to the columella breakpoint. Tip projection is the distance of the nasal tip from the vertical facial plane when measured from the level of the alar-facial groove. The normal tip projection should be two thirds of the ideal dorsal length.

TRIPOD THEORY

The tripod theory of Anderson regarding tip projection, support, and rotation helps to comprehend the technique of tip plasty.[2]

Two lateral crura form two legs of the tripod, and two conjoined medial crura act as the third leg. When the medial crura are strengthened by a columellar strut, or septocolumellar suture, the medial leg of the tripod

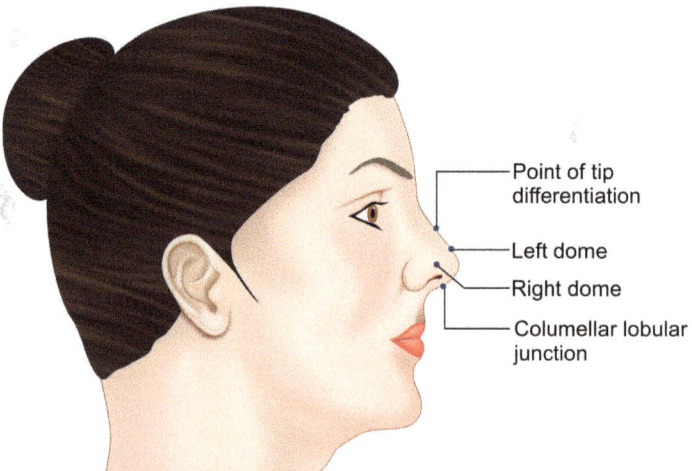

Fig. 1: Four essential landmarks of nasal tip.

becomes the dominant leg, leading to tip rotation superiorly. When the medial leg is shortened, the tip will deproject and rotate downward. Shortening the lateral legs will cause deprojection and rotation (upward rotation) of the tip. If the medial and lateral crura are shortened, deprojection of the tip occurs and if they are lengthened, projection is attained.

Lateral crural steal suture produces tip projection and rotation (upward rotation). Conversely, resection and overlay of the lateral crura (lateral crural flap or overlay technique) create rotation with deprojection. This is usually done in long and overprojected nose. If only deprojection and no rotation is required, an equal amount of overlapping in both medial and lateral crura can be performed. Division and overlap of the medial crura create derotation (downward rotation) and deprojection of the tip.

Skin thickness is an important factor in rhinoplasty. The combination of thick skin and plenty of subcutaneous tissue makes tip plasty difficult and may not produce the desired result with the popular techniques such as cephalic trimming and dome scoring. The caudal margin of the lower lateral cartilage and the alar rim do not run parallel. The distance between the caudal margin of the lower lateral cartilage and the alar rim varies in different areas of alar rim. So, before making the marginal incision, the caudal edge should be palpated to prevent injury to the lower lateral cartilage.

TIP SUPPORT MECHANISM

The major tip support mechanisms that keep the tip in proper position are as follows:
- Aponeurotic junction of the upper lateral and lower lateral cartilages
- Attachment of the footplate of the medial crura to septal cartilage
- Shape, size, and strength of the lateral crura
- Accessory cartilages and their attachments to the piriform aperture. Three to four accessory cartilages are scattered in the fibrous tissue connecting the lateral crura to the piriform aperture.
- Interdomal fibrous attachment
- Fibrous sling (Sling of Pitanguy) from the dorsal septum and nasal skin to the posterior margins of the domes of the lower lateral cartilages.

TYPES OF NASAL TIP DEFORMITIES

- *Tip with inadequate projection:* Normally, tip should be the highest point of the nose. Here, the nasal tip is below the level of the normal dorsal line. The tip seems to be pulled in toward the nasal spine having a downward inclination. It may be due to a short columella.
- *Overprojecting tip:* This is often caused by a combination of three factors:
  1. A large nasal spine
  2. Long medial and lateral crura
  3. A high nasal septum

- *Malposition of the lower lateral cartilages:* It is diagnosed by broad and flat nasal tip, vertical grooves around the tip, notched alar rims, and a square appearance of the basal part of nose.
- *Broad tip:* The normal distance between both tip-defining points is about 5–6 mm, with a distance of >6 mm being considered as a broad tip.[3]
- *Bulbous tip:* In contrast to the broad tip, which is more apparent in the frontal view, the bulbous tip is more prominent in the lateral view. This is due to the high rounded cephalic portion of the lateral crus, which forms the highest point of the tip profile.
- *Bifid tip:* Here the divergent angle of the domes is wide and the domes are rounded, forming a bilobular tip.
- *Hanging tip:* Here, the nasal tip is either too long or lacks columellar support. When the nasal tip falls below the horizontal line at the subnasale, the nose is considered long. A columella of adequate length that lacks skeletal support will cause the tip to rotate downward leading to a "hanging tip". When it is associated with a hump, it is called "parrot beak nose" **(Fig. 2)**.
- *Asymmetrical tip:* This may be due to the asymmetry of the tip cartilages or indirectly due to caudal dislocation of septum.
- *Plunging tip:* This may be associated with columellar retraction, a lack of columellar base support and a short upper lip.

  This is caused by a long unsupported nasal tip which is pulled down by powerful depressor nasi muscles.
- *Cleft lip nasal tip deformity*

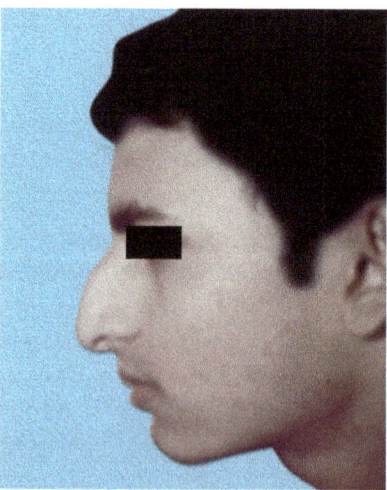

Fig. 2: "Parrot beak nose" with hump and hanging tip.

APPROACHES TO THE TIP

Patients present with different varieties of tip deformities require different planning for every patient to achieve good result.

Cartilage Splitting Approach

The approach is done via intracartilaginous incision. Here, the vestibular skin and lateral crus of lower lateral cartilage are incised 6–8 mm cephalic to the caudal border of the lateral crus. The incision avoids the nasal valve area. The cephalic part of lateral crus which is present above the incision can be excised (cephalic trimming). The dorsum of the nose can be approached through this incision with no chance to damage the soft triangle area. This approach is useful for uncomplicated tip plasty and it preserves the natural shape of the tip.

Delivery Approach

It is also called internal approach or closed technique. Many surgeons prefer delivery approach over external approach as there is less postoperative tip edema and no chance of transcolumellar scar. Adequate exposure is obtained for various tip modifications.

Bilateral intercartilaginous incisions are made with a number 15 blade. It will help in retrograde dissection between the skin and lateral crura by curved Fomon scissors. Marginal incisions are made on both sides caudal to the caudal border of lower lateral cartilage. The marginal incision should avoid the soft triangle area. Through the marginal incision, undermining and dissection between the skin and lateral crura can be done. The lateral crus, dome, and upper part of the medial crus are completely freed from the overlying skin. Through the intercartilaginous incision, a long plain dissecting forceps is introduced and the forceps brings out the nose between the caudal margin of the lower lateral cartilage and overlying skin and the alar cartilage is delivered like a bucket handle. The fibrofatty tissue over the lateral crus is removed with the help of fine scissors and toothed dissecting forceps. The excessive fibrofatty tissue between two domes and upper ends of medial crura are removed. The cephalic part of the lateral crus is excised after stripping the cartilage from the underlying vestibular skin (cephalic trimming). Injury to the vestibular skin is avoided to prevent subsequent stenosis.

Cephalic Trimming

Cephalic trimming causes:
- Rotation (upward rotation) of the tip
- Narrowing of the lobule
- Formation of the nasoalar crease.

Cephalic trimming of lateral crus should be done in such a manner that a strip of cartilage of at least 6–8 mm in width is left behind and maintains the continuity of the lateral crus **(Figs. 3 to 5)**. Preservation of 6–8 mm rim strip permits insertion of any sutures and maintains adequate support for the nostril rim and prevents retraction of ala. The caudal margin of the lateral crura is followed, tapering the excision at both ends. The domal notch area is not narrowed. The underlying mucosa of the lateral crura is infiltrated with local anesthesia for hydrodissection. The cartilage is then held with forceps and a number 15 blade is used to excise the cephalic part. The removed cartilage can later be used as a tip graft.

Lateral Crural Turn-in Flap

Cephalic trimming is not done when significant concavity is found in the lateral crura that can be corrected by folding or flipping the crura (lateral crural turn-in flap). This technique is usually done in patients with wide lateral crura that

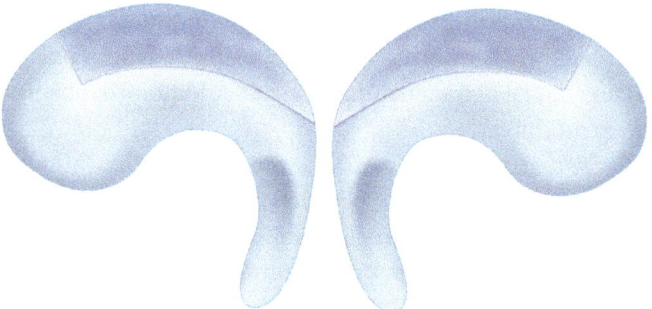

Fig. 3: Area of excision during cephalic trimming.

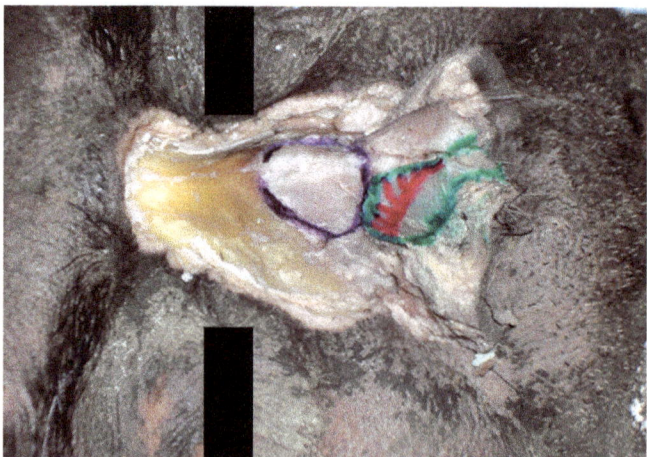

Fig. 4: Nasal bones, upper lateral cartilage (blue), lower lateral cartilage (green) and area of cephalic trimming in lateral crus of lower lateral cartilage (red) shown on cadaver after removal of skin.

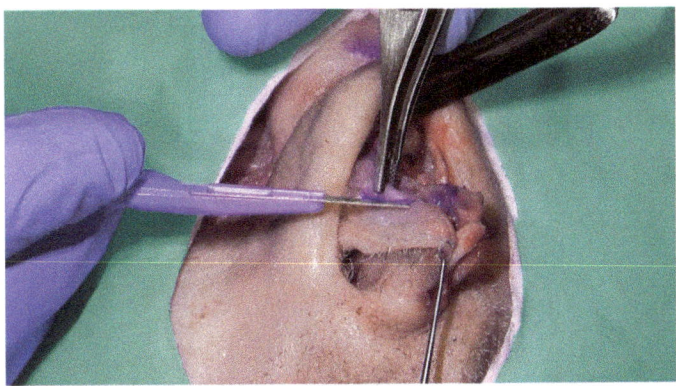

Fig. 5: Cadaver dissection showing cephalic trimming.

are thin and lack support. The amount of cartilage that otherwise would be trimmed is marked, folded under the cephalic margin, and sutured in place by 5-0 PDS. This turn-in flap gives extra structural support to the lateral crural area and prevents postoperative supra-alar pinching.[4]

External Approach

This open approach is done by Rethi Goodman incision. Here, bilateral marginal incisions and transcolumellar incision are made.

Indications of external approach are the following:
- It can be done in all rhinoplasties.
- Difficult tip rhinoplasty
- Complicated septal deviations
- Secondary rhinoplasty
- For teaching purposes
- Cleft lip nasal deformity.
- Repair of septal perforation.[5]

External approach for tip plasty permits the placement of sutures with exact symmetry and various techniques of tip plasty can be done more easily, more symmetrically, and with better outcome **(Fig. 6)**.[6]

Rarely, external scar may occur at columella. Adamson et al. (1990) reviewed 100 consecutive rhinoplasties by external approach and reported only 2.5% incidence of columellar scar.[7] Postoperative tip edema due to transection of lymphatics of columella may be another problem. Tip edema may take as long as 6 months to subside. External approach may cause hypoesthesia of the tip and prolongs the surgical procedure itself.[8]

SUTURE TIP PLASTY

Transection of the domes usually does not result in an ideal tip definition and sometimes causes irregularities, particularly in noses with thin skin. Instead of

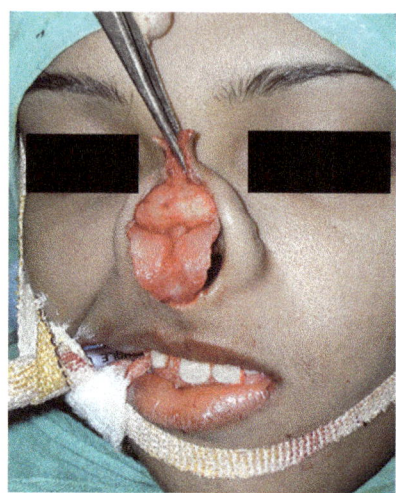

Fig. 6: Mobilization of soft tissues exposing the lower lateral cartilages and nasal dorsum during tip plasty by external approach.

excising and repositioning of the tip cartilages, the lateral crus can be preserved and tip cartilage modification can be done through precise suture placement and tension control and one is able to preserve or enhance nasal tip contour, projection, and rotation.[9]

The suture material should be 5-0 PDS. The surgeon should use only as many sutures as required to attain the perfect tip. Sutures should be tied properly, neither too loose nor too tight. Undermining of the mucosa is not needed before inserting the suture; one can simply penetrate the cartilage without damaging the underlying mucosa. The underlying mucosa can be infiltrated with local anesthesia before placement of suture to avoid penetration by the needle.

The suture techniques used in tip plasty are: (1) Columellar strut and suture, (2) domal creation suture and transdomal suture (TDS) for tip definition, (3) domal equalization suture or, interdomal suture (IDS) to control tip width, (4) lateral crural steal (LCS), (5) tip-positioning suture to create a supratip break, (6) lateral crural mattress suture (LCMS) to reduce convexity of lateral crus, (7) columella-septal suture, and (8) intercrural sutures.[10-12]

Suture techniques, however, are not a substitute for cartilage grafts in case of gross deformity when major changes are to be made in the tip.[13,14]

1. *Columellar strut and suture:* Columellar strut provides stability, projection, and shape of the columella. It prevents drooping of the tip. The columellar strut is usually 20 mm long, 2.5 mm wide, and 1.5 mm thick, but the actual shape can vary depending upon the need. The graft is usually taken from the vomerine septal cartilage because of its thickness and rigidity. A vertical suture of 5-0 PDS is placed through the columella, which holds the strut between the medial crura **(Figs. 7 and 8)**.

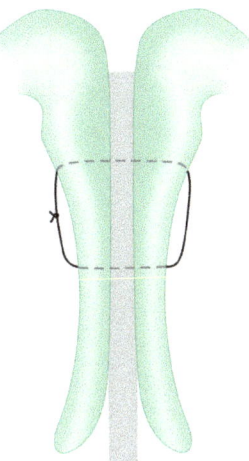

Fig. 7: Columellar strut and suture.

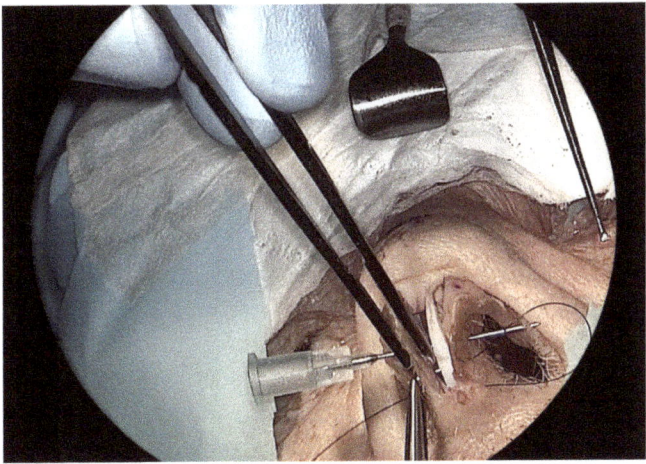

Fig. 8: Suturing of columellar strut in cadaver.

If the columellar strut is placed directly against the nasal spine or, it overlaps the caudal septum, a postsurgical displacement from the midline may occur. If a piece of soft tissue is not placed in between the columellar strut and nasal spine, the patient may get a clicking sensation during smiling.

2. *Domal creation suture or, transdomal suture (TDS):* The domal creation suture produces tip definition. After locating the domal notch, the domal segment is gently held by an Adson-Brown forceps and a horizontal mattress suture is inserted across the domal segment from medial to lateral with the knot tied medially. The suture is gradually tightened until the ideal domal convexity and dome-defining points are attained **(Fig. 9)**. Too tight or too loose sutures are avoided. Unlike tip grafts, tip sutures attain definition without graft visibility, or atrophy of the graft.

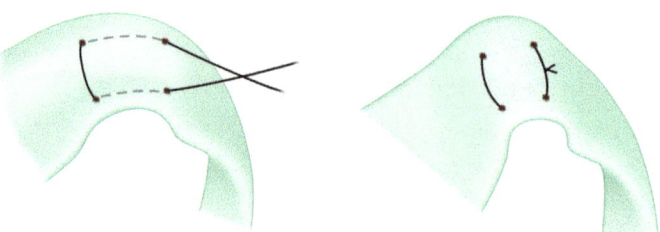

Fig. 9: Domal creation suture.

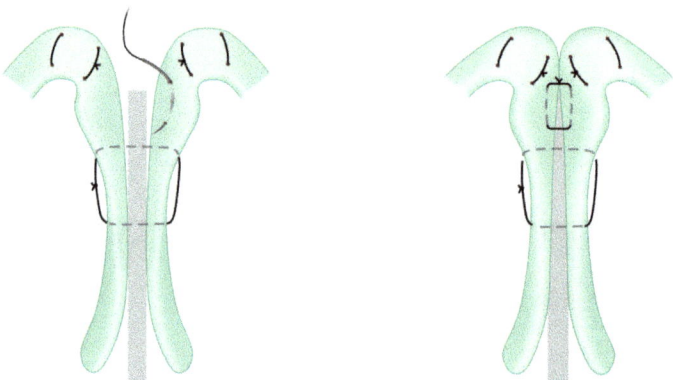

Fig. 10: Domal equalization or interdomal suture.

3. *Domal equalization suture or, interdomal suture (IDS):* The interdomal suture modifies width at the domes and in the infralobule. The normal angle of domal divergence is approximately 30°.

   It is a vertical suture that enters just below the transdomal suture on the left side and exits just above the columellar suture. Then, it enters the right crura across the medial crura and exits just below the transdomal suture. The suture is usually done 2–3 mm behind the caudal margin of the crura. The suture is gradually tightened to diminish the interdomal distance until the desired width is attained **(Fig. 10)**.

   As the transdomal suture and columellar suture are already done, inserting the interdomal suture is easy. If the suture is placed near the caudal border of the crura, then too much narrowing of the columella occurs. The columella narrows at its midpoint, flares at its base, and gradually widens in the infralobule. So, too much narrowing of the infralobular columella should be avoided.

   A broad nasal tip can be corrected by removing interdomal soft tissue, sometimes combined with cephalic trimming. The interdomal distance may be further decreased with interdomal suture. A fibrofatty tissue flap may be formed with the interdomal soft tissue instead of removing it. It is sutured to the center area and is fixed to the tip graft.[15]

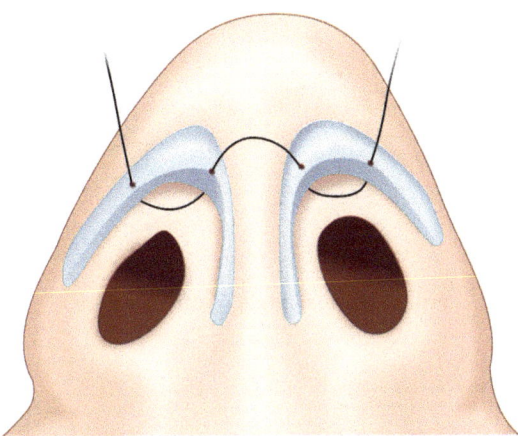

Fig. 11: In lateral crural steal (LCS), the lateral crura are moved on to the domes and sewn together.

4. *Lateral crural steal suture:* Lateral crural steal suture increases projection and rotation, and refines the nasal tip. It is done to correct amorphous, underrotated, and underprojected nasal tip. Here, horizontal mattress sutures of 5-0 PDS are placed just medial to or at the dome and then into the lateral crura and sewn together. This will lengthen the middle crura at the cost of the lateral crura **(Fig. 11)**. Further narrowing and refinement may be done by interdomal and transdomal sutures.[16]
5. *Tip-positioning suture or tip anchoring suture:* This suture prevents tip ptosis and helps to achieve the final tip position. A bite is taken from one dome, going from inside out and then through the anterior septal angle and coming out through the other dome from inside out. The knot is secured on the dorsum and thus fixing and positioning of the tip is done.
6. *Lateral crural mattress suture (LCMS):* It is a transverse mattress suture placed at the most convex area of the lateral crura. It is done in the treatment of wide and broad tips. The needle is inserted about 1 mm from the caudal border and exits 1 mm from the cephalic border. Then another bite is taken 6–8 mm laterally in the similar way from the cephalic to the caudal border. The convexity is flattened when the suture is gradually tightened. To avoid penetrating the mucosa, infiltration of local anesthesia is done under the convex area before suturing **(Fig. 12)**.
7. *Medial crura-septal suture* causes increase of tip projection, rotation of the tip, and retraction of the columella.
8. *Suturing the medial crural footplates* causes approximation of the footplates, narrowing of the columella base, and improves undesirable nostril shape.

Previously, it was believed that permanent sutures are necessary to have a permanent effect on the cartilage shape. But that has not been proved true. Polydioxanone (PDS) sutures work like permanent sutures and have the benefit of not causing stitch reactions or microabscesses.[12]

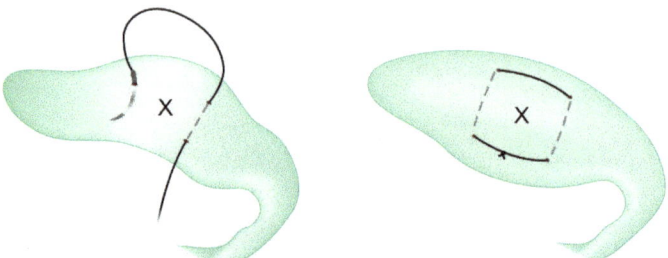

Fig. 12: Lateral crural mattress suture.

CORRECTION OF DIFFERENT TIP DEFORMITIES

Tip with Inadequate Projection

Lower lateral cartilages are exposed either by delivery technique or external approach. Cephalic trimming of lateral crura is done to sharpen the lobule if required.

Lateral crural steal is an effective technique to increase projection and rotation simultaneously.[17] Tip projection can be increased by 2–4 mm, depending on the size of the lower lateral cartilage. The skin under the dome can be separated before the suturing of the lower lateral cartilage. The suturing technique provides versatility and can be revised during operation until the ideal tip is attained. The underlying skin, if not separated acts as a spacer under the dome and prevents too much narrowing of the dome. So, some surgeons do not separate the vestibular skin from the lower lateral cartilage before suturing.

Septocolumellar suture is an effective technique to increase tip projection by about 2–4 mm, depending on the situation. However, if it is exaggerated, a web may form at the subnasale and the upper lip can move upward.[18]

Tongue-in-groove technique achieves long-term tip projection. Here, the tip becomes firmly fixed wherever it is positioned during operation. But the major problem of this procedure is the resultant stiffness of the tip.[19,20]

In cases of deformed, or weak medial crura, placement of columellar struts helps to strengthen the medial crura and increases tip projection.[21] The columellar strut should be quite long (25 mm) and rigid. The alar cartilages are pulled vertically on the columellar strut and fixed by sutures. Then, transdomal sutures are done. The columellar strut can be anchored to spreader grafts along with the caudal septum. A caudal septal extension graft can be placed to increase projection in cases where the caudal septum is deficient, weak, or deviated.[22] An L-shaped graft can also be placed when the dorsocaudal segment of the cartilaginous septum is deficient, crooked, or overresected from a previous surgery.[23]

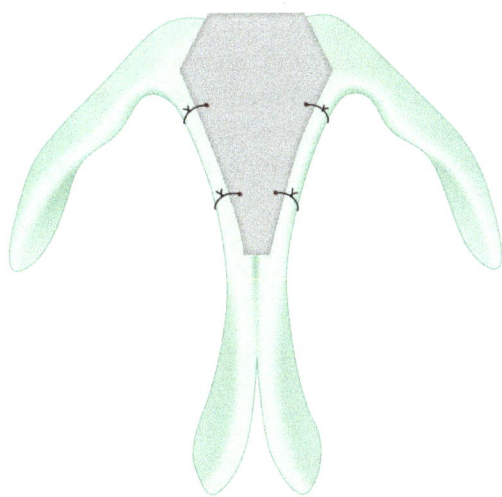

Fig. 13: Shield graft sutured at the tip.

Caudal septal extension graft may lead to deviated nasal tip if it is sutured to the caudal septum in overlapping fashion. To prevent deviated nasal tip, the caudal septal graft can be placed end to end with existing caudal septum and anchoring it to extended spreader grafts and the anterior nasal spine.

Autogenous cartilage is the preferable graft material for tip plasty.[24] There are four general types of tip grafts: Cap or buttress graft at tip area behind the shield graft, onlay tip graft (Peck graft), infratip lobular graft (shield graft) **(Fig. 13)**, and columellar tip graft.[25]

Shield-shaped tip grafts can be used to increase tip projection and change tip contour.[26] They also can camouflage tip asymmetries.

Shield grafts are mainly made from harvested septal cartilage or excised cephalic part of lateral crura. The length of the shield graft is 8-15 mm and width 8-12 mm at the leading edge. The graft should be thicker at the leading edge and thinner at the base. The graft is secured at the caudal margins of the medial crura with 5-0 PDS sutures.

A shield graft should project 1-2 mm above the existing domes normally. But, in patients with underprojected tip, the shield graft should project 2-4 mm above the existing domes. When the projection is increased by 3 mm or more, then the shield graft should be supported by lateral crural grafts for a smooth transition from tip to lateral crura. Additionally, a cap or buttress graft may be placed behind the leading edge of the shield graft and sutured to the graft and both domes to make a better transition from the edge of the tip graft to the supratip area.[27] The cap graft also prevents backward bending of the tip graft and loss of projection. The edges of the shield grafts should be beveled to prevent its visibility in patients with thin skin.

Onlay tip grafts are very versatile to increase tip projection. They can be placed in single or multiple layers. Tip grafts can also be sutured on top of a long columellar strut making an "umbrella graft" as described by Peck.[28] Tip grafts can be camouflaged by soft tissue to prevent visibility.

In noses with thick skin, Goldman's technique can be done. In this technique, the lateral crura are divided on either side lateral to the dome and the medial crura along with the parts of the domes are sutured together to increase the projection of the tip.[29] But this technique is not used because of the undesirable aesthetics.

Overprojecting Tip

An overprojected tip can be reduced by performing a full transfixion incision causing loss of a major tip support mechanism, but this method has not been found to be predictable.[30]

By external approach, septocolumellar suture technique can be done to correct an overprojected tip. A tongue-in-groove procedure can also be done when the caudal septum is long. Here, the medial crura can be attached anywhere on the caudal septum according to the need.

When the medial crura are longer than usual, the crura can be cut either segmentally with the cut margins joined end to end[31] or with the margins overlapped and sutured without any resection.[32] The medial crus is divided 4-5 mm below the dome and overlapping of the fragments about 2-5 mm is done according to the amount of deprojection required and sutured with 5-0 PDS. A columellar strut is placed and a septocolumellar suture is done for additional support.

When the lateral crura are unusually longer, lateral crural overlay can be done to shorten the lateral crura.[33] Hydrodissection is done before the dissection of the cartilage from the vestibular skin. The lateral crura is cut 1 cm lateral to the dome and the lateral segment is overlapped by the medial segment. A 2-5-mm overlap is usually done. A lateral crural strut graft can be placed to provide rigidity to the lateral crura. Lateral crural turn-in flap can also be done along with lateral crural overlay technique. In lateral crural turn-in flap, the cephalic portion is turned inward as a flap and stabilized with 5-0 PDS mattress sutures **(Fig. 14)**.

In another technique where the tip is broad, cephalic trimming is done first. Vertical transection is made on the lower lateral cartilage medial to the dome. Posteriorly based pedicled chondral flaps are made on both sides by separating the underlying vestibular skin **(Figs. 15 to 17)**. Vertical dome scoring is done on the chondral flaps. To reduce overprojection, upper parts of the medial crura are excised. Now the posteriorly based chondral flaps are pulled medially and sutured with the medial crura by 5-0 PDS.[34] The newly made domes may be approximated by inverting mattress sutures.

When the overprojection is quite great (>6 mm) with deformities of the lower lateral cartilages, modification by sutures is difficult. After cephalic

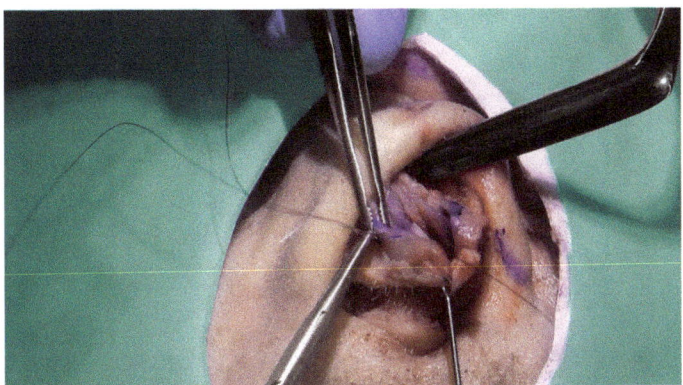

Fig. 14: Suturing of lateral crural turn-in flap in right side in cadaver.

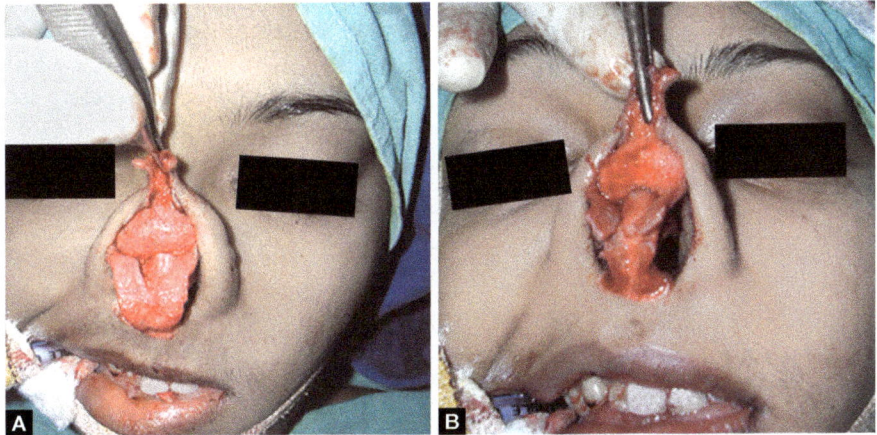

Figs. 15A and B: Cephalic trimming of lower lateral cartilages (A) and posteriorly based bilateral pedicled chondral flaps after cutting the lower lateral cartilages medial to domes (B) during tip plasty by external approach.

trimming, the middle crura is cut and the lateral crura is undermined submucosally. Around 4–8 mm of domal segment is excised, which reduces projection considerably. The cut fragments are sutured with 5-0 PDS. Then, a columellar strut and tip graft are sutured into place.

Broad Tip

Factors on which the result of tip plasty depends include skin thickness, inherent strength and position of the lower lateral cartilage, tip and caudal septal support, domal structure, and contraction during the healing process.[35] A retracted soft triangle facet may require placement of rim graft once the ideal tip projection is achieved. Alar flaring and alar width may need simultaneous correction.

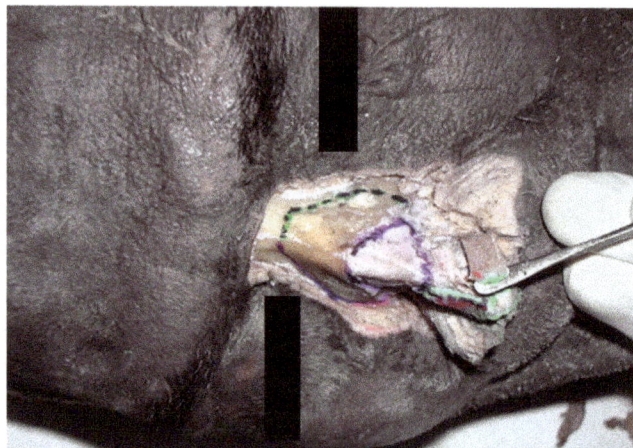

Fig. 16: Cadaver dissection showing posteriorly based pedicled chondral flap after cephalic trimming following transection of the lower lateral cartilage medial to dome.

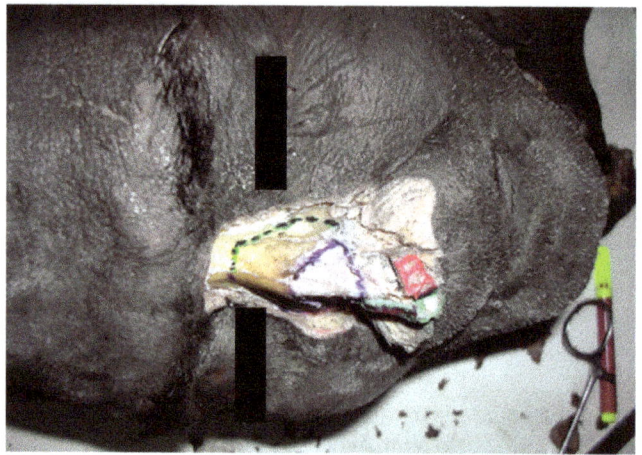

Fig. 17: Cadaver dissection showing fully mobile posteriorly based pedicled chondral flap (red).

Frontal and basal views are required to study tip shape, whereas for projection and tip position, lateral and basal views are required. After exposure, excess fibrofatty tissue is removed over lateral crura, interdomal area, and beneath the skin flap. The vascularity of the skin of nasal tip should be protected.[36] There should be a thick uniform cobblestone appearance to the soft tissue left behind after removal of fibrofatty tissue from undersurface of the tip skin.

Cephalic trimming is done. The lower lateral cartilage is transected vertically medial to the dome and posteriorly based pedicled chondral flaps are made in both sides by separating the underlying vestibular skin. Multiple vertical half-thickness incisions (dome scoring) are made over anterior part of the chondral flaps. After removing intercrural fibrofatty tissue, the upper ends of the medial crura may be sutured by a PDS mattress suture. To increase tip projection, a small piece of septal or chondral cartilage may be placed over the upper ends of medial crura beneath the pedicled chondral flaps **(Figs. 18 and 19).**

In patients with thin skin, transection of alar cartilage near dome is avoided and continuity of lower lateral cartilage is maintained to prevent postoperative tip irregularities. In these patients after removing excess fibrofatty tissue, cephalic trimming is done. Domal creation sutures are done to increase domal definition, and lateral crural mattress sutures are done to decrease lateral crural convexities. To narrow the interdomal area, interdomal suture can be done by 5-0 PDS. If the lower lateral cartilages are rigid or overprojected, then tip graft, columellar strut, and domal segment excision are necessary. Domal segment excision corrects the broad tip, while tip graft makes new tip-defining points.

Cephalic malposition of the lateral crura is defined as lateral crura that are situated 30° or less from the midline. Here, the lateral crus is directed toward the medial canthus instead of the lateral canthus leading to a vertical fullness of the nasal tip that disturbs the dorsal aesthetic lines.[37] A broad tip with malposition of the lower lateral cartilages in cephalic position is corrected by delivery of the entire lateral crura and repositioning in normal position with or without lateral crural strut grafts.

Hanging Tip or Plunging Tip

After exposure of the lower lateral cartilages, fibrofatty tissue is removed. Cephalic trimming is done as usual. To rotate the tip upward, a triangular piece of septal cartilage (with the base of the triangle toward the dorsum) is excised.

In parrot beak nose, hump is removed. A columellar strut is placed in between two medial crura and sutured together **(Figs. 7 and 8).** The strut is prepared from harvested septal cartilage, and, when necessary, from auricular cartilage or rib cartilage. The strut measures 8–12 mm in length and 3–4 mm in width. The strut is inserted in a space created between the medial crura, and extends from 2 mm above the anterior nasal spine to the angle between the medial and middle (intermediate) crura, preferably leaving some soft tissue between the strut and the nasal spine.[38] "Laughing strut" occurs when the columellar strut clicks across the nasal spine only when the patient laughs spontaneously, not when he smiles or talks. Asymmetry of the tip may occur if the medial crura are asymmetrically sutured to the strut, or if a too long strut extends beyond the nasal spine and shifts to one side of the nasal spine resulting in a deviated nasal tip. An umbrella graft may be placed in columella and tip region. Another method is to place a T-graft made from septal cartilage just behind the columella. The vertical portion of the T-graft is placed between the two skin surfaces of the membranous septum immediately posterior to the medial crura and the broad part of the cartilage is placed at the base of the columella.

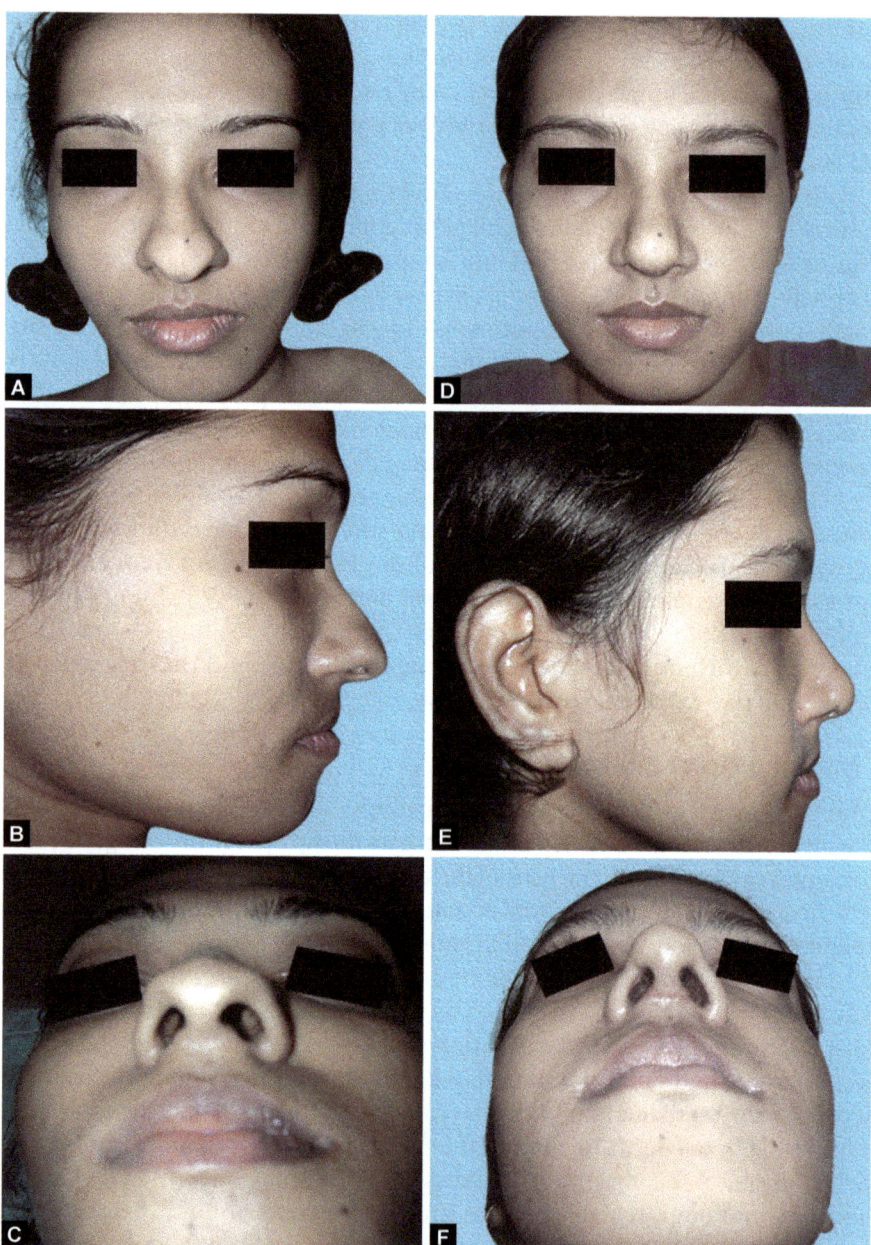

Figs. 18A to F: (A to C) Preoperative; (D to F) Postoperative views of tip plasty in a case of broad tip. Cephalic trimming, section of the lower lateral cartilage medial to the dome, bilateral posteriorly-based pedicled chondral flaps and scoring of the flaps were done by external approach. Both medial crura were sutured by 5-0 PDS.

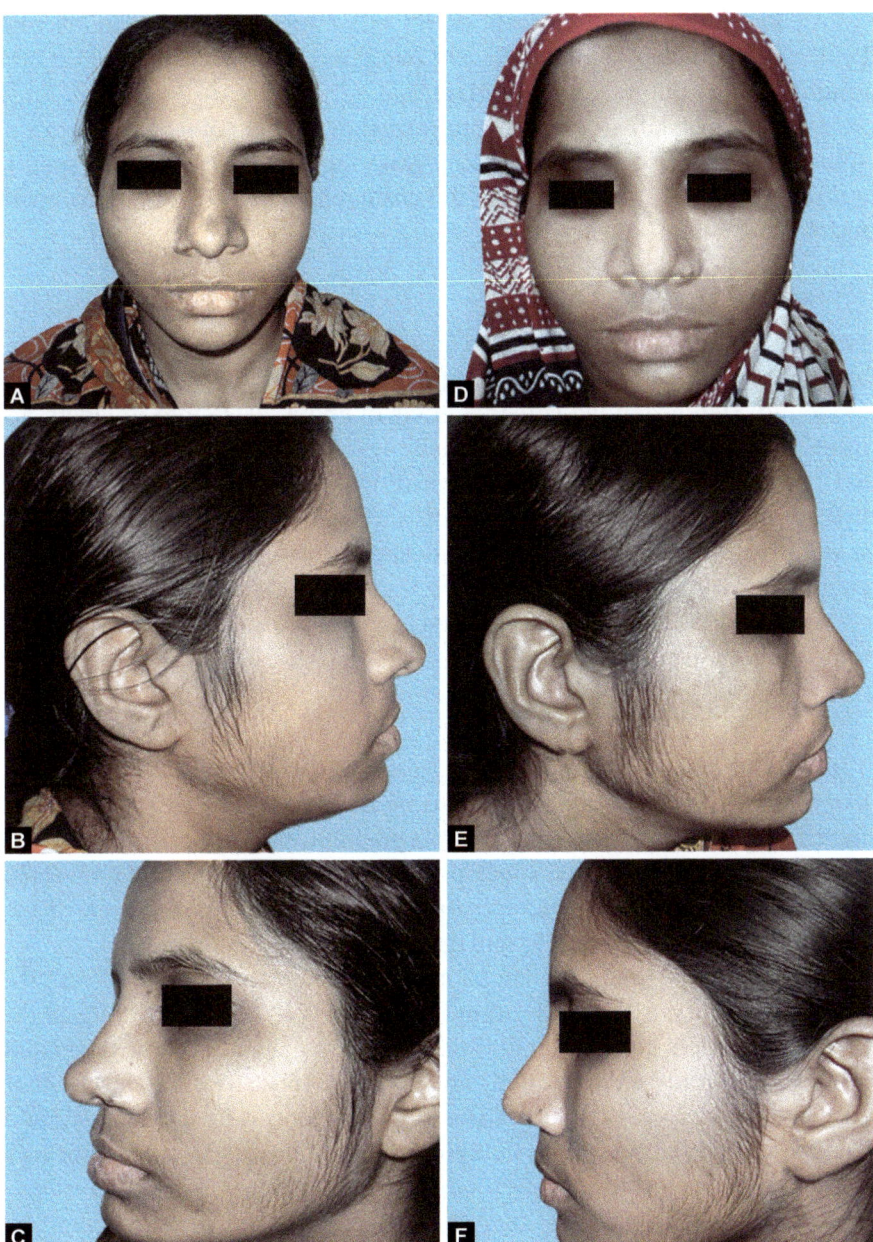

Figs. 19A to F: (A to C) Preoperative; (D to F) Postoperative views of a case of bulbous tip with supratip depression and deviated nasal septum (DNS). Septoplasty and augmentation of the supratip area were done with a single layer of septal cartilage. Tip plasty was done by cephalic trimming, cutting of the lower lateral cartilage medial to dome, bilateral posteriorly based pedicled chondral flaps, and suturing of the medial crura by external approach. Subcutaneous soft tissue was removed from the tip area.

Another useful technique to rotate the tip is a shortening of the lateral crura by division and overlapping of the cut fragments and securing by a 5-0 PDS mattress suture (lateral crural overlay).[39]

In acute nasolabial angle due to retrusion of the caudal septum/nasal spine, columellar strut and plumping grafts can be used. Plumping graft is a piece of cartilage graft placed in the nasolabial angle to correct the acute nasolabial angle.

Upwardly Rotated Tip

In short noses with upwardly rotated tip, a prominent dorsum with a nasofacial angle >40°, and wide nasolabial angle due to a prominent caudal septum are found. Here extended spreader grafts of about 20–25 mm in length are used. The spreader grafts extend caudally beyond the anterior septal angle by 6–10 mm. A triangular columellar strut with a wide base dorsally is inserted in between the extended spreader grafts and anchored into place by 5-0 PDS. It will push the columella downward. Then, tip suturing is done onto the columellar strut.

Septal extension graft can be placed instead of columellar strut. Tip grafts may be necessary.

Alar Malposition

These cases have a deformed tip, large-sized nostrils, and collapse of the external valves. Alar malposition can be defined as any displacement of the lateral crura from its usual parallel position with the nostril rims. The treatment is done by alar transposition and lateral crural strut grafts. Cephalic trimming, elevation of the lateral crura off the underlying mucosa, placement of columellar strut, tip sutures, and tip grafts are also required.

In alar transposition, the lateral crura is divided at its junction with the accessory cartilage and undermining of the whole lateral crura up to the domal segment is done. Then the lateral crura is transposed from a cephalic position to a more caudal position parallel with the nostril rim. Once the lateral cartilage is transposed, columellar strut is placed and tip suturing is done. Then the lateral crural strut graft is placed in a lateral pocket after suturing it to the lateral crura **(Fig. 20)**.

Cleft Lip Nasal Tip Deformity

This type of deformity is the most difficult to correct. Here, commonly the lower lateral cartilage is poorly developed on the side of unilateral cleft lip which has already been repaired. There may be gross deviation of nasal septum to normal side, asymmetry, and inadequate projection of tip, acute nasolabial angle, asymmetric retrodisplaced nostril, displaced lateral crus, and flattened ala **(Figs. 21 and 22)**.[40] There is hypoplasia and retroposition of the maxilla at the

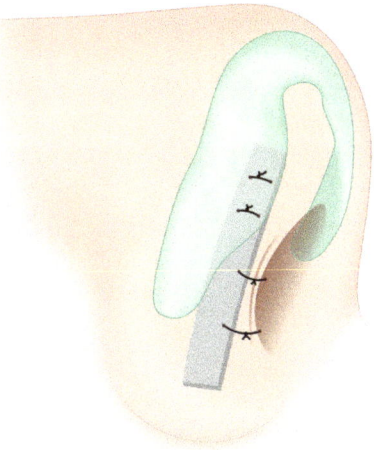

Fig. 20: Alar transposition with lateral crural strut graft.

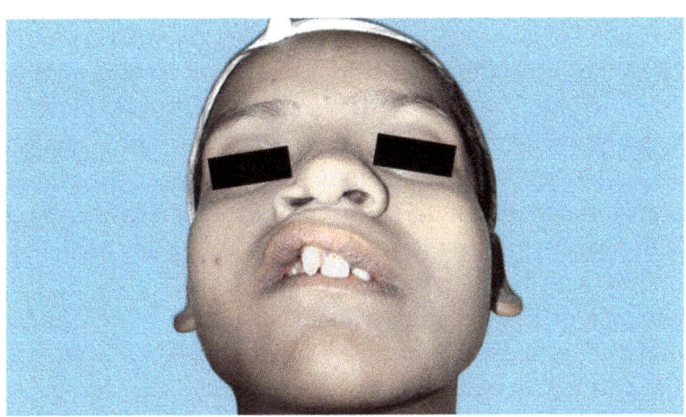

Fig. 21: Cleft lip nasal deformity with flattened and underdeveloped ala in right side, asymmetric nostrils, acute nasolabial angle, asymmetry and inadequate projection of tip and deviated nasal septum (DNS) in a case of unilateral repaired cleft lip (in right side).

cleft side, leading to a lack of maxillary support. In mild cases, a cartilage graft can be placed to give a foundation for the alar base. In severe cases, maxillary advancement is done. External approach should be done for proper exposure. The following grafts are usually required for the rhinoplasty: (a) Shield graft or onlay tip graft for tip definition, (b) columellar strut, (c) dorsal graft, and (d) premaxillary graft for maxillary support. Autogenous septal or conchal cartilage grafts are used. Septoplasty is done by hemitransfixion incision. The anterior nasal spine is repositioned from the noncleft side to the midline by horizontal osteotomy and fixation by sutures. Usually, the lateral crus is larger at the noncleft side; so, to maintain symmetry cephalic trimming is done. The small piece of cartilage obtained after cephalic trimming can be used as a tip graft

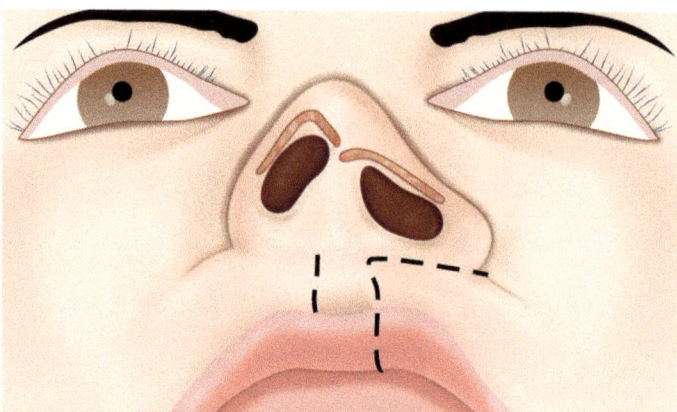

Fig. 22: Cleft lip nasal deformity showing hypoplastic lower lateral cartilage in left side.

to make the dome prominent at the cleft side. The vestibular skin is separated from the lateral crus at the cleft side. The whole lateral crus at the cleft side is now placed upward and more medially for an augmented symmetric dome. It is fixed with the lower lateral cartilage on the normal side by mattress sutures (5-0 PDS). Sometimes, the lateral crus is dissected free of its lateral attachment to have better repositioning. Transdomal sutures are done. A columellar strut is inserted in between two medial crura. The suturing of the cephalic border of the lower lateral to the caudal border of the upper lateral cartilage is done to bring the lower lateral into a normal upward rotating position. The alar base of the cleft side is reallocated medially.[41]

A shield graft or onlay tip graft is placed to attain the ideal projection and definition. Usually, the lateral crura on the cleft side is distorted needing a lateral crural strut graft and sometimes a composite graft for the nostril rim. There may be thick vestibular scars both in the lateral wall and floor which are repaired by removal of scar tissue and placement of composite graft harvested from concha.

In another method of repair, septoplasty is done first. Then cephalic trimming of lateral crus is done on the healthy side. On the affected side, a posteriorly based unilateral chondral flap is made after transecting the medial crus about 0.5 cm medial to the dome. Columellar strut is placed in between two medial crura. On the affected side, the dome is elevated and the upper part of transected medial crus is sutured with the dome on the healthy side by mattress suture. Onlay cartilage grafts may be placed over the lateral crus on the cleft side and over the tip area **(Figs. 23A to D)**.

Pinocchio Nose

Pinocchio, an animated puppet, is punished for each lie that he tells by undergoing further growth of his nose.

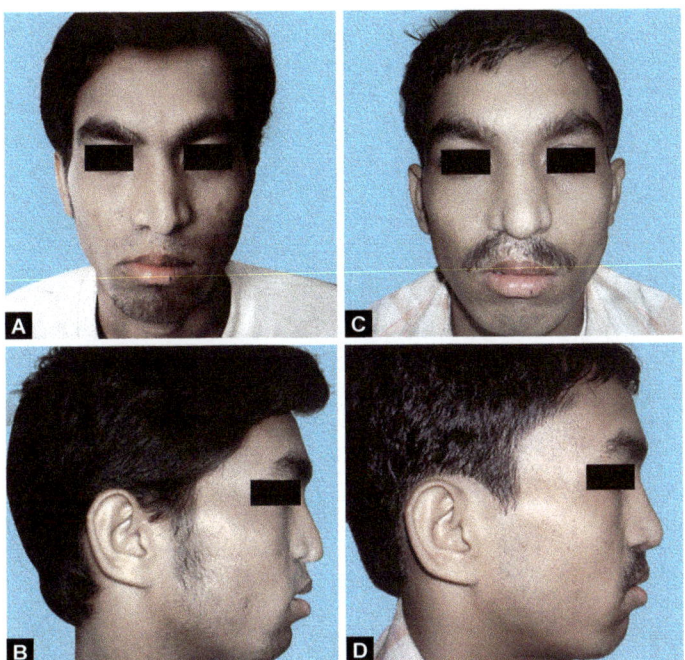

Figs. 23A to D: (A and B) Preoperative; (C and D) Postoperative views of cleft lip nasal deformity with poorly developed lower lateral cartilage in right side and gross deviated nasal septum (DNS). External approach was done. Septoplasty, cephalic trimming in left side, posteriorly based chondral flap after transecting medial crus medial to dome in right side, columellar strut in between two medial crura and suturing of two medial crura were done. Onlay cartilage grafts were placed over lateral crus in right side and over tip.

The "Pinocchio" nose is a variant of the oversized nose characterized by a forward projection of the nasal tip. It is the result of an excessive overgrowth of the lower half of the nose. The medial and lateral crura of the lower lateral cartilages are unusually long and form the framework of a too long columella.[42]

The overprojected tip is corrected by medial and lateral crural overlay. Cephalic trimming and tip sutures are done. Alar resection and sill excision are done.[43] Septoplasty, hump reduction, and osteotomies are done if required **(Figs. 24A to D)**.

Tension Nose

Tension nose is described by a high nasal dorsum, with stretching of the skin and soft tissue of the nose over a highly arched and narrowed nasal vault. There is excessive growth of the septum which exerts a "pedestal effect" by pushing the lower lateral cartilages forward. Overprojection of the tip cartilages, blunting of the nasolabial angle, and shortening of the upper lip may all be seen in this deformity. By open rhinoplasty, excessive elements of the septal cartilage and anterior nasal spine are reduced, resulting in tip deprojection.

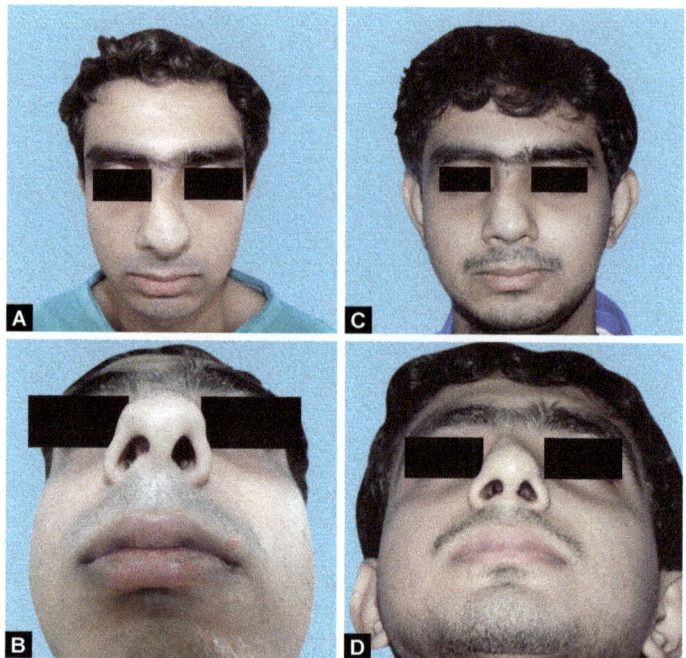

Figs. 24A to D: (A and B) Preoperative; and (C and D) Early postoperative views of a case of Pinocchio nose with overprojected and broad tip and hanging columella. Septoplasty with 'tongue in groove' technique, segmental excision of dome, cephalic trimming, osteotomies, rasping of bony dorsum and tip suturing were done by external approach.

Then reprojection of the tip is achieved by using cartilage grafts and suturing techniques to build strength, support, and elegance into the nasal tip.[44]

Cocaine Nose

Cocaine causes gradual erosion of nasal septum and the nasal mucous membrane, penetrates the maxillary sinuses, and can damage the upper lateral cartilages. Rhinoplasty in cocaine noses is difficult, requiring an osseocartilaginous dorsal graft to correct severe midvault collapse and intraoral mucosal flaps to correct severe intranasal lining contracture.

Before surgical correction, the patient should avoid cocaine for at least 1 year. Septal perforation is not repaired. The nasal mucous membrane is released high up under the bony vault and then pulled down leaving the donor area to heal by secondary intention. In severe cases, the heavily scarred mucosa can be excised under the upper lateral cartilages to allow derotation of the tip. Cartilaginous rib graft is used for the dorsum and columellar strut is inserted. The lower lateral cartilages are advanced over the strut. Tip grafts are used. Suturing of the columellar incision can be difficult and may need V-Y techniques and even skin grafts. Vestibular stenosis and nostril collapse require alar batten grafts and composite grafts. Peripyriform augmentation can be done by diced cartilage grafts.

Pug Nose

Pug nose means a short nose with an upturned tip. Saddle-nose deformity is also called "pug nose" or "boxer's nose". "Pug nose" was first described by John Orlando Rose in 1887. The deformity is characterized by a distinctive scooped out appearance of the nasal dorsum resembling a horse saddle. The shape is due to a collapse of the intrinsic cartilaginous and/or bony support structures of the nose. Characteristics include a loss of dorsal height, middle vault and dorsal depression, diminished tip support and definition, columellar retraction, shortened vertical length, overrotation of tip, and retrusion of anterior nasal spine.

Bossae

Knuckling of the lower lateral cartilages in the domal area forms "bossae". When excess cephalic trimming and inadequate narrowing of the domes are done in bifid tip with strong alar cartilages and thin skin, "bossae" may occur.[4,5] Postoperative scar contracture in this area is the cause of the deformity. It is treated by trimming of the knuckled areas with suturing of the lower lateral cartilages. Minor residual deformity can be corrected by camouflage graft.

REFERENCES

1. Leach JL, Athre RS. Four suture tip rhinoplasty: a powerful tool for controlling tip dynamics. Otolaryngol Head Neck Surg. 2006;135:227-31.
2. Anderson JR. The dynamics of rhinoplasty. Presented at: Proceedings of the 9th International Congress of Otorhinolaryngology. In: Excerpta Medica; 1969.
3. Rohrich RJ, Adams WP Jr. The boxy nasal tip: classification and management based on alar cartilage suturing techniques. Plast Reconstr Surg. 2001;107:1849-63.
4. Murakami CS, Barrera JE, Most S. Preserving structural integrity of the alar cartilage in aesthetic rhinoplasty using a cephalic turn-in flap. Arch Facial Plast Surg. 2009;11(2):126-8.
5. Goodman WS, Streszlow VV. The surgical closure of nasoseptal perforations. Laryngoscope. 1982;92(2):121-4.
6. Goodman WS. Surgery of the nasal tip by external rhinoplasty. J Laryngol Otol. 1980;94:485-94.
7. Adamson PA, Smith O, Tropper GJ. Incision and scar analysis in open rhinoplasty and head and neck surgery. Archives of Otolaryngology. 1990;116:671.
8. Bafaqeeh SA, al-Qattan MM. Alterations in nasal sensibility following open rhinoplasty. Br J Plast Surg. 1998;51(7):508-10.
9. Mao GY, Yang SL, Zheng JH, Liu QY. Aesthetic Rhinoplasty of the Asian Nasal Tip: A Brief Review. Aesth Plast Surg. 2008;32:632-7.
10. McCollough EG, English JM. A new twist in nasal tip surgery. An alternative to the Goldman tip for the wide or bulbous lobule. Arch Otolaryngol. 1985;111: 524-29.
11. Tardy ME, Cheng E. Transdomal suture refinement of the nasal tip. Facial Plastic Surg. 1987;4:317-26.

12. Gruber RP, Weintraub J, Pomerantz J. Suture Techniques for the Nasal Tip. Aesthetic Surg J. 2008;28:92-100.
13. Gunter JP, Landecker A, Cochran CS. Frequently used grafts in Rhinoplasty Nomenclature and Analysis. Plast Reconstr Surg. 2006;118:14e.
14. Cardenas-Camarena L, Guerrero MT. Improving nasal tip projection and definition using interdomal sutures and open approach without transcolumellar incision. Aesthetic Plast Surg. 2002;26:161-6.
15. Wang T, Xue Z, Yu D, Zhang H, Tang X, Wang J, et al. Rhinoplasty in Chinese: management of lower dorsum and bulbous nasal tip. Chin Med J. 2009;122(3):296-300.
16. Kridel RWH, Konior RJ, Shumrick KA, Right WK. Advances in nasal tip surgery. The lateral crural steal. Arch Otolaryngol Head Neck Surg. 1989;115:1206-12.
17. Kridel RW, Konior RJ. Controlled nasal tip rotation via the lateral crural overlay technique. Arch Otolaryngol Head Neck Surg. 1991; 117(4):411-5.
18. Porter JP, Toriumi DM. Surgical techniques for management of the crooked nose. Aesthetic Plast Surg. 2002;26(Suppl 1):S1.
19. Kridel RW, Scott BA, Foda HM. The tongue-in-groove technique in septorhinoplasty. A 10-year experience. Arch Facial Plast Surg. 1999;1(4):246-56.
20. Guyuron B, Varghai A. Lengthening the nose with a tongue-and-groove technique. Plast Reconstr Surg. 2003;111(4):1533-9.
21. Rohrich RJ, Hoxworth RE, Kurkjian TJ. The role of the columellar strut in rhinoplasty: indications and rationale. Plast Reconstr Surg. 2012;129(1):118e-25e.
22. Toriumi DM. Caudal septal extension graft for correction of the retracted columella. Op Tech Otolaryngol Head Neck Surg. 1995;6:311-8.
23. Toriumi DM. Subtotal reconstruction of the nasal septum: a preliminary report. Laryngoscope. 1994;104(7):906-13.
24. Maas CS, Monhian N, Shah SB. Implants in rhinoplasty. Facial Plast Surg. 1997;13:279-90.
25. Nahai F, Gruber RP, Bogdan MA, Friedman GD. Changing the convexity and concavity of nasal cartilages and cartilage grafts with horizontal mattress sutures: part II clinical results. Plast Reconstr Surg. 2005;115:595-606.
26. Johnson CM, Toriumi DM. Open structure rhinoplasty. Philadelphia: WB Saunders; 1990.
27. Toriumi DM, Johnson CM. Open structure rhinoplasty: featured technical points and long-term follow-up. Facial Plast Surg Clin North Am. 1993;1:1-22.
28. Peck GC Jr, Michelson L, Segal J, Peck GC Sr. An 18-year experience with the umbrella graft in rhinoplasty. Plast Reconstr Surg. 1998;102(6):2158-65.
29. Goldman IB. Surgical tips on the nasal tip. Eye Ear Nose Throat Mon. 1954;33:583-91.
30. Tardy ME Jr, Walter MA, Patt BS. The overprojecting nose: anatomic component analysis and repair. Facial Plast Surg. 1993;9(4):306-16.
31. Lipsett EM. A new approach to surgery of the lower cartilaginous vault. Arch Otolaryngol. 1959;70:42-7.
32. Soliemanzadeh P, Kridel RW. Nasal tip overprojection: algorithm of surgical deprojection techniques and introduction of medial crural overlay. Arch Facial Plast Surg. 2005;7(6):374-80.
33. Kridel RW, Konior RJ. Controlled nasal tip rotation via the lateral crural overlay technique. Arch Otolaryngol Head Neck Surg. 1991;117(4):411-5.
34. Lipsett EM. A new approach to surgery of the lower cartilaginous vault. Arch Otolaryngol Head Neck Surg. 1959;70:42.
35. Daniel RK. Middle eastern rhinoplasty in the United States: part I. Primary rhinoplasty. Plast Reconstr Surg. 2009;124(5):1630-9.
36. Toriumi DM, Mueller RA, Grosch T, Bhattacharyya TK, Larrabee WK Jr. Vascular anatomy of the nose and the external rhinoplasty approach. Arch Otolaryngol Head Neck Surg. 1996;122:24.

37. Toriumi DM, Asher SA. Lateral crural repositioning for treatment of cephalic malposition. Facial Plast Surg Clin North Am. 2015;23:55-71.
38. Daniel RK. The nasal tip: anatomy and aesthetics. Plast Reconstr Surg. 1992;89(2):216-24.
39. Foda HM. Management of the droopy tip: a comparison of three alar cartilage modifying techniques. Plast Reconstr Surg. 2003;112(5):1408-17.
40. Bardach J, Cutting C. Anatomy of the unilateral and bilateral cleft lip and nose. Multidisciplinary management of cleft lip and palate. Philadelphia: WB Saunders Co; 1990. pp. 150-9.
41. Nolst Trenite GJ. Rhinoplasty: a practical guide to functional and aesthetic surgery of the nose. The Hague, Netherlands: Kugler Publications; 2005.
42. Fredricks Simon. Tripod resection for "Pinocchio" nose deformity. Plast Reconstr Surg. 1974;53(5):531-33.
43. William ES, Giancario FZ. Management of the overprojected nose and ptotic nasal tip. Aesthetic Surg J. 2009;29:253-8.
44. Johnson CM Jr, Godin MS. The tension nose, Open structure rhinoplasty approach. Plast Reconstr Surg; 1995;95(1):43-51.
45. Sykes JM, Senders CW. Surgery of the cleft lip nasal deformity. Operat Tech Otolaryngol Head Neck Surg. 1990;1:2119-224.

CHAPTER 14

Sutures and Dressing

Before closing the incisions, the nose is inspected and palpated again for any final corrections. Pressure is given over the nose gently by a gauze piece from above downward to squeeze out the blood beneath the soft tissues.

At the transcolumellar incision, the suturing is done in the following manner: at first, the midline suture at the apex of the inverted V-shaped incision is done for alignment; then, sutures are done at the lateral corners for redraping of the skin; and lastly, sutures are done at the columellar pillar by 5-0 Vicryl or prolene. Additional sutures may be done if required. The transfixion incision is closed with 2–3 sutures of 4-0 plain catgut. The intercartilaginous incisions may not be sutured as the open intercartilaginous wound helps in drainage of blood if any.

Nasal cavities are packed with lubricated 1-cm broad ribbon gauze loosely on both sides. Anterior nasal packing is done to prevent bleeding and hematoma formation, to ensure good tissue apposition, and to prevent synechia and displacement by splinting.

The packing is usually removed after 24 hours. Venous and lymphatic drainage may be hampered by very tight and prolonged packing. To avoid prolonged packing, septal suturing can be done. Tight intranasal pack after osteotomies may cause splaying out of the bony segments of the mobilized lateral walls. Light nasal packing little beyond the vestibule is sufficient in case of rhinoplasty without septoplasty.

External nasal dressing is done to prevent hematoma and swelling, to fix the skin on the underlying structure, to prevent displacement by external injury and to prevent splaying of the lateral walls by intranasal packing and edema. The skin of the nose is swabbed with Tincture Benzoin before the application of paper tape.[1]

Micropore is applied over the skin of the nose because it causes minimal skin reaction. Micropore tapes that are 1 cm broad are placed in the following sequence:
- A longitudinal tape is applied around the lobule at the upper part of columella extending along the sides of the bridge of the nose.
- Three slightly overlapping tapes are applied transversely over the dorsum from the level of nasion to supratip. The adhesive tapes will help in redraping of the skin and will prevent hematoma formation and malpositioning of the underlying structure.

Splinting can be done with a six-layered plaster of Paris, soaked in tepid water and applied over the nose till it dries. This splint is fixed over the nose

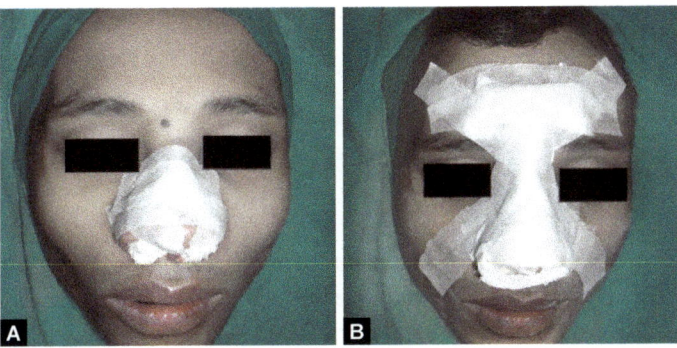

Figs. 1A and B: (A) Adhesive tapes to drape and fix the nasal skin; (B) Plaster of Paris splint fixed over the adhesive tapes on the nose.

with micropore tapes **(Figs. 1A and B)**. The size of the plaster splint should be according to the size of the nose. If it is too big, it will be displaced while smiling and chewing. The splint is replaced on the 4th postoperative day with a new one if it gets loosened due to subsidence of edema. Aluminum splints are also good and can be used. The splint is removed after 7–10 days.

Though rhinoplasty is not so sterile operation, infections occur in <1% of all interventions.[2-4] The risk of infection increases, when rhinoplasty is combined with sinus surgery in presence of purulent sinusitis.[5]

In about 50% of all healthy people, *Staphylococcus aureus* is found in the nasal vestibule. However, bacteremia following septoplasty is rare.[6] Exotoxin of *Staphylococcus* can cause toxic shock syndrome in presence of nasal packings.[7,8]

REFERENCES

1. Nolst Trenite GJ. Rhinoplasty: a practical guide to functional and aesthetic surgery of the nose. The Hague, Netherlands: Kugler Publications; 2005.
2. Abifadel M, Real JP, Servant JM, Banzet P. Apropos of a case of infection after esthetic rhinoplasty. Ann Chir Plast Esthet. 1990;35(5):415-7.
3. Hetter GP. Infection after rhinoplasty. Plast Reconstr Surg. 1983;71:439-40.
4. Cabouli JL, Guerrissi JO, Mileto A, Cerisola JA. Local infection following aesthetic rhinoplasty. Ann Plast Surg. 1986;17(4):306-9.
5. Millman B, Smith R. The potential pitfalls of concurrent rhinoplasty and endoscopic sinus surgery. Laryngoscope. 2002;112:1193-6.
6. Silk KL, Ali MB, Cohen BJ, Summersgill JT, Raff MJ. Absence of bacteremia during nasal septoplasty. Arch Otolaryngol Head Neck Surg. 1991;117(1):54-5.
7. Holt GR, Garner ET, McLarey D. Postoperative sequelae and complications of rhinoplasty. Otolaryngol Clin North Am. 1987;20(4):853-76.
8. Thumfart WT, Volklein C. Systemic and other complications. Fac Plast Surg. 1997;13(1):61-9.

CHAPTER 15

Postoperative Care

The patient should have prior information regarding postoperative swelling of the eyelids, nasal blockage due to mucosal edema and nasal dressing. Oral and written advice is helpful to the patient to reduce the postoperative complications.

Postrhinoplasty advice given to the patients is as follows:
- To use a saline nasal spray
- To sleep with the head elevated for the first week after surgery
- Not to sleep on the side of the face but rather sleep on the back of the head for the first 2 weeks after surgery
- Not to blow his nose for 7 days after surgery as it can hamper proper healing and cause bleeding
- To wipe his nose gently with tissues, if necessary
- To keep his mouth open while sneezing
- To avoid alcohol and aspirin for 2 weeks
- Not to do vigorous physical exercise and should avoid excessive physical exertion, lifting heavy objects, or straining for 6 weeks after his surgery as these activities will hamper wound healing and cause bleeding.[1]
- To avoid injury to his nose
- Not to wear regular glasses for at least 3 weeks. He may tape the glasses to his forehead. He can wear contact lenses 2 days after surgery.
- To avoid direct exposure of nose to sunlight for 6 weeks after surgery.[2] Exposure to sun will slow down the healing process and will cause swelling in the nose.
- To avoid foods that require prolonged chewing
- To avoid excessive facial movements or smiling for 1–2 weeks
- To avoid getting the nasal cast wet during washing the face
- To avoid washing hair for 1 week unless some other person helps to do it for the patient
- To brush the teeth gently with a soft toothbrush
- To avoid excessive movement of the upper lip to keep the nose at rest
- To wear clothing that opens in front or back for 1 week
- To avoid swimming for 1 month
- To avoid smoking for at least 2 weeks as smoking delays healing.

The patient should not be concerned if, after removal of dressing, the nose, eyes, and upper lip show some swelling and discoloration. Postoperative scleral hemorrhage may last for 3–6 weeks. Facial swelling and ecchymosis around eyes usually subside within 3 weeks after surgery but tip edema following external rhinoplasty may take 6 months to 1 year to subside.

The time taken for gradual reduction of swelling over nose is 3 months at bony dorsum, 6 months at cartilaginous dorsum, 9 months at supratip area, and 12 months at tip.

The nasal surface may become somewhat insensitive after rhinoplasty. Full sensation usually comes back within 3 months after surgery.

It is usual to accept the result after 1 year as final outcome.[3]

REFERENCES

1. Nolst Trenite GJ. Rhinoplasty: a practical guide to functional and aesthetic surgery of the nose. The Hague, Netherlands: Kugler Publications; 2005.
2. Sheen JH, Sheen AP (Eds). Aesthetic Rhinoplasty (reprint of 1987 edition), 2nd edition. St. Louis: Quality Medical Publishing; 1998.
3. Tardy ME Jr. Rhinoplasty: the Art and the Science. Philadelphia, Pennsylvania: WB Saunders Company; 1997.

CHAPTER 16

Augmentation Rhinoplasty

INTRODUCTION

Nowadays, the most common cause of depressed nasal dorsum or saddle nose is trauma. It may affect either bony or cartilaginous or both parts of dorsum. Saddle deformity may be associated with wide dorsum. The dorsum of nose is usually studied by the frontal and lateral views. On frontal view, the dorsal aesthetic lines, bony width and inclination of the side walls are studied. The supraorbital ridge lines become narrow at the radix and then descend vertically along the sidewalls of the nose to the tip-defining points as the parallel dorsal aesthetic lines. The normal width of the dorsal aesthetic lines is 8–10 mm in males and 6–8 mm in females.

Common causes of saddle nose are trauma, septal hematoma or abscess, extensive septal surgery, overreduction of dorsal hump, ethnic and some chronic inflammatory conditions of nose. The thickness of the skin-soft tissue envelope and the vascularity of the recipient bed are important factors for the long-term result of the surgery. Thin and scarred skin makes rhinoplasty difficult.

CLASSIFICATION OF SADDLE NOSE DEFORMITY (DANIEL RK, BRENNER KA)[1]

Type 0: Pseudosaddle: Depression of the cartilaginous vault relative to the bony vault

Type I: Supratip depression and columellar retraction

Type II: More advanced depression, with reduction of tip projection and septal support

Type III: Total loss of cartilaginous dorsal integrity and depression of the nasal lobule

Type IV: Severe depression with involvement of the bony dorsum

Type V: "Catastrophic" defects with skin contracture, loss of nasal lining and extreme shortening of nose.

To augment a saddle nose implantation of some substance is required. Biomaterial is defined as any material used for augmentation and replacement of tissue, whether natural or synthetic.[2]

Characteristics of a good biomaterial are the following:

Macroscopic:
- Compatible physical properties
- Nonresorbable
- Remains stable in position
- Can be removed easily
- Retains constant shape and volume
- Exchangeable
- Can be modified
- Easy availability
- Moderately priced

Microscopic:
- No/minimal inflammatory reaction
- No/minimal surface contamination
- Resistant to infection
- Not carcinogenic
- No transmission of disease
- Not degradable[3,4]

However, every biomaterial available is deficient of some of these listed properties.

TYPES OF IMPLANTS

The implants may be either natural or synthetic:

Natural Grafts

- *Autografts:* Autologous material is the best graft material in nasal surgery, in spite of its limited quantity and the additional harvesting procedure. Autografts include cartilage, fascia, and dermis. Autologous cartilage is the most commonly used material for augmentation of nose.[5] Incidence of infection and resorption of autologous cartilage grafts is very rare.[6,7] Unlike synthetic implant, autologous cartilage can be grafted in areas with deficient soft tissue envelope.[8]
- *Homografts (allografts):* These are taken from different individuals of the same species. These are preserved or irradiated cartilage. Homografts are preserved in 70% alcohol or formalin. Septal cartilage homograft is usually used. The matrix of the homograft cartilage is invaded and replaced by adjacent connective tissue and often shows mild resorption over time. Homograft cartilage is rarely used as there is unpredictable result, relatively high rate of infection, incidence of warping and the fear of disease transmission.[9,10] Welling et al. (1988) reviewed 42 patients implanted with irradiated homologous cartilage grafts and found that 100% of the grafts were absorbed when in place longer than 10 years.[11]

Acellular dermis (AlloDerm) is an acellular allograft dermal matrix. This is prepared from fresh human cadaveric skin. Partial resorption of this graft may occur. AlloDerm can be used to camouflage minor irregularities of the dorsum. Since AlloDerm is acellular, there is a very low risk of viral transmission.
- *Xenografts (heterologous):* These are taken from different species. Commonly used xenografts are porcine or bovine collagen.

Synthetic Grafts (Alloplasts)

Commonly used alloplasts are silicone, polytetrafluoroethylene (Teflon, Proplast, Gore-tex), porous polyethylene (Medpore), mersilene and supramid mesh, titanium, and hydroxyapatite. Although most patients do well with synthetic implants, some of them develop complications like redness and ulceration of the skin over the implant, infection, extrusion, displacement, translucency of the implant, and long-standing pain.[12,13] Easy availability, no donor site morbidity, adaptability, excellent initial results, as well as low cost and requirement of minimal surgical skills made alloplasts popular, but they do not become fixed to the nasal skeleton and displacement is a common problem due to vulnerability of the nose for trauma.

The first alloplast to have widespread use in rhinoplasty was solid silicone.[14] It is not porous and on the nasal dorsum it does not remain fixed. A dead space is usually present between the implant and the surrounding fibrous capsule, leading to increased rate of infection and expulsion.

Mersilene (polyethylene terephthalate) is a polyester fiber mesh which is chemically inert. It can be molded and sutured easily, having a natural feel and good stability, but provides no support to nasal framework. As there is extensive tissue ingrowth, total removal after healing is very difficult.

Though Beekhuis (1974) mentioned Supramid mesh as an ideal material for dorsal augmentation; the late results were very bad with disappearance of the graft due to degradation.[15]

Medpore or high-density polyethylene is relatively flexible and compressible. It is well incorporated into the surrounding tissue due to presence of large pores in it, which permit ingrowth of connective tissue.[16]

Although Gore-tex is the current alloplast of choice, there is also chance of infection and other long-term diverse problems. Gore-tex is an expanded polytetrafluoroethylene polymer having many pores, which allow limited connective tissue ingrowth with minimal capsule formation. It is biocompatible and the limited soft tissue ingrowth provides adequate stability to the implant with easy removal.[17,18] It is felt like soft tissue and can be resterilized if not used. It fits nicely into precise pockets. Though Gore-tex has less extrusion and infection rate than other alloplasts,[19] one of the disadvantages of it for dorsal augmentation is its lack of structural rigidity. It should not be placed on the tip of the nose. Conrad et al. (2008) found Gore-tex to be a safe, inexpensive, and predictable alternative to autografts.[20]

However, for the patient's best interest, autografts should be the first choice.

Autografts

Solid dorsal grafts have problems of visibility, sharp margins, or warping. Fascia is used for minimal augmentation (0.5–1.5 mm). Diced cartilage in fascia can also be used for dorsal augmentation (1–8 mm). Bone grafts are not used nowadays because of their tendency to be resorbed.

The following autografts are commonly used:
- *Minor augmentation:* Septal or conchal cartilage, fascia, dermis—Dermis is not preferred because of the high rate of absorption. A straight segment of septal cartilage having the size of 35 mm in length and 5–6 mm in width is the ideal graft for dorsal augmentation.
- *Moderate augmentation (dorsal augmentation 1–4 mm):* Septal or conchal cartilage in layers—Several cartilage pieces are sutured together with 3-0 Vicryl to make a larger graft **(Fig. 1)**. Septal and conchal cartilages may be combined. Septal cartilage is a better graft than conchal cartilage because it is thicker and easily obtained. Rib cartilage may be used.
- *Major augmentation (dorsal augmentation 4 mm or greater):* Rib cartilage, diced cartilage in fascia—Conchal cartilage may be taken from both auricles. Calvarial or cranial bone has a lower resorption rate because of its membranous origin than endochondral bone grafts, such as iliac crest and rib.[21] Cranial bone grafts have a resorption rate of about 20–30%.[22] Although calvarial bone can be used for augmentation, it has some disadvantages

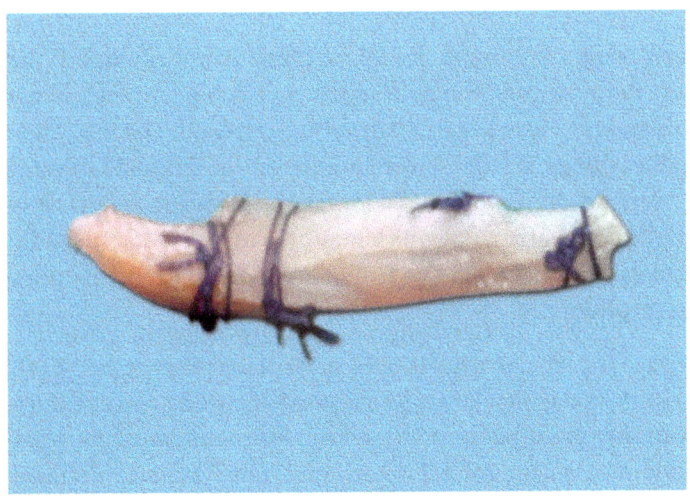

Fig. 1: Pieces of conchal cartilage sutured with 4–0 Vicryl to make a dorsal graft for augmentation.

such as difficult harvesting, limited thickness and scar over scalp area.[23] During harvesting of calvarial bone, there is a risk of intracranial injuries.[24-26] However, bone grafts are very rarely used in rhinoplasty nowadays.

Rib cartilage is the best material for the correction of severe saddle deformities.[27,28]

Temporal fascia: For minor augmentation under the skin, temporal fascia is preferred. It is used to correct volume deficiency or to camouflage dorsal irregularities.[29,30] A 5 × 5 cm sheet of fascia is rolled and sutured along its seam. With the help of a percutaneous suture, the graft is inserted into the dorsal pocket up to the radix and then sutured distally near the tip. Temporal fascia may be used to cover the cartilage grafts to avoid possible irregularities or sharp margins.[31] Temporal fascia interposition graft may be used in patients with traumatized or thin skin.[32] There is temporary swelling of the graft in the immediate 1-2 months of the postoperative period, but after shrinkage, the graft maintains 80% of its original volume.[29]

Autologous cartilage is the first choice for grafting. Its absorption rate is minimum, needs no blood supply for survival, and it is easy to shape. Cartilage graft survives by diffusion of plasma from surrounding tissue and is the ideal graft in secondary rhinoplasty.

Septal cartilage: Harvesting of septal cartilage is done, leaving a caudal and dorsal strut of at least 1.5 cm intact in the nasal septum to maintain the structural integrity of the nose. Unlike conchal and rib cartilage, septal cartilage graft is usually straight and strong and warping of the cartilage does not occur. It can be easily shaped and very lightly crushed to change its thickness and can be used for support, contouring, or filling.

Conchal cartilage: If enough septal cartilage is not obtained, the conchal cartilage is the next preference. Harvested conchal cartilage is not straight, is less strong, and more fragile than septal cartilage. The size and thickness of conchal cartilage are not same in different individuals. Its stiffness and pliability depend on its thickness. Perichondrium can be preserved in one surface of the conchal cartilage, as it may help in rapid fixation of the cartilage graft. Cartilage grafts if crushed to facilitate contouring tend to undergo higher rates of resorption.

Rib cartilage: The rib cartilage is used in virtually every aspect of rhinoplasty and is the preferred graft when rigid support is necessary. Dorsal augmentation with rib cartilage grafts has proven useful in the secondary rhinoplasty patients and in patients with congenital deformities, posttraumatic deformities, or in primary rhinoplasty patients who require a significant amount of structural support.

Rib cartilage has a tendency to curl postoperatively. To prevent distortion, the rib cartilage is trimmed on opposing surfaces (balanced cross section). A straight piece of the eighth or ninth rib is harvested from right side and then shaped like a boat discarding the peripheral parts. The rib cartilage has adequate length and thickness for major augmentation. Harvesting of rib cartilage is usually painful and rarely pneumothorax may occur as a complication. In elderly patients, due to gradual calcification of the rib cartilage, there is less tendency for warping but sculpturing the rib cartilage becomes difficult.

Diced cartilage in fascia: Many surgeons prefer diced cartilage over a solid piece of cartilage because of its flexibility and there is almost no chance of warping. Peer (1943) first described the technique of diced cartilage in reconstructive surgery.[33] Then Erol (2000) developed a technique and termed "Turkish Delight," where he wrapped finely diced cartilage in one layer of Surgicel moistened with an antibiotic (rifamycin).[34] But in many cases, severe resorption of the graft with high rate of inflammation and foreign body reaction due to Surgicel was reported. Thereafter, the concept of wrapping in temporal fascia was started. There is less chance of infection to fascia and it has a good survival rate. It is also easy to shape and suture. Wrapping of the diced cartilage in fascia results in smooth surface of the graft with no irregularities or visible edges. Sometimes diced cartilage pieces are mixed with tissue glue to make it a solid graft and used as a dorsal graft without wrapping it in fascia.

Diced cartilage in fascia is a useful graft for dorsal augmentation. The cartilage is diced into small pieces (<0.5 mm) which are introduced into a fascial sleeve that is placed over the dorsum.

A large sheet of temporal fascia graft is harvested. Cartilage is diced into small pieces (<0.5 mm) using excised cartilage, septum, concha, or rib with number 11 blade. A 1-mL tuberculin syringe is taken and diced cartilage pieces are kept into it. Then the plunger is introduced and the cartilage pieces are pushed by the plunger. The cartilage pieces are so small that they can pass through the hub and thus there is no need to cut the hub from the syringe.

The dorsal defect is measured. The fascia is folded into an 8–10 mm wide × 20–35 mm long sleeve. The free edge is trimmed and sutured with 4-0 Vicryl. The syringe is introduced into the open end of the sleeve and it is filled to make a graft of adequate thickness. The graft is fixed with 4-0 plain catgut at the cephalic end. The percutaneous suture is inserted at the nasion level and the graft is placed over the dorsal defect. After packing the nasal cavities, the dorsum is covered with micropore tapes. Removal of the cast is done after 1 week and if necessary, gentle molding helps to make a smooth dorsum. The molding of the graft can be done up to 2 weeks. The patient is advised not to wear glasses for 6 weeks.

Harvesting of Conchal Cartilage

Conchal cartilage is a high-quality graft which is available in substantial amounts. It is the material of choice when septal cartilage is lacking and provides an excellent smooth, convex dorsal contour. Harvesting a large piece of conchal cartilage is technically easier by the anterior approach than the posterior approach, but there is a chance of visible scar. To facilitate the dissection, 2% lignocaine in combination with 1:100,000 adrenaline is injected in the subperichondrial plane at the anterior or concave surface of the concha and in the supraperichondrial plane at the posterior or convex surface. The incision is made on the posterior surface of the concha, 3–4 mm lateral to the postauricular crease. The anterior perichondrial layer is preserved for the donor site, and the posterior layer remains attached with the resected graft. The attached perichondrium ensures the survival of the cartilage graft. At the anterior surface, the dissection is done in the subperichondrial plane with the Freer elevator. During dissection, there should not be any fracture or tear of the conchal cartilage. The entire conchal cartilage can be taken out after dissection at the posterior surface with a curved Joseph scissors. During the posterior approach, to mark the cartilage incision, several needles are pushed through the pinna from the anterior surface just medial to the antihelix, along the lateral margin of the concha. After meticulous hemostasis, the skin incision is repaired with 4-0 nylon suture. Hematoma is prevented by placing cotton wool on each side of the concha and sutured in place with a 3-0 nylon through-and-through suture which is removed after 3 days **(Figs. 2 to 4)**.[35]

Harvesting of Rib Cartilage Graft

From rib cartilage, we get sufficient amount of cartilage for moderate or major dorsal augmentation. Limited computed tomography scan of the sternum and ribs with coronal reconstructions should be done in older patients where ossification of the cartilaginous rib is suspected.

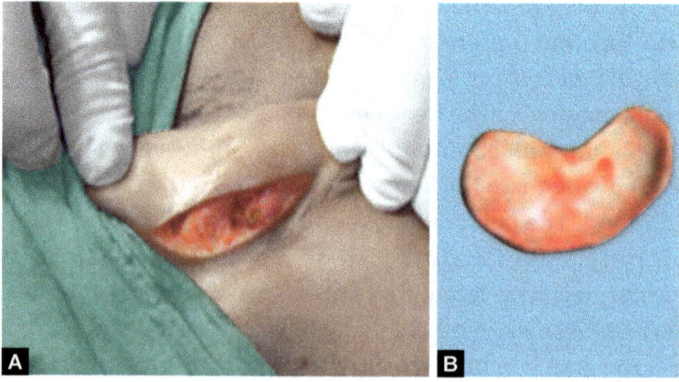

Figs. 2A and B: Harvesting of conchal cartilage.

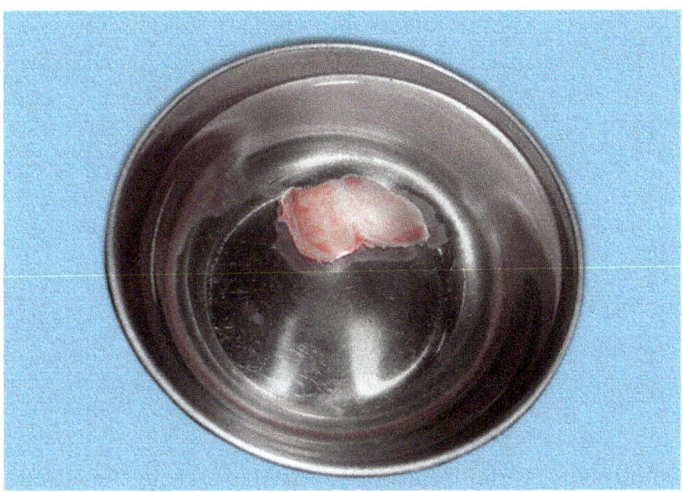

Fig. 3: Conchal cartilage in normal saline.

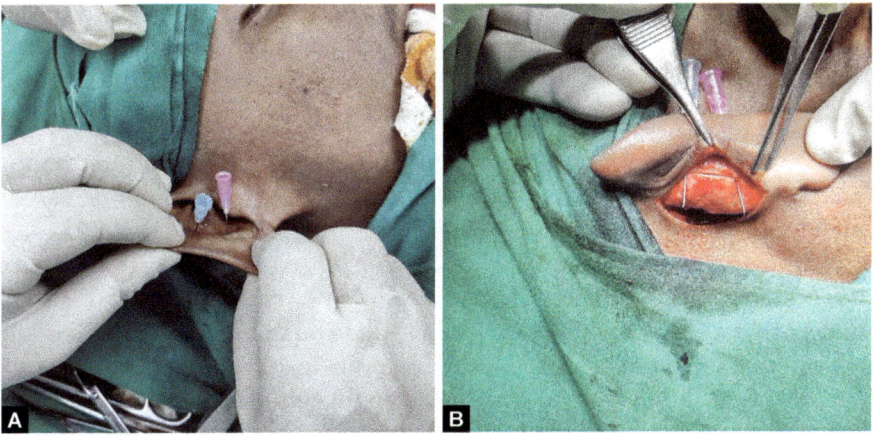

Figs. 4A and B: To mark the cartilage incision, several needles are pushed from the anterior surface just medial to the antihelix. It will prevent deformity of the antihelix during harvesting of the cartilage.

Chest is palpated to determine the preferred rib **(Fig. 5)**. Cartilage graft is taken from the 8th or 9th rib by subcostal incision. Extra cartilage may be harvested from the tenth rib. Bone graft may be harvested from the 9th rib. The 5th or the 6th rib may also be taken by an inframammary incision. The 5th rib is straighter and not fused to any other ribs but it tends to be smaller. The 6th rib is longer but more curved than the 5th rib and it tends to fuse to other ribs. The graft is taken from the right side to avoid postoperative left-sided chest pain which may be confused with cardiac pain.[35]

Inframammary approach: In this approach, the inframammary fold is marked in the sitting posture of the patient. The patient should be warned that if she

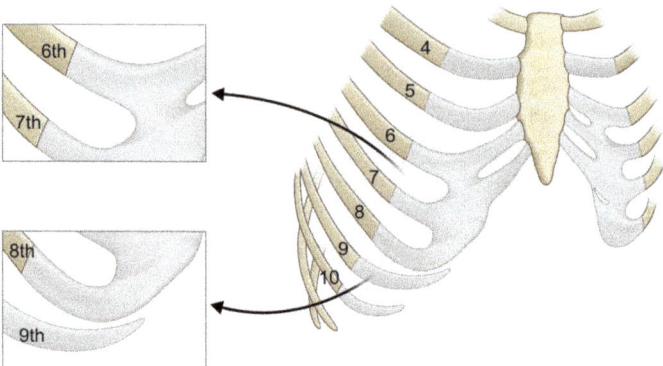

Fig. 5: Costal cartilage harvest.

has breast implant, it may rupture. The patient lies in the supine position with the back elevated at about 10° and the neck remains in slightly extended position. An incision of about 3.5 cm is made, medial to the midclavicular line and 2–3 mm below the inframammary fold to harvest 5th costal cartilage. It is preferable to harvest 5th costal cartilage as it is rarely connected to the 6th rib. But in about 95% of the patients, the 6th rib is connected to the 7th rib. This cartilage fusion should be carefully divided to harvest the rib.

Subcostal approach: In this approach, about 3.5-cm long skin incision is made along the length of the rib. In a thin patient, a smaller incision can be made.

The muscles are separated by dissection with a hemostat. To minimize the postoperative pain, the muscle fibers are not cut but bluntly dissected to expose the costal cartilage. Incision is made on the perichondrium of the rib and the perichondrium is elevated from the cartilaginous part of the rib circumferentially with care so that no damage occurs to the underlying pleura. The perichondrium from the anterior surface of the rib can be harvested as a separate graft. It can be used later to cover the nasal dorsum in patients with thin skin. The perichondrium is elevated from the under surface of the rib cartilage carefully. If the perichondrium remains intact over the pleura, there will be less chance of pneumothorax. An incision is made just medial to the osteochondral junction. Then a medial incision is made according to the required length of cartilage. The portion of the costal cartilage is removed and kept in normal saline **(Figs. 6A to C)**. A standard, layered soft tissue closure is done without a drain. There is a potential risk of pleural injury. Before suturing the wound area, pleura is checked for any tears. After saline irrigation into the surgical area, the anesthesiologist can be requested to raise intrathoracic pressure, when bubbles will appear if a leak is present. A chest X-ray can be done for confirmation.

If the pleural leak is detected on the table, it can be repaired by the following method. The exact site of the hole in the parietal pleura is identified. If the

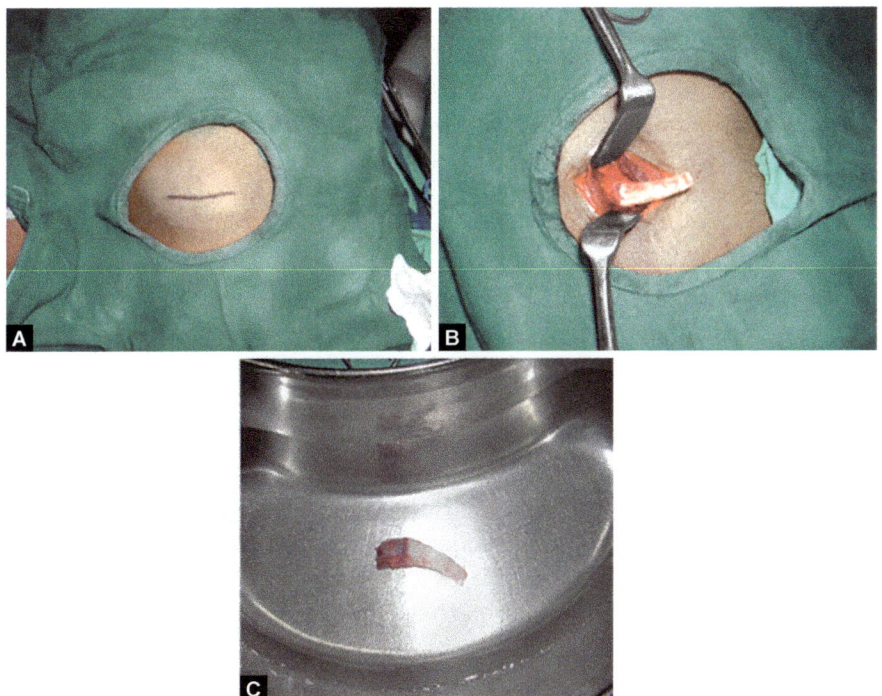

Figs. 6A to C: Harvesting of rib cartilage: (A) Incision along the length of the rib; (B) Delivery of the rib cartilage; (C) Rib cartilage with bone graft in normal saline.

patient is hemodynamically stable, then a rubber catheter is introduced through the hole in the chest wall for a few centimeters into the pleural space. A 2-0 Vicryl purse-string suture at the wound around the rubber catheter is kept ready. The suture is tightened as Valsalva is done by the anesthesiologist and forces the air out of the pleural space and out through the catheter. The rubber catheter is then withdrawn from the wound and the suture is further tightened.

Rib cartilage has a tendency to warp. To prevent warping, a boat-like configuration is given to the graft by balanced cross-section. Balanced cross-section involves amputation of an equal amount of cartilage from both sides to minimize warping of the graft. The core part of the rib is used discarding the peripheral pieces. The prepared rib segment may be soaked in saline for 10 minutes to detect any acute warping before implantation. Fixation of the graft after placing the graft over dorsum may also reduce the tendency to warp.

Patients are advised to refrain from exercise or other strenuous activity for 2–3 weeks after surgery and not to lift objects heavier than 10–15 pounds for 6–8 weeks after surgery.

Harvesting of Iliac Crest Bone Graft

It is almost of historical interest because very few surgeons use iliac crest bone graft in rhinoplasty. Autogenous bone from the iliac crest is harvested as corticocancellous blocks, which require significant dissection of soft tissues. A large amount of bone can be harvested from the iliac crest for major dorsal augmentation. According to the required augmentation, the piece of bone can be shaped with an electric drill or rasp. As iliac crest graft is a endochondral bone, there is a chance of postoperative resorption of the graft to some extent. There is a high chance of resorption if the graft is not immobilized properly, not placed beneath the periosteum and there is no proper bone-to-bone contact over the nasal dorsum. Bone grafts should never be used for augmentation in patients having atrophic rhinitis. Keeping in mind the possible resorption of iliac crest graft, about 30% overcorrection should be done during placement of the graft.

During operation, the right hip is raised by placing a sand bag under it. A 2.5-inch long incision is made from about 0.5 inch behind the anterior iliac spine going posteriorly along the outer margin of the crest with a convexity downward. The periosteum is exposed and then incised along the inner margin of the crest and elevated from the underlying bone. Parallel cuts are made over the iliac crest with a 12-mm osteotome and a corticocancellous block of bone is removed **(Figs. 7 and 8)**. Alternatively, after lifting the cortical part of the bone, cancellous bone graft may be taken from the iliac crest as cancellous bone has a very low resorption rate. The cortical bone part is replaced and the periosteum is sutured. Common complications of iliac bone harvesting are gait disturbance, pain, excessive blood loss, infection, and paresthesia.

Harvesting of Calvarial Bone

Calvarial bone, being a membranous bone, is less likely to resorb. A horizontal incision (4–6 cm) is made superior to the temporal line to harvest parietal bone in the nondominant side. The periosteum is incised and elevated for proper exposure. The graft is outlined by drilling (graft size: 1–1.5 cm × 4–4.5 cm). Drilling is done through the outer table up to the diploe. A sharp osteotome is used to cut the graft carefully without injuring the inner table and dura. The donor site can be filled with hydroxyapatite. The incision is closed in multilayer. Dural injury, although rare, is a known risk. Powell and Riley reviewed calvarial bone grafts in 170 patients and found resorption rates of as high as 30%. Because of this problem and the increased morbidity of harvesting bone grafts, most surgeons prefer using cartilage grafts.[20]

Banking of the Cartilage

The leftover cartilage piece can be banked beneath the scalp in the temporal region, when temporal fascia graft was taken or in the postauricular mastoid area. Extra costal cartilage can be kept in the sub costal donor area. Small piece of residual costal cartilage harvested from the inframammary site can be kept in the temporal region. The grafts usually retain their rigidity, volume,

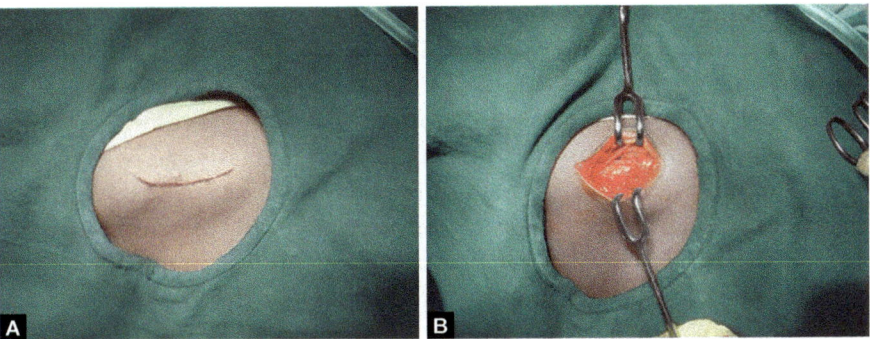

Figs. 7A and B: Harvesting of iliac crest bone graft: (A) Incision; and (B) Exposure of bone.

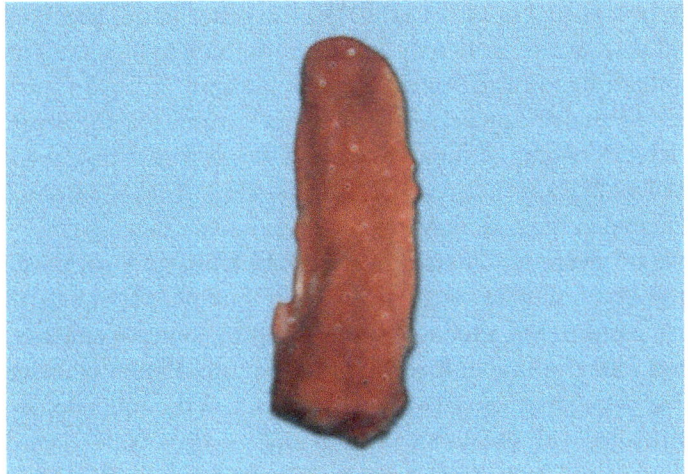

Fig. 8: Iliac crest bone graft.

and shape even up to 6 years. Banked cartilage is a readily available source of graft material.

MANAGEMENT OF SADDLE NOSE

In most cases of saddle nose deformities, tip plasty is usually required along with augmentation of the saddle defect. There are various approaches for correction of saddle nose deformities. When wide exposure is required for extensive reconstruction and grafting, external rhinoplasty is a better approach than internal approach. For minor or moderate augmentation, intercartilaginous incision, cartilage-splitting incision or marginal incision can be made for graft insertion. Midcolumellar approach is a direct midline approach. Here, a vertical incision is made between two medial crura. Grafts can be placed in precise pockets with minimal undermining but there is a chance of postoperative columellar scar.

External approach has several advantages over endonasal approach for graft placement. Infection can spread to the grafts via intranasal incision. External rhinoplasty provides easy access and a symmetrical pocket can be made by elevating the nasal bone periosteum under direct vision. In external rhinoplasty, lateral nasal wall augmentation and tip plasty can be done with better exposure and the graft lies away from the incision site reducing the risk of extrusion through the incision site. Depth perception and measurement of the amount of reduction or augmentation are difficult in closed approach. Greater visualization and more working area are the benefits of the open approach.

Adequate skin-soft tissue envelope is very important for graft placement. The graft should be placed in a supraperichondrial and subperiosteal plane. Too big graft puts pressure on the overlying soft tissue leading to ischemia, necrosis, and extrusion of the graft. On the other hand, postimplantation mobility due to smaller graft may lead to continuing tissue injury resulting in chronic inflammation and displacement of the graft.

Pieces of septal or conchal cartilage may be sutured together with 3-0 Vicryl to make a block of graft of suitable size and shape. The graft is prepared with great care avoiding any sharp edges. The preservation of a small amount of soft tissue attached to the graft may help in fixation of cartilage grafts.

In case of severe saddle deformity with lack of septal support, extended spreader grafts should be placed in between the upper lateral cartilages and the dorsal septum. For adequate septal support, septal extension graft can be sutured with the caudal margin of the septum. Before placement of the spreader grafts, extramucosal tunnels are made at the junction of the upper lateral cartilages with the dorsal septum and the upper lateral cartilages are carefully separated from the dorsal septum with scissors. The spreader grafts are then secured in place by 5-0 PDS sutures. When septal extension graft has not been placed, a columellar cartilage strut is sutured in between two medial crura and the upper end of the columellar strut is fixed with the spreader graft. Alternatively, L-shaped supporting cartilage graft may be used and sutured at the anterior nasal spine before placing the dorsal graft. Rib cartilage can be placed for dorsal augmentation. Diced cartilage in fascia can also be used for augmentation. Appropriate contouring of the rib graft is done by making the undersurface concave and the superior surface convex. The cephalic and caudal ends of the graft are made slightly tapered. Cold or powered instruments are used for contouring.

Bone grafts are very rarely used nowadays. A larger-sized bone graft than the actual size required is always inserted because there will be resorption of the graft to some extent. After insertion of the graft the dorsal skin should not be under tension. The chance of survival of the bone graft is more if there is good bone-to-bone contact with the nasal bones. The edges of the grafts must be beveled and smooth to avoid undue visibility of the graft **(Figs. 9A to D)**.

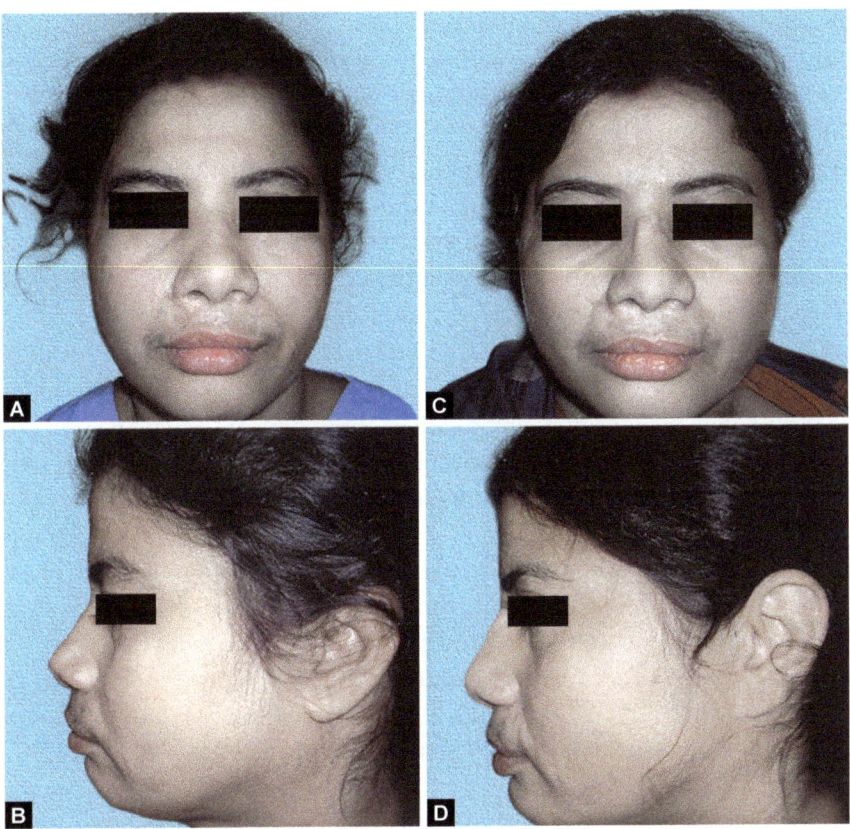

Figs. 9A to D: (A and B) Preoperative; and (C and D) Postoperative views of a posttraumatic case with low dorsum, broad tip and columellar retraction. There is scarring over face. Augmentation rhinoplasty was done with pieces of conchal cartilage by external approach. Columellar cartilage strut was placed. Cephalic trimming, transection of lower lateral cartilages medial to domes and posteriorly based chondral flaps were done in both sides. Medial crura were sutured with 5-0 PDS and a tip shield graft was placed. There is some visibility of the edge of the graft in right side.

Minor supratip depression can be corrected by rotating two medially based rectangular cephalic flaps from the lateral crura of the lower lateral cartilages (after cephalic trimming) and suturing in midline (Kazanjian technique).

When alloplastic materials are used, special precautions are required to prevent contamination. At first, the dissection plane is prepared and then the implant is removed from its sterile packaging. The implant is inserted after it is soaked in antibiotic solution and the recipient bed is irrigated. The site of incision should be far away from the graft to minimize the bacterial contamination.[36] To prevent the spread of infection from nasal cavity, it is better to avoid medial osteotomy and separation of the junction of the upper lateral cartilages with the dorsal septum during augmentation rhinoplasty. Dissection should not be done beyond the radix area because it will cause unwanted cephalic displacement of the implant. In an open approach, the implant should be fixed to the soft tissue by suturing in the desired location. If small holes are made on the implant, it will prevent caudal migration of the implant by fibrous ingrowth into the holes. The chance of extrusion of the implant is increased if the implant is tight on the recipient bed and when the implant is placed near the nasal tip. Adhesive paper tapes applied over nasal skin will prevent hematoma formation by removing dead space. External splint is applied for protecting the implanted area and removed after 1 week **(Figs. 10 to 23)**.

Common Problems of Grafts

- *Absorption of the graft:* More in case of endochondral bone, e.g., iliac crest bone. Minimum absorption occurs in the case of autologous cartilage grafts. Cartilage grafts should be used in atrophic rhinitis and secondary rhinoplasty.
- *Displacement of the graft:* To avoid displacement, the graft should always be inserted subperiosteally and the size of the recipient pocket should not be too big. The graft may be fixed by sutures.
- *Necrosis of the skin:* Necrosis occurs if the skin is tight over the graft. The blanching of the skin indicates that the graft is bigger than the pocket. A bigger pocket can be made by undermining the skin over the sides of the nose.
- *Hematoma:* Adhesive paper tapes are applied over nasal dorsum to prevent dead space and subsequent hematoma formation.
- *Infection:* Strict aseptic procedures should be followed during surgery.
- *Graft visibility:* This occurs in patients with thin skin. The graft may be wrapped with temporal fascia before insertion.
- *Warping of the graft:* This may occur in rib cartilage if trimming of the graft is not done by balanced cross section.
- *Extrusion of the graft:* This may occur in cases of augmentation by synthetic grafts.

NONSURGICAL RHINOPLASTY

Nonsurgical rhinoplasty offers a quick, minimally invasive, financially feasible option for those seeking cosmetic nasal contouring. Though the procedure is temporary, this can be used for patients who are not medically, mentally, or economically prepared for surgery or those who would like a trial before an operation.

Here injectable fillers, most commonly hyaluronic acid or calcium hydroxyapatite, are used to change the shape of the nose without any invasive technique.[37,38]

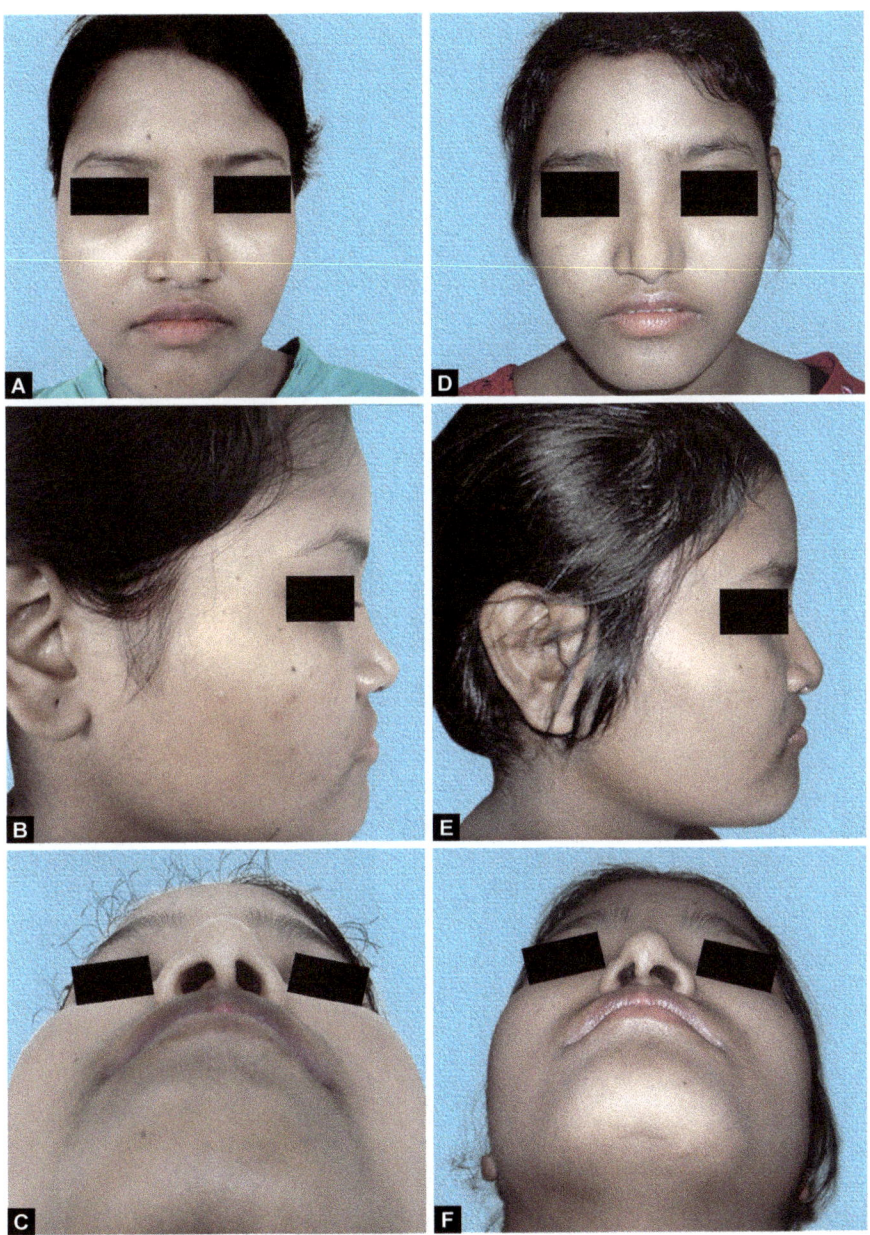

Figs. 10A to F: (A to C) Preoperative; and (D to F) Postoperative views of a saddle nose. Augmentation rhinoplasty was done by layered conchal cartilage and tip plasty was done by cephalic trimming, scoring of domes, interdomal suturing, and onlay tip graft by external approach.

American physician Alexander Rivkin (2002) started to use injectable fillers such as hyaluronic acid and calcium hydroxyapatite to improve the contours of the patients' noses.

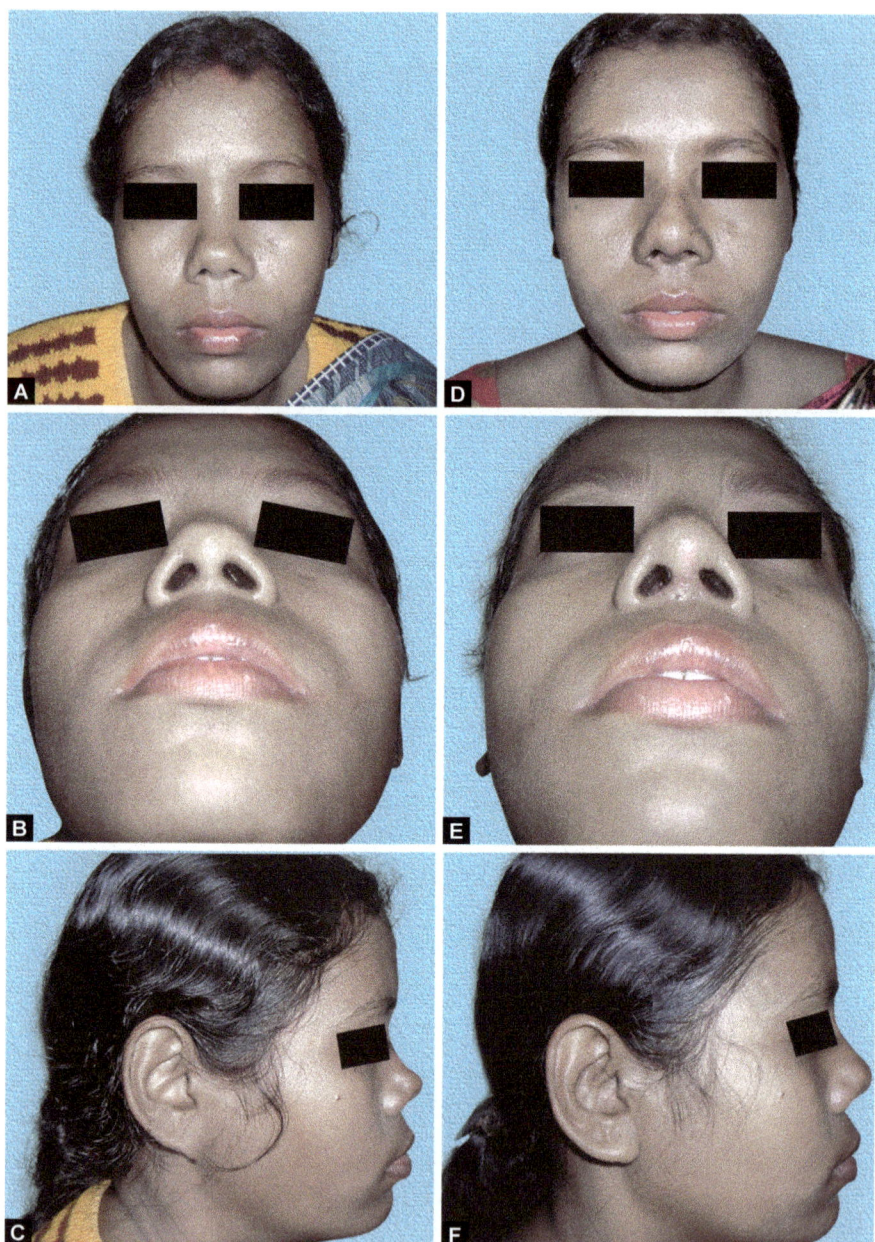

Figs. 11A to F: (A to C) Preoperative; and (D to F) Postoperative views of a case of saddle nose with broad tip. Augmentation was done by layered conchal cartilage taken from right pinna. Tip plasty was done by interdomal suture and dome scoring. Columellar strut was placed in between medial crura and a tip shield graft was sutured by external approach.

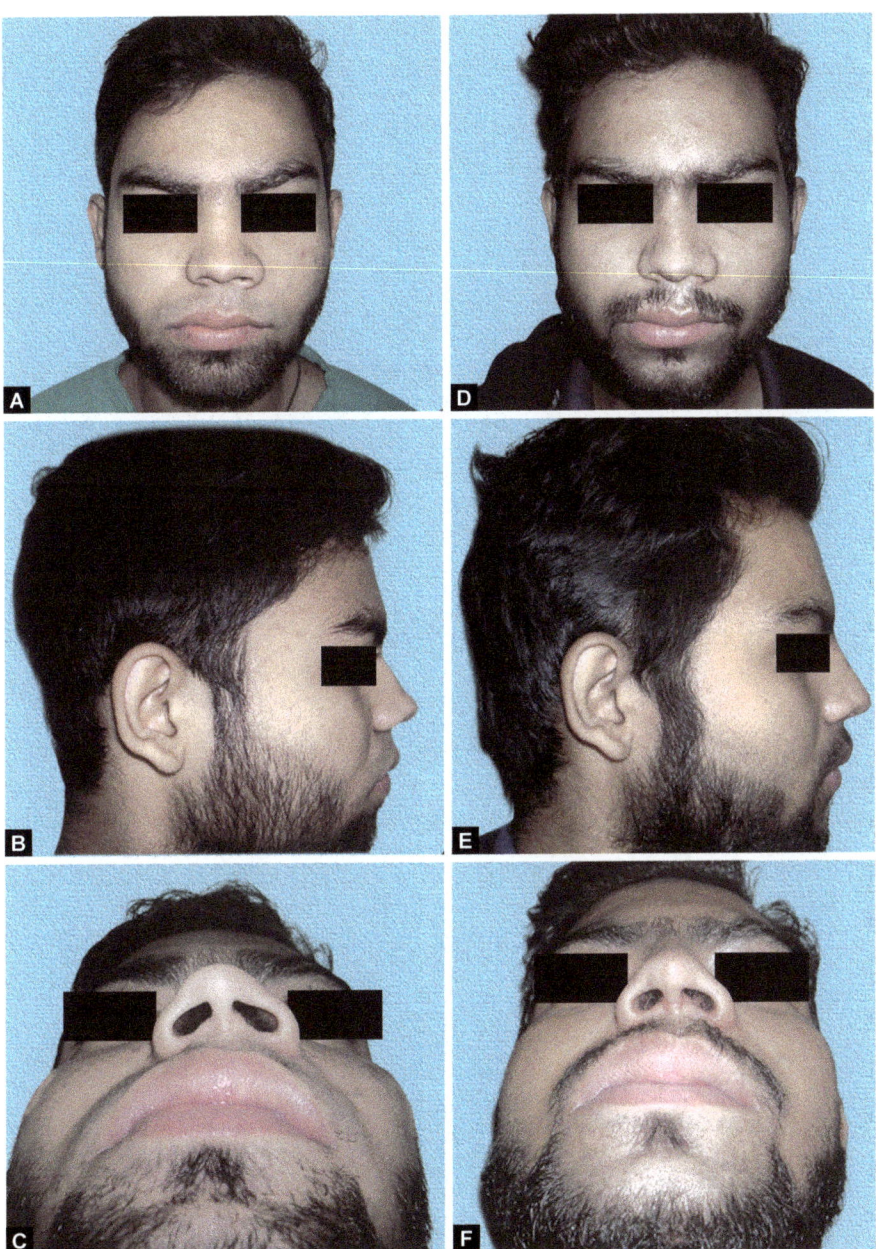

Figs. 12A to F: (A to C) Preoperative; and (D to F) Postoperative views of saddle nose with alar asymmetry. Augmentation was done with layered conchal and septal cartilage. Cephalic trimming was done more in left side. Tip plasty was done by posteriorly based chondral flaps, columellar strut and tip graft by external approach.

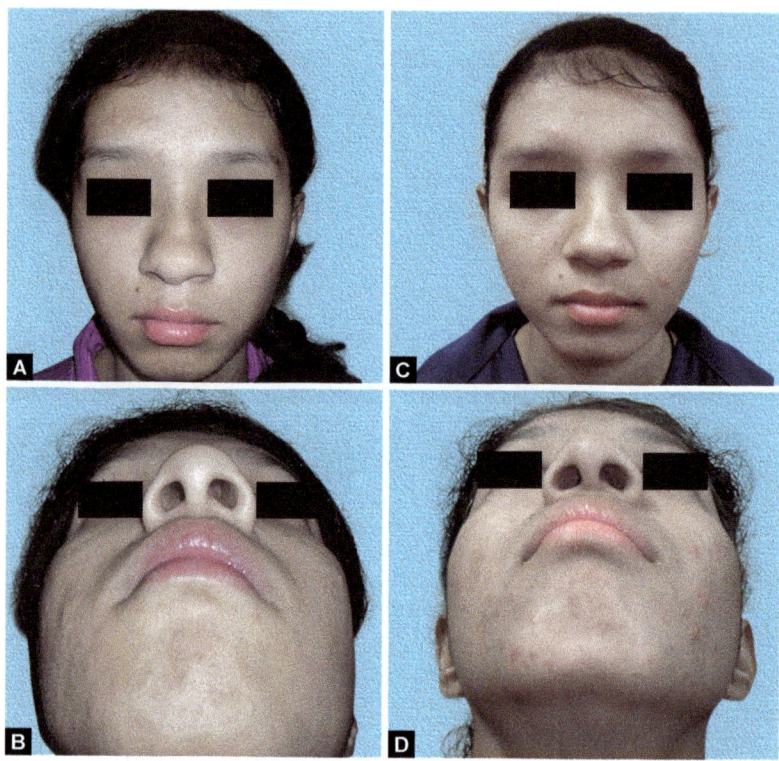

Figs. 13A to D: (A and B) Preoperative; and (C and D) Postoperative views of a case of saddle nose with caudal deviation of septum to left side. Septoplasty and augmentation rhinoplasty were done by layered conchal and septal cartilage by closed technique.

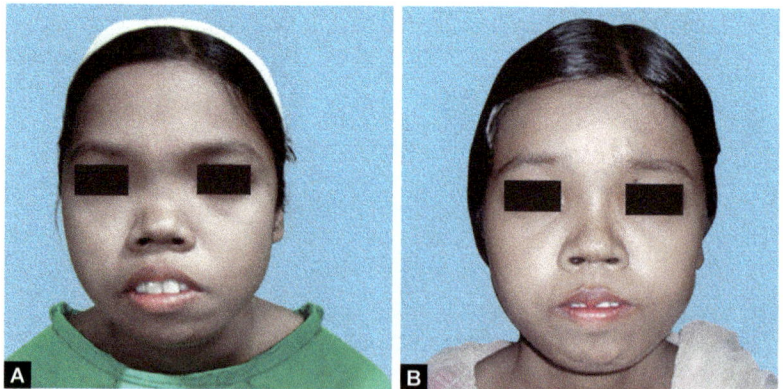

Figs. 14A and B: (A) Preoperative; and (B) Postoperative views of a case of severe saddle deformity. Augmentation was done by layered conchal cartilage.

Australian physician Andrew Tuan-Anh Le (2005) reported good results after injecting polyacrylamide gel (PAAG), a hydrophilic colloid, known commercially as Aquamid.[39]

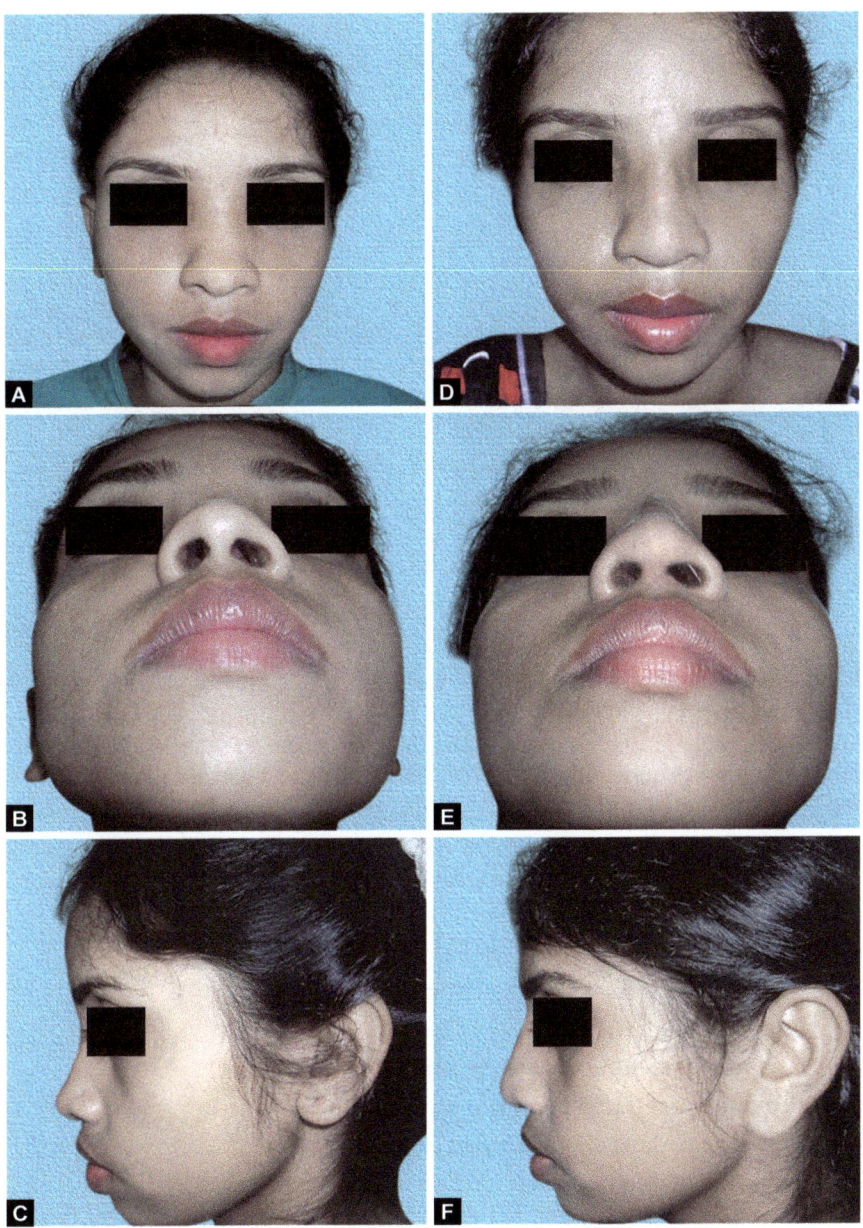

Figs. 15A to F: (A to C) Preoperative; and (D to F) Postoperative views of low dorsum. Dorsal augmentation was done with layered conchal cartilage by external approach. Columellar strut and shield graft were placed and interdomal suturing was done.

Bruising and swelling are mild as it is not an invasive procedure. The procedure cannot decrease the size of the nose or correct functional defects.

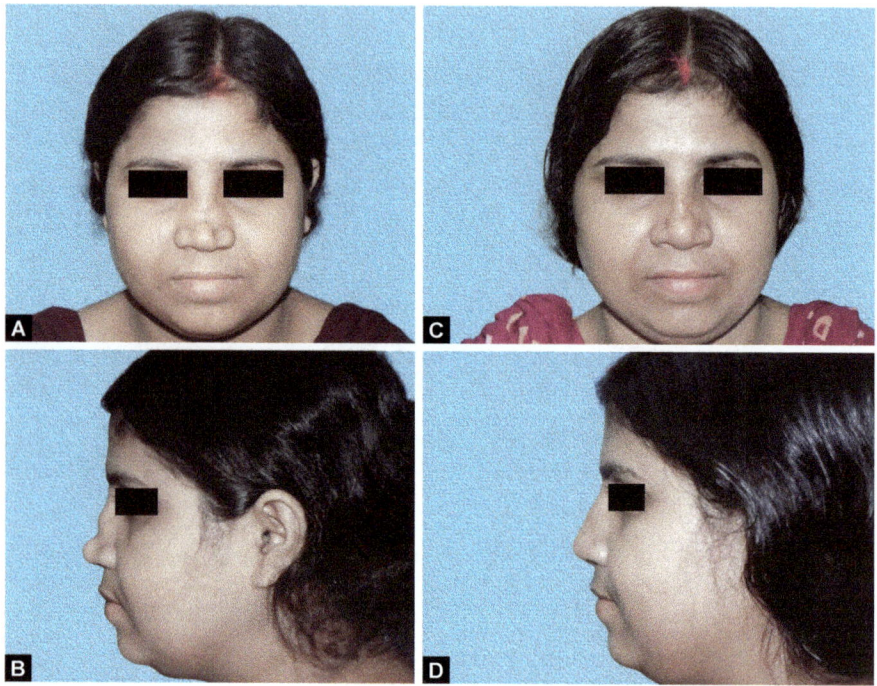

Figs. 16A to D: (A and B) Preoperative; and (C and D) Postoperative views of a case of saddle nose with retracted columella. Spreader grafts and columellar strut were placed. Augmentation was done with layered conchal cartilage and domal equalization suture was done by external approach.

The indications of the nonsurgical rhinoplasty are the following:
- To augment a flat nasal bridge
- Correction of retracted columella
- To increase the nasal tip projection
- Minimal reduction of the size of nostril
- Perceptual lessening of nasal hump
- Correction of retracted anterior nasal spine
- To fill a small depression at nasal sidewall
- Correction of a saddle nose
- Traumatic nasal injury
- To conceal the margins of tip grafts
- To correct bifid tips

First, the nose is marked. Then the area is anesthetized using xylocaine without adrenaline. Adrenaline is avoided to inspect blanching of the skin when there is vascular compromise. Local infiltration anesthesia, if injected in large amount can obscure the area being injected. Small amounts are injected in the tip, usually 0.1–0.2 mL, and slightly more in the dorsum. Some physicians

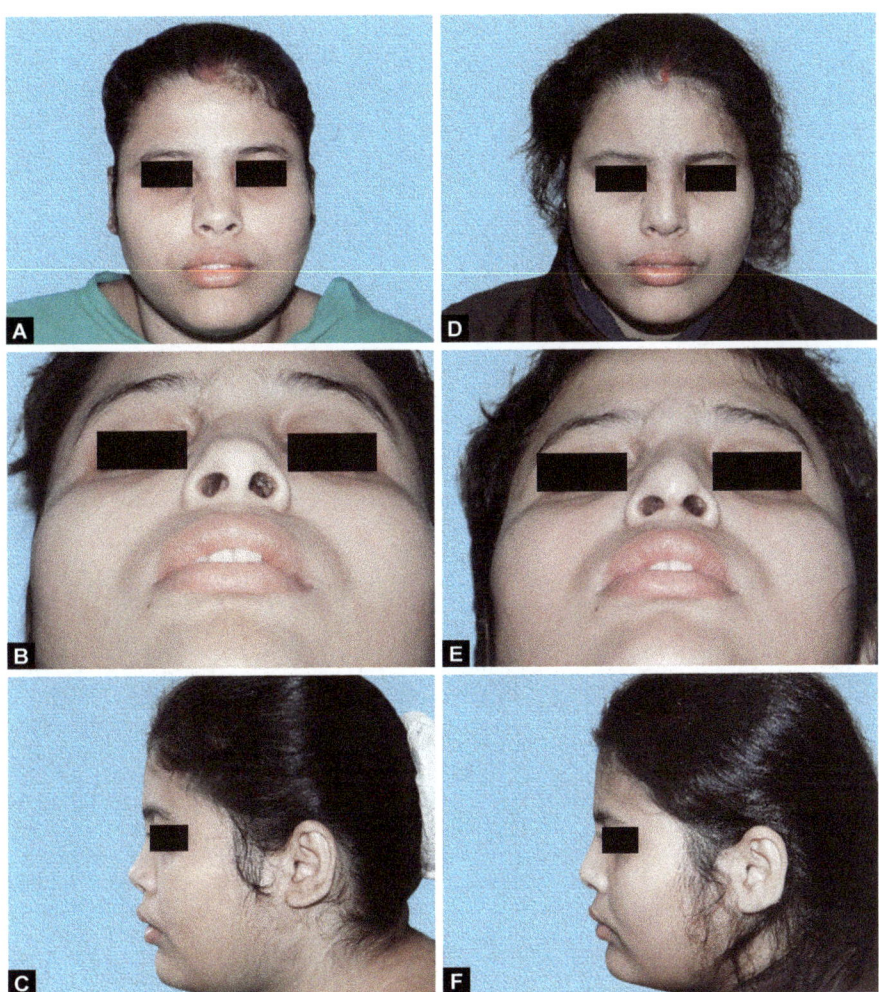

Figs. 17A to F: (A to C) Preoperative; and (D to F) Postoperative views of a post-traumatic case of saddle nose deformity with DNS. Septoplasty was done. Augmentation was done with layered septal and conchal cartilage by external approach. Columellar strut and tip graft were placed and domal creation and domal equalization sutures were done with 4-0 PDS.

do the procedure by topical anesthesia after applying topical cream over skin. But topical anesthetic creams usually cause vasoconstriction of skin and thus, should not be used. Since the face has excellent blood supply, patients are advised to stop medicines such as aspirin, a week before the procedure.

For injection of the fillers, the physician uses a prepackaged sterile syringe containing the material and a hypodermic needle (e.g., 27-G, 25 mm) to inject the filler beneath the nasal skin, in the deep subcutaneous tissues, superficial to the periosteum. Immediately after the injection, digital pressure is applied to position the implant properly. Hemostasis is done by giving mild pressure

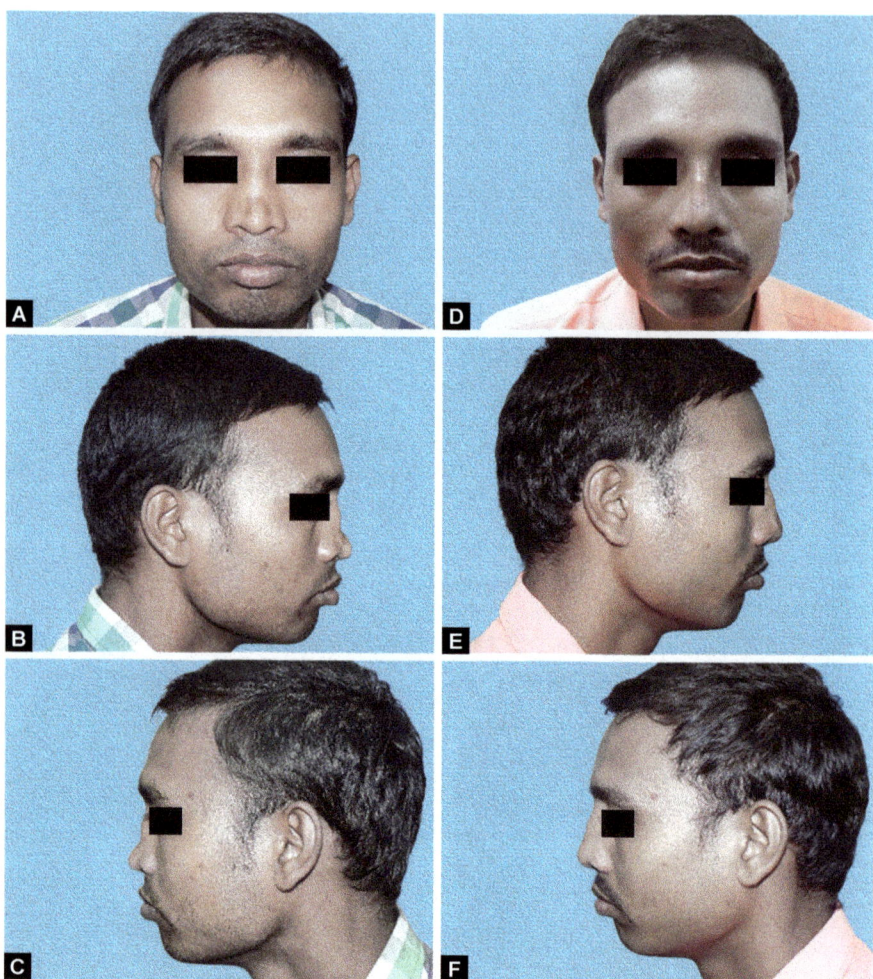

Figs. 18A to F: (A to C) Preoperative; and (D to F) Postoperative views of a case of saddle nose with septal perforation. Rib cartilage was harvested. Osteotomies, placement of spreader grafts and columellar strut were done by external approach. Dorsal augmentation was done with rib cartilage. Tipplasty was done with cephalic trimming, domal equalization suture and tip grafts.

with cotton. Ice packs can be applied to minimize bruising and edema. There may be some swelling, redness, and tenderness for 1–2 days. If blanching occurs, due to vascular compromise, digital massage is done to disperse the filler and open the blood vessels.

The procedure takes about 10–30 minutes to perform as an office procedure. The patient can start normal work after completion of the procedure.

If a good correction is obtained with hyaluronic acid without any adverse reaction, then a longer lasting material like calcium hydroxyapatite can be used the next time.

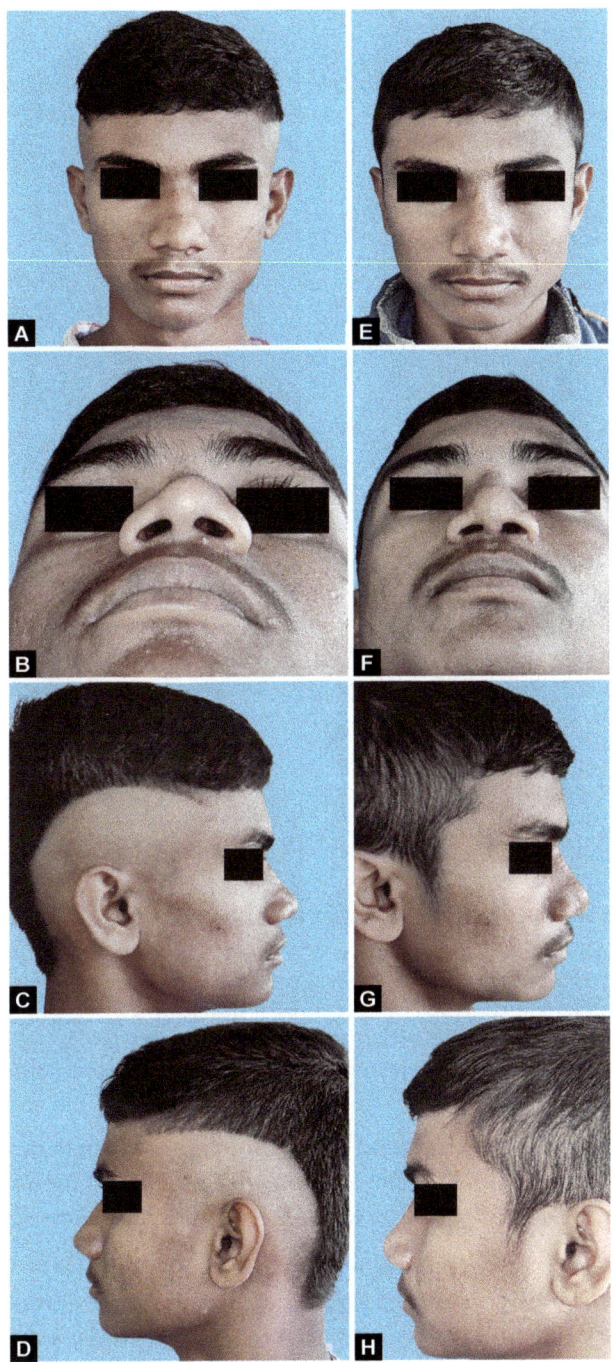

Figs. 19A to H: (A to D) Preoperative; and (E to H) Postoperative views of saddle nose with alar asymmetry. Augmentation was done with layered conchal and septal cartilage by external approach. Alar resection was done in left side. Cephalic trimming and placement of columellar strut were done. Tipplasty was done with interdomal suture.

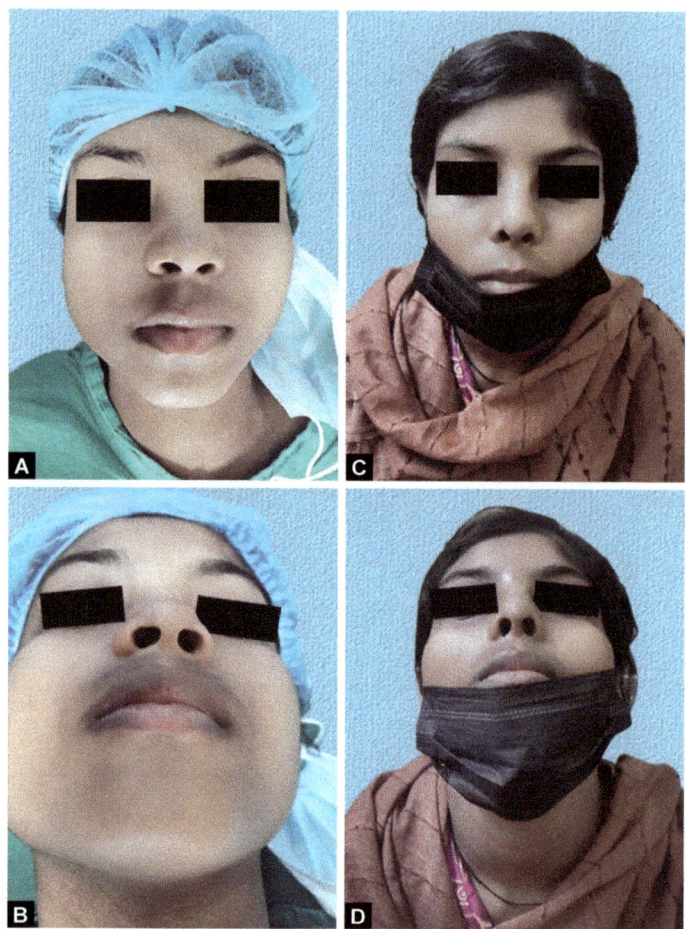

Figs. 20A to D: (A and B) Preoperative; and (C and D) Postoperative views of a case of saddle nose following septal abscess. Costal cartilage was harvested. By external approach, bilateral spreader grafts and columellar strut were sutured with 4-0 PDS. Dorsal augmentation was done with diced costal cartilage in temporal fascia. Cephalic trimming, placement of shield graft and tip plasty by domal creation (transdomal) suture were done.

Vascular compromise is more common in areas having scarred and thin skin. Injection of 0.1 mL filler per scarred area is sufficient for any correction. Repeated injections can be done at 4–6 weeks intervals if necessary.

Soft-tissue filler agents are the following:

- *Hyaluronic acid (Juvederm, Restylane):* This is a safe and nonallergenic temporary filler. It lasts for 6–10 months. This material can be dissolved with injections of hyaluronidase.[40] The duration of hyaluronic acid depends on the subsite. It lasts longer in the tip and alar bases than in the loose tissues of the radix and proximal dorsum. Duration may be as long as 3 years in the tip and 1 year in the radix.

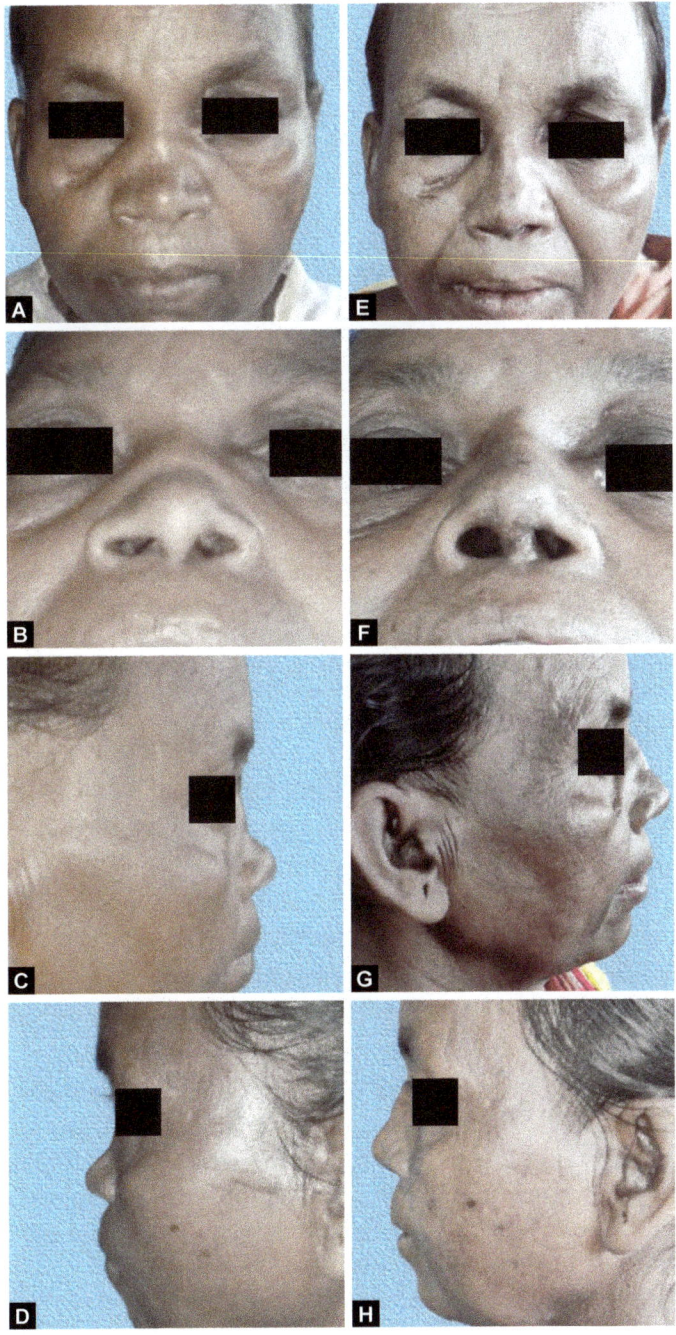

Figs. 21A to H: (A to D) Preoperative; and (E to H) Postoperative views of a saddle nose deformity with septal perforation. Conchal cartilages were harvested from both the ears. Spreader grafts and septal extension graft were sutured by external approach. Dorsal augmentation was done with layered conchal cartilage. Cephalic trimming and tip plasty by domal creation (transdomal) suture were done.

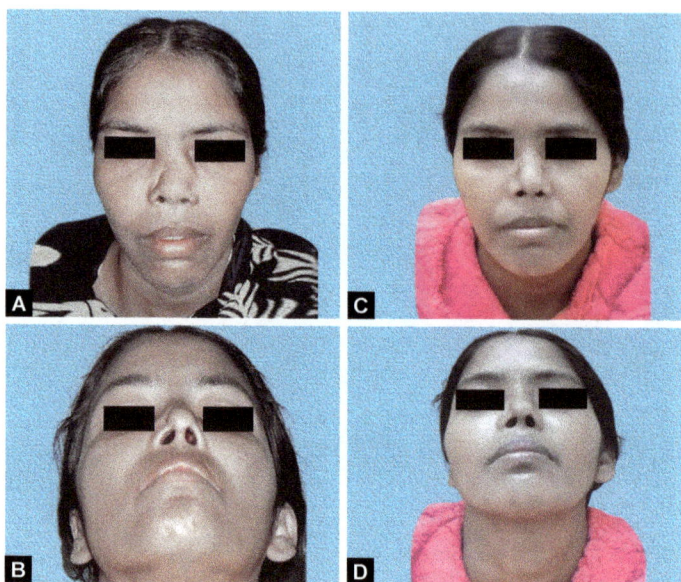

Figs. 22A to D: (A and B) Preoperative; and (C and D) Postoperative views of a depressed and crooked nose with scarring and collapse of the right lateral wall of nose. Septoplasty, osteotomies and dorsal augmentation by layered conchal cartilage were done by external approach. Cephalic trimming in left side and placement of alar batten and rim grafts were done in right side. Columellar strut was placed.

- *Calcium hydroxyapatite (Radiesse):* This is a calcium based, non-allergenic filler that lasts for 10–14 months. It is not reversible.
- *Polymethylmethacrylate (Artefill):* This is a permanent filler made from inert, microscopic surgical plastic beads. This is injected over several treatment sessions. A skin test is required prior to treatment.[41]
- *Liquid silicone:* A permanent filler used in a microdroplet technique.
- *Polyacrylamide gel (PAAG or Aquamid):* This is a permanent filler. Complications have been reported with the use of Aquamid.[42]

Complications of the procedure are discomfort, hematoma, infection, structural asymmetry, skin necrosis due to arterial embolism, pressure necrosis from over injection at nasal tip, osteophyte from periosteal injection and rarely foreign body granuloma.[38] Injection at the radix and upper third of the nose should be done medially to avoid the dorsal and lateral nasal arteries. Aspiration must be done before injection. Intravascular filler injection may cause arterial embolization and necrosis of skin[43] or retinopathy.[44] The dorsal nasal artery anastomoses with the ophthalmic, infratrochlear, and angular arteries, and the embolism through the connected vasculature manifests as widespread skin necrosis. It is also a branch of ophthalmic artery, so propagation of the filler embolus may cause blindness. Prompt anticoagulation and hyaluronidase injection may help in reducing complications.[45]

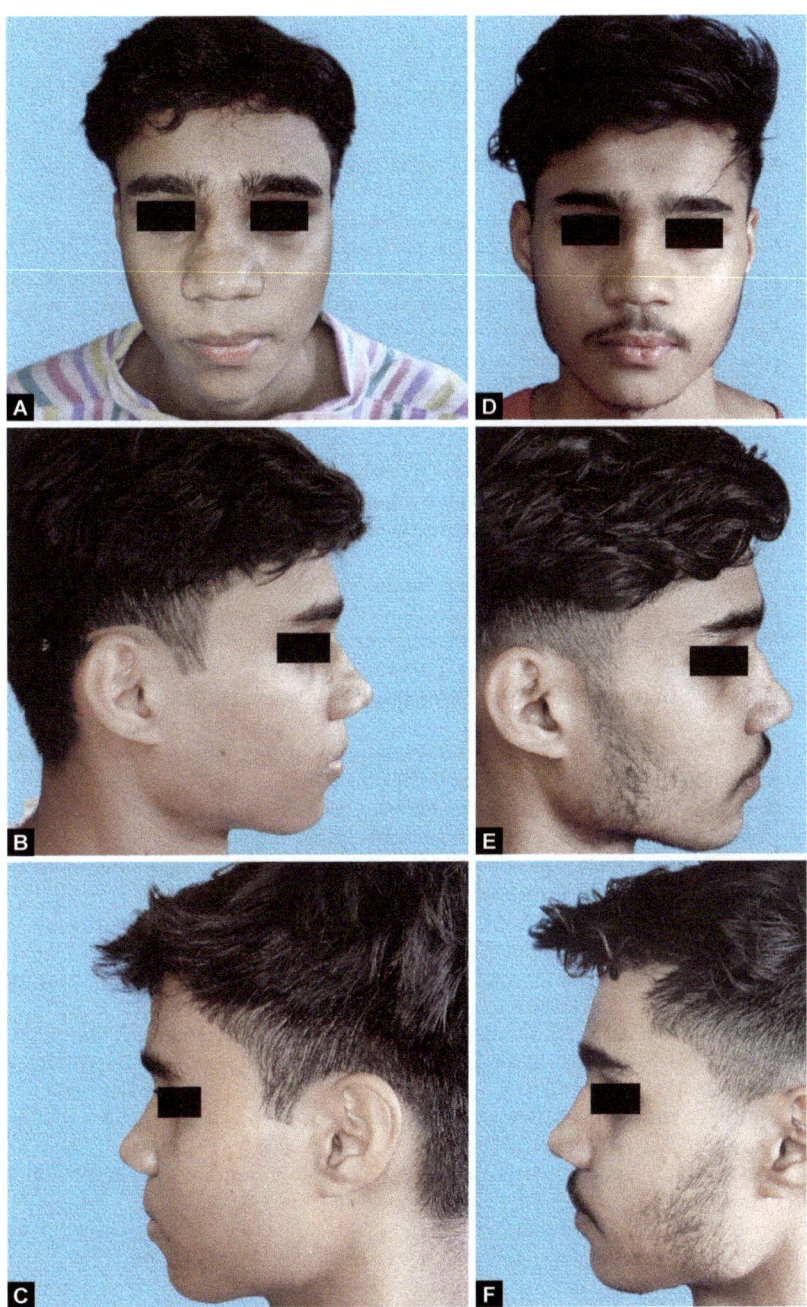

Figs. 23A to F: (A to C) Preoperative; and (D to F) Postoperative views of a post-traumatic saddle nose deformity. Conchal cartilages were harvested from both the ears. Medial, transverse and lateral osteotomies were done. Septal extension graft was sutured by external approach. Dorsal augmentation was done with layered conchal cartilage. Cephalic trimming and tipplasty by domal creation (transdomal) and domal equalization sutures were done. Shield graft was placed.

REFERENCES

1. Daniel RK, Brenner KA. Saddle nose deformity: a new classification and treatment. Facial Plast Surg Clin North Am. 2006;14(4):304.
2. Constantino PD, Freedman CD. Soft tissue augmentation and replacement in the head and neck: General considerations. Otolaryngol Clin N Am. 1994;27:1-12.
3. Holt RG. Implants in facial, head and neck surgery. In: Bailey BJ (Ed). Head and Neck Surgery Otolaryngology. Philadelphia: JB Lippincott; 1993:1923-36.
4. Scales JT. Tissue reactions to synthetic materials. Proc Roy Soc Med. 1953;46:647-52.
5. Stucker FJ, Gage-White L. Survey of surgical implants. Fac Plast Surg. 1986;3:141-4.
6. Sheen JH. Secondary rhinoplasty. In: Maccarthy JG (Ed). Plastic Surgery. Vol 3, The Face, part II. Philadelphia: WB Saunders Co; 1990;1895-923.
7. Ortiz-Monasterio F, Olmedo A, Oscoy LO. The use of cartilage grafts in primary aesthetic rhinoplasty. Plast Reconstr Surg. 1981;67:597-605.
8. Vuyk HD, Adamson PA. Biomaterials in rhinoplasty. Clinical Otolaryngol. 1998;23:209-17.
9. Wellings DB, Maves MD, Schuller DE, Bardach J. Irradiated homologous cartilage grafts: long- term results. Arch Otolaryngol Head Neck Surg. 1988;114:291-5.
10. Leykovits G. Irradiated homologous costal cartilage for augmentation rhinoplasty. Ann Plast Surg. 1990;25:317-27.
11. Welling DB, Maues MD, Schuller DE, Bardach J. Irradiated homologous cartilage grafts: Long-term results. Arch Otolaryngol Head Neck Surg. 1988;114:291.
12. Pak MW, Chan ES, van Hasselt CA. Late complications of nasal augmentation using silicone implants. J Laryngol Otol. 1998;112(11):1074-7.
13. Parker PJ. Grafts in rhinoplasty: alloplastic vs autogenous. Arch Otolaryngol Head Neck Surg. 2000;126(4):558-61.
14. Brown BL, Neel HB, Kern EB. Implants of supra-mid, proplast, plasti-pore, and silastic. Arch Otolaryngol Head Neck Surg. 1979;105:605-9.
15. Beekhuis GJ. Saddle nose deformity. Etiology, prevention and treatment: augmentation rhinoplasty with Polyamide. Laryngoscope. 1974;84:2.
16. Romo T 3rd, Sclafani AP, Jacono AA. Nasal reconstruction using porous polyethylene implants. Facial Plast Surg. 2000;16(1):55-61.
17. Schoenrock LD, Reppucci AD. Correction of subcutaneous facial defects using Gore-tex. Fac Plast Surg Clin N Am. 1994;2:373-88.
18. Waldman SR. Gore-tex for augmentation of the nasal dorsum: a preliminary report. Ann Plast Surg. 1991;26:520-5.
19. Godin MS, Waldman RS, Johnson CM. The use of expanded polytetrafluoroethylene (Gore-tex) in rhinoplasty, a 6-year experience. Arch Otolaryngol Head Neck Surg. 1995;121:1131-6.
20. Conrad K, Torgerson CS, Gillman GS. Applications of Gore-Tex implants in rhinoplasty reexamined after 17 years. Arch Facial Plast Surg. 2008;10(4):224-31.
21. Zius JE, Whitaker LA. Membranous versus endochondral bone: implications for craniofacial reconstruction. Plast Reconstr Surg. 1983;72:778-85.
22. Powell NB, Riley RW. Facial contouring with outer table calvarial bone. A 4-year experience. Arch Otolaryngol Head Neck Surg. 1989;115(12):1454-8.
23. Daniel RK. Rhinoplasty and rib grafts: evolving a flexible operating technique. Plast Reconstr Surg. 1994;94:597-609.
24. Jackson IT, Choi HY, Clay R, Bevilacqua R, Terkonda S, Celik M, et al. Long-term follow-up of cranial bone graft in dorsal nasal augmentation. Plast Reconstr Surg. 1998;102:1869-73.
25. Frodel JL, Marentette LJ, Quatela VC, Weinstein GS. Calvarian bone graft harvest, techniques, considerations and morbidity. Arch Otolaryngol Head Neck Surg. 1993;119:17-23.

26. Kline RM, Wolfe SA. Complications associated with the harvesting of cranial bone grafts. Plast Reconstr Surg. 1995;95:5-20.
27. Gibson T, Davis WB. Distortion of autogenous rib grafts: its cause and prevention. Br J Plast Surg. 1957;10:247-74.
28. Agaoglu G, Erol OO. In situ split costal cartilage graft harvesting through a small incision using a gouge. Plast Reconstr Surg. 2000;106(4):932-5.
29. Miller PA. Temporalis fascia graft for facial and nasal contour augmentation. Plast Reconstr Surg. 1988;81:524-33.
30. Baker TM, Courtiss EH. Temporalis fascia grafts in open secondary rhinoplasty. Plast Reconstr Surg. 1994;93:802-10.
31. Guerrero Santos J. Tempoparietal free fascia grafts in rhinoplasty. Plast Reconstr Surg. 1984;74:465-74.
32. Guerrero Santos J. Nose and paranasal augmentation: autogenous fascia and cartilage. Clin Plast Surg. 1991;18:65-86.
33. Peer LA. Extended use of diced cartilage grafts. Plast Reconstr Surg. 1954;14:178-85.
34. Erol OO. The Turkish delight: a pliable graft for rhinoplasty. Plast Reconstr Surg. 2000;105:2229-49.
35. Toriumi DM, Benjamin Swartout. Asian Rhinoplasty. Facial Plast Surg Clin N Am. 2007;15:293-307.
36. Stucker FJ. Use of implantation in facial deformity. Laryngoscope Sl. 1977;1523-27.
37. Beer KR. Nasal reconstruction using 20 mg/ml cross-linked hyaluronic acid. J Drugs Dermatol. 2006;5(5):465-6.
38. Rokhsar C, Ciocon DH. Nonsurgical rhinoplasty: an evaluation of injectable calcium hydroxylapatite filler for nasal contouring. Dermatol Surg. 2008;34(7):944-6.
39. Le Andrew Tuan-anh. Rhinoplasty using injectable polyacrylamide gel – a patient study. Australasian J Cosmetic Surg. 2005.
40. Rivkin A. Nonsurgical Injection Rhinoplasty with Calcium Hydroxylapatite in a Carrier Gel (Radiesse): A 4-year, Retrospective Clinical Review. Cosmetic Dermatol. 2009;22(12):619-24.
41. Rivkin A. New fillers under consideration: What is the future of injectable aesthetics? Facial Plastic Surgery. 2009;25(2):120-3.
42. Rivkin A, Kontis TC. The history of injectable facial fillers. Facial Plastic Surgery. 2009;25(2):67-72.
43. Shanz S, Schippert W, Ulmer A, Rassner G, Fierlbeck G. Arterial embolisation caused by injection of hyaluronic acid (Restylane). Br J Dermatol. 2002;146:928-9.
44. Peter S, Mannel S. Retinal branch occlusion following injection of hyaluronic acid (Restylane). Clin Experiment Opthalmol. 2006;34:363-4.
45. Glaich A, Cohen J, Goldberg I. Injection necrosis of the glabella: protocol for prevention and treatment after use of dermal fillers. Dermatol Surg. 2006;32:276-81.

Rhinoplasty in Atrophic Rhinitis

INTRODUCTION

Atrophic rhinitis is a chronic inflammatory disease, which is characterized by progressive atrophy of the mucous membrane and turbinate bones and is associated with a fetid smell originating from the nose. There is a presence of viscid secretion, which rapidly dries up forming foul smelling crusts. This fetid odor is also known as ozena.[1] The nasal cavities are abnormally patent.

Atrophic rhinitis may be primary or secondary.

The etiology of primary atrophic rhinitis still remains obscure. This is common in China, India, and Middle East.

The incidence of primary atrophic rhinitis (ozena) has diminished markedly in recent times and this may be due to effective control of chronic nasal infections by antibiotics. About 0.3-1% of the population are affected with primary atrophic rhinitis in countries with a high prevalence.[2]

The incidence of atrophic rhinitis is less in the natives of equatorial Africa. Family history may be positive in about 15-30% of the cases.[2]

Poor nutrition is considered to be one of the factors in the development of atrophic rhinitis.

Estrogen deficiency is also mentioned as a cause by some authors.[3] The incidence of atrophic rhinitis is more in girls during puberty, and there is aggravation of symptoms during menstruation and pregnancy. Improvement of symptoms has been seen in some cases with estrogen therapy.

Mucosa and submucosa undergo ischemic atrophy and metaplasia of normal ciliated columnar epithelium into stratified squamous epithelium occurs. Chronic cellular infiltration, granulations, and fibrosis are seen in submucosa.

Atrophy of mucosal glands and cilia results in a pale mucosa and thick scanty secretions. The secretions dry and form crusts. The secondary infection by *Coccobacillus* foetidus ozaenae, *Klebsiella ozaenae, Bacillus* mucosus, and diphtheroids produces typical fetid smell.[4] Terminal arterioles show periarteritis and endarteritis obliterans. Nerves become atrophied. Olfactory nerves are atrophied causing anosmia.

The disease is more common in females. It usually starts shortly after puberty. The disease is mostly seen among patients from lower socioeconomic groups.[5,6] Foul smell makes the patient a social outcast. But the patient does not get the foul smell from his nose (merciful anosmia).

A rarefying osteitis of the turbinates is seen. Taylor and Young[7] observed a positive alkaline phosphatase reaction in the endothelial cells of the capillary walls that indicated active bone resorption.

Nasal obstruction is usually the main symptom. The patient becomes unable to perceive the air current in the nose due to loss of sensation of the nasal mucosa. Large crusts also cause mechanical obstruction to air flow.

Extensive nasal surgeries, chronic rhinosinusitis, tuberculosis, syphilis, lupus vulgaris, leprosy, atrophic stage of rhinoscleroma, and radiation exposure may cause secondary atrophic rhinitis. Extensive turbinate surgeries may lead to "empty nose syndrome" in which the patient complains of nasal obstruction in the absence of an obstructive cause.[8,9] The pathophysiology is unclear but probably involves altered nasal receptor sensitivity.

Investigations are necessary to rule out secondary causes of atrophic rhinitis. These include hematological studies, computed tomography (CT) scan, and biopsy.

If primary atrophic rhinitis does not respond to conservative treatment, Young's operation can be done. In young's operation closure of one or both nasal cavities is done. In this operation, skin folds are raised by a circular incision in the vestibule and suturing of these folds together is done to close the nasal cavities. After a period of 6-12 months when the nasal cavities are opened up, the mucosa of the nasal cavities are found to be healed.[10] It is better to perform the surgery in a staged manner, while waiting for one nose to heal before attempting on the other side **(Figs. 1A to C)**.[11] The advantages of Young's operation are the following: It gives rest to the nasal mucosa; a medium with the CO_2 and pH is created which helps to bring about regeneration of normal mucosa; and finally, closure of the nostril produces a negative postchoanal pressure leading to vasodilatation within the cavity.[12]

Saddle deformity may be associated with some cases of primary atrophic rhinitis. This is due to less development of the nasal bones. Major depression of nasal bridge is due to absorption and/or weakening of the nasal bones or the septal cartilage. Raised level of alkaline phosphatase in atrophied nasal mucosa may lead to absorption of cartilage and bone.[13] Rhinoplasty in atrophic rhinitis may be dangerous as there is more chance of postoperative infection and graft failure. But with adequate precautions, rhinoplasty can be done with minimum dissection in atrophic rhinitis patients. With rhinoplasty, there may be a change in direction of nasal airflow, affecting the disease favorably. However, rhinoplasty can be combined with Young's operation.[14]

All the patients are treated conservatively by alkaline nasal douche, instillation of 25% anhydrous glucose in glycerin in nasal cavities, systemic antibiotics, and iron and vitamins as usual, before performing rhinoplasty. Alkaline nasal douche mixture contains 28.4 g of sodium bicarbonate (helps in loosening the crusts), 28.4 g of sodium biborate (antiseptic), and 56.7 g of sodium chloride (makes the solution isotonic). One teaspoonful of this

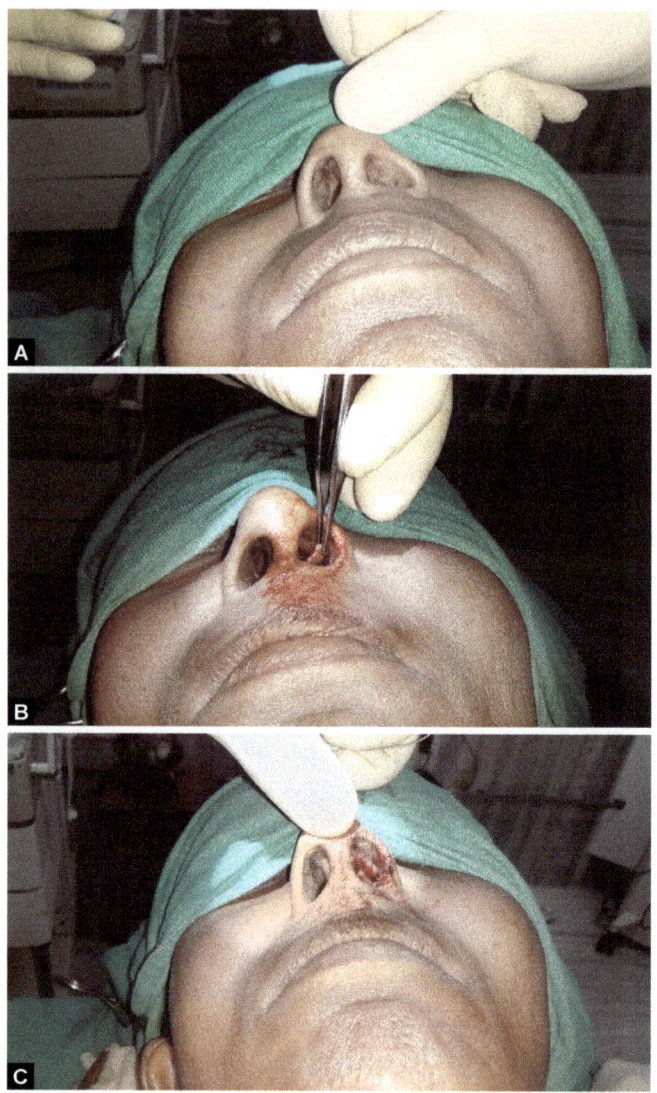

Figs. 1A to C: (A) Closure of left nostril by Young's operation done 1 year back; (B and C) Opening of Young's operation done by elevation of a skin flap and removal of thick scar tissue from the undersurface of the flap. The elevated flap is sutured in its new place at the defect of the lateral nasal wall with 5-0 Vicryl. The defect at the floor of the vestibule is covered with a full-thickness postauricular skin graft and sutured with 5-0 Vicryl.

mixture is dissolved in half pint (280 mL) of warm water and is used to clean the nasal cavities.

Crusts are removed by suction clearance and infection is controlled by giving systemic antibiotics 1 week before the surgery.

The principle of minimum dissection to get maximum result should be followed in rhinoplasty in atrophic rhinitis. Patients should be counseled about how much of the deformity can be successfully corrected.[15] In long-standing atrophic rhinitis, the skin is usually adherent to the underlying structures and mobilization of skin-soft tissue envelope is difficult during rhinoplasty. Extra care and patience are needed to avoid buttonhole formation during elevation of the skin. Synthetic implants and bone grafts are not used in these patients as there is a high chance of extrusion of the implants and there is also high incidence of absorption of bone grafts.[16] For minor or moderate augmentation, autologous conchal cartilage is the best material and is used in two or three layers. For major augmentation, rib cartilage graft can be used. The grafts are placed under the nasal bone periosteum to avoid displacement and minimize absorption of the graft. Warping of rib cartilage is minimized by doing balanced cross section of the graft. Septoplasty is performed with limited elevation of mucoperichondrium and limited removal of septal cartilage and bone **(Figs. 2 to 4)**.

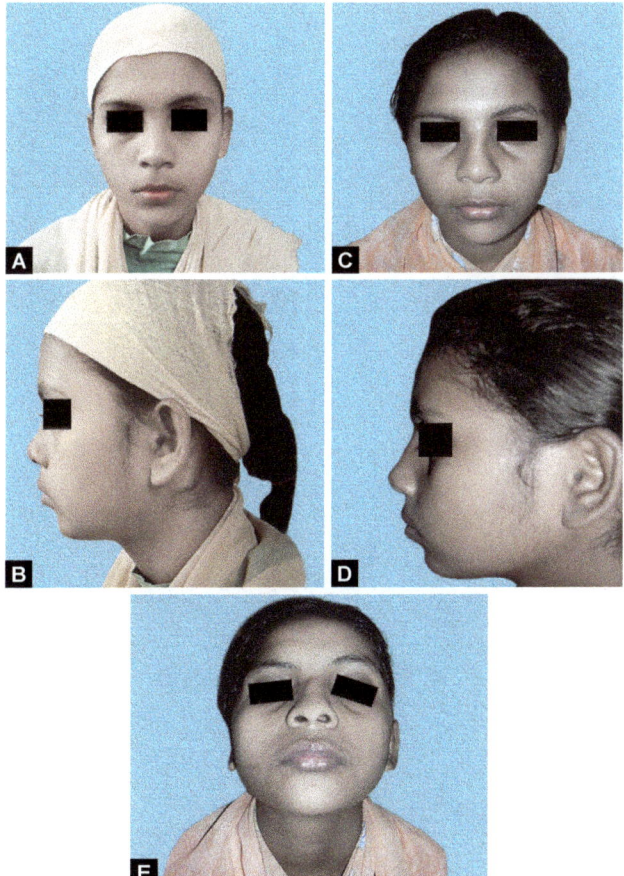

Figs. 2A to E: (A and B) Preoperative; and (C to E) Postoperative views of a case of saddle nose in atrophic rhinitis. Augmentation was done by layered conchal cartilage by closed technique and Young's operation was done in left side.

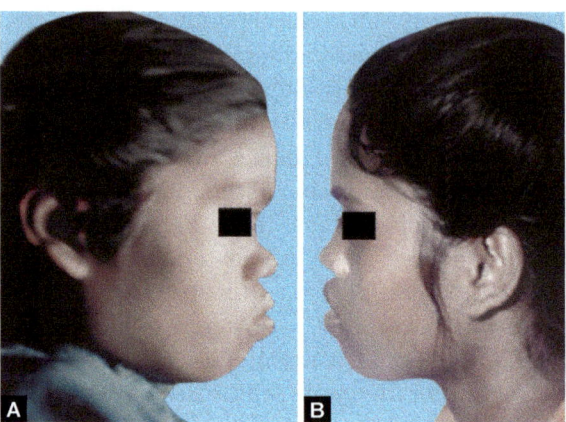

Figs. 3A and B: (A) Preoperative; and (B) Postoperative views of a case of severe saddle deformity in atrophic rhinitis. Augmentation was done by rib cartilage by external approach.

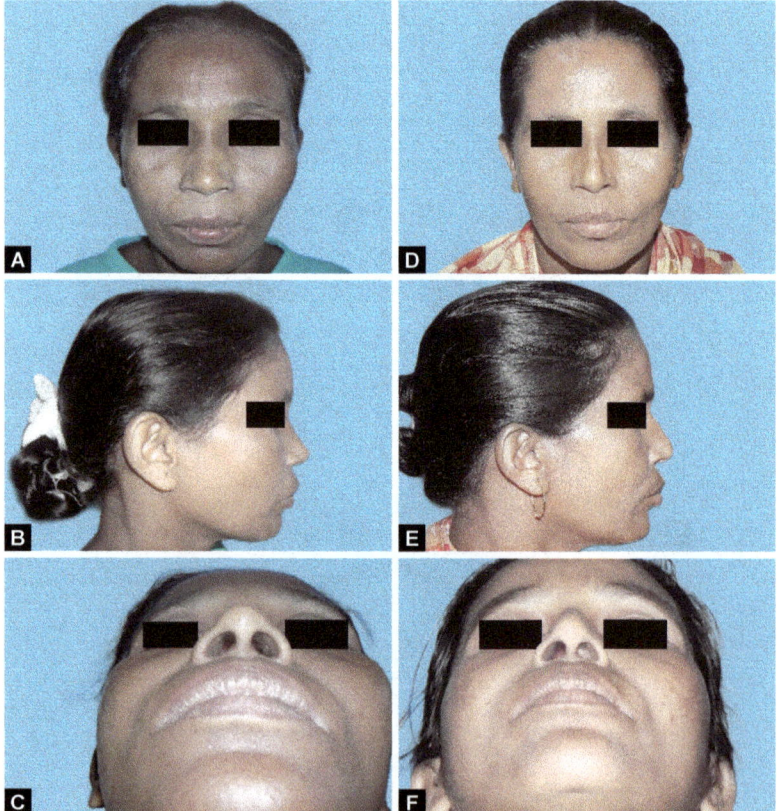

Figs. 4A to F: (A to C) Preoperative; and (D to F) Postoperative views of a case of saddle nose in atrophic rhinitis. Augmentation was done with layered conchal cartilage. Columellar strut and tip graft were placed and tip suturing was done by external approach. Young's operation was done in the left side.

REFERENCES

1. Zohar Y, Talmi YP, Strauss M, Finkelstein Y, Shvilli Y. Ozena revisited. J Otol. 1990;19:345-9.
2. Dutt SN, Kameswaran M. The aetiology and management of atrophic rhinitis. J Laryngol Otol. 2005;119:843-52.
3. Barbary AS, Yassin A, Fouad H. Histopathological and histochemical studies on atrophic rhinitis. J Laryngol Otol. 1970;84:1103-12.
4. Dudley JP. Atrophic rhinitis: antibiotic treatment. Am J Otolaryngol. 1987;8:387-90.
5. Dutt SN, Kameswaran M. The aetiology and management of atrophic rhinitis. J Laryngol Otol. 2005;119(11):843-52.
6. Bunnag C, Jareoncharsri P, Tansuriyawong P, Bhothisuwan W, Chantarakul N. Characteristics of atrophic rhinitis in Thai patients at the Siriraj Hospital. Rhinology. 1999;37(3):125-30.
7. Taylor M, Young A. Histopathological and histochemical studies on atrophic rhinitis. J Laryngol Otol. 1961;75:574-90.
8. Wang Y, Liu T, Qu Y, Dong Z, Yang Z. Empty nose syndrome (in Chinese). Zhonghua Er Bi Yan Hou Ke Za Zhi. 2001;36:203-5.
9. Moore Eric J, Keru Eugene B. Atrophic rhinitis a review of 242 cases. Am J Rhinol. 2001;15(6):355-61.
10. Young A. Closure of the nostrils in atrophic rhinitis. J Laryngol Otol. 1967;81(5):515-24.
11. Young A. Closure of the nostrils in atrophic rhinitis. J Laryngol Otol. 1971;85:715-8.
12. Thiagarajan B. Atrophic rhinitis: A review. Rhinology; 2012.
13. Girgis I. Surgical treatment of ozaena by dermofat graft. J Laryngol Otol. 1966;80:615-27.
14. Ghosh SK, Saha AK, Ranjan R. Rhinoplasty and Young's operation in atrophic rhinitis. IJO and HNS. 2006;58(4):352-4.
15. Deka RC. Some aspects of rhinoplasty. Indian J Otolaryngol. 1996;48:34-40.
16. Baser B, Grewal DS, Hiranandani NL. Management of saddle nose deformity in atrophic rhinitis. J Laryngol Otol. 1990;104:404-7.

CHAPTER 18

Surgery of the Crooked Nose

INTRODUCTION

A "crooked" nose generally means a nose that lacks continuous "brow-tip aesthetic lines." These lines descend from the medial ends of the eyebrows vertically along the sidewalls of the nose and end at the sides of the nasal tip **(Fig. 1)**.

To appreciate a patient's dorsal deviation better, a straight midline vertical line can be drawn from the center point between the pupils or medial canthi.[1]

Correction of the crooked nose is one of the most challenging procedures in rhinoplasty. However, there is no universal standard of aesthetic ratios of the nose and the shape of the nose should be in harmony with individual gender, appearance, and character.[2]

The crooked or twisted nose is caused by a complex deformity of the bony pyramid, the upper and lower cartilaginous vaults, and the septum, and leads to functional and aesthetic problems.[3]

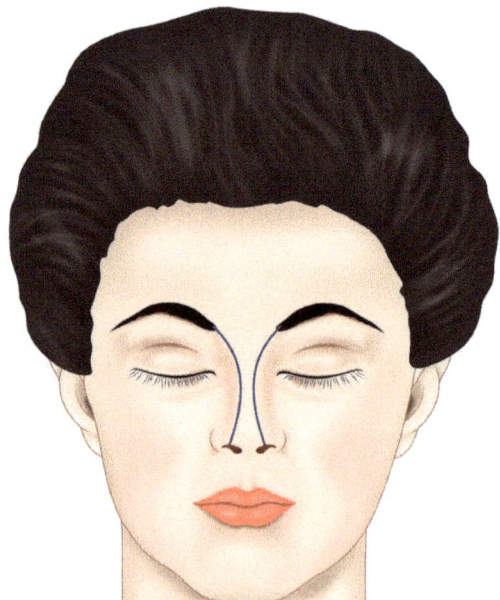

Fig. 1: Dorsal aesthetic lines originate on the supraorbital ridges and end at the tip-defining points.

Any nasal trauma in adults or childhood trauma is a common cause of a crooked nose. It may be congenital or may occur following any nasal surgery. Childhood trauma may result in the developmental asymmetry of the nasal vault. The nasal bone may be bigger and more convex on one side than the other.

Asymmetry in the face may be associated with crooked nose. To assess the asymmetry, two lines are drawn: a vertical line from the midpoint between two medial canthi, and a horizontal line passing through both medial canthi. These two reference lines can indicate facial asymmetries.[3]

A crooked nose is usually associated with septal deviation. Deviation of the central part of the septum causes more nasal obstruction than external nasal deformity. If the dorsal caudal "L" part of the septum is deviated, greater septal contribution is made to the crooked nose deformity.

Crooked nose can be subdivided into three types:
1. *True crooked nose:* In a true crooked nose, the nasal dorsum is deviated in a "C"- or "S"-shaped manner crossing the midline.
2. *Deviated nose:* In a deviated nose, the nasal dorsum is deviated to one side of the midline.
3. *Asymmetric nose:* In an asymmetric nose, the dorsum is in midline but it is irregular and asymmetric.

In rhinoplasty for the crooked nose, both aesthetic and functional goals should be achieved in one surgery because the external deformity is often associated with the functional problem due to deviated septum.

Preoperative photographs with frontal, lateral, oblique, and basal views are taken in all patients. The frontal view helps in assessment of the nasal deformities and its relationship to facial asymmetries. Full correction of nasal asymmetries is not possible if these are secondary to asymmetries of the facial skeleton. The basal view is taken for assessment of tip deviation, deviation of caudal septum, and asymmetries of the nostrils.

The surgeon should have an open discussion with the patient about what can be really achieved when performing rhinoplasty. Sometimes, it becomes difficult to create a perfectly straight and symmetric nose. Patient's expectations should be known preoperatively to avoid dissatisfaction postoperatively.[4]

Straightening a crooked nose is difficult because the deviated cartilage and bone have a certain level of memory such that the nose tends to drift back toward its preoperative position unless the deviation is corrected carefully. Correction of a crooked nose involves repositioning the septum and nasal bones. If the deviated septum is not made straight, it will push the nose to the deviated side.

Reduction of the fractured nasal bones is done within 2 weeks after the trauma. If not treated, the bones will heal in a crooked position. The resetting process takes about 3 months. After that time, rhinoplasty can be done.

Rohrich and Adams (2000) commented that the incidence of postreduction deformity requiring subsequent septorhinoplasty ranges from 14 to 50%. They attributed this high revision rate to unrecognized to uncorrected septal deviation.[5]

Before making a surgical plan for rhinoplasty, a careful physical examination is done to evaluate the nose and facial aesthetics. Skin type and age of the patient are important factors that must be considered. Thick skin restricts the degree of tip narrowing.[6] External nose is examined to locate the deformity at the different levels of the nose. The intranasal examination is done to view the nasal septum and turbinates. Any nasal bone irregularities and deformities are evaluated. The anterior septal angle is located, and tip support is evaluated. The condition of the internal and external nasal valves is seen. If a positive Cottle test, done by pulling the skin of the cheek laterally, relieves obstruction, internal valve narrowing is suspected. The relationship of the caudal septum and nasal spine is examined.

In camouflaging technique, a graft is inserted into a deformity, creating an illusion of correction. Camouflaging is useful in localized deformities without nasal obstruction; but there is a risk of residual deformities and visible grafts in this technique. Minor residual asymmetries following septoplasty and osteotomies can be corrected by camouflaging techniques.

Camouflaging onlay grafts are used for treating irregularities over nasal dorsum. Via intercartilaginous incisions, dorsal onlay grafts are placed at the supraperichondrial or subperiosteal plane. If the graft is placed too superficially, malposition of the graft may occur and the graft may be visible and palpable. One must be careful during revision rhinoplasty or posttraumatic cases, when correct tissue planes may be obscured. Transcutaneous sutures may be used to make the graft stable. The suture is done by 5-0 Vicryl and is tied over a gauze piece. The suture is removed after 1 week.

SPREADER GRAFT

Common indication of placement of spreader grafts is a deviated nose with narrowed internal nasal valve.

Spreader grafts are strut-shaped cartilage grafts, usually harvested from septal cartilage. A typical dimension is $24 \times 8 \times 2$ mm. However, the size can vary considerably. The grafts are inserted into submucoperichondrial pockets created in between the superior parts of upper lateral cartilages and dorsal septum **(Fig. 2)**. The spreader graft widens the angle of the internal nasal valve

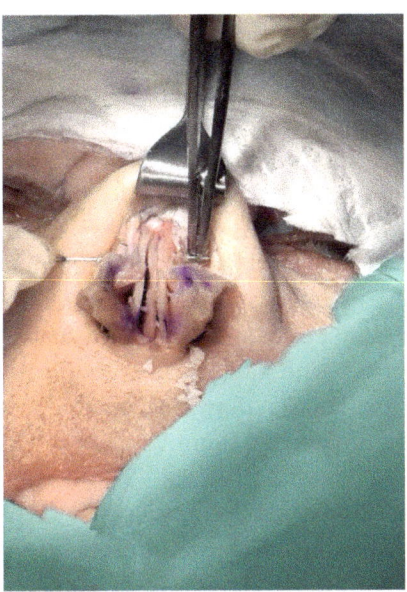

Fig. 2: Placement of spreader grafts in cadaver.

and opens the nasal airway. It also increases dorsal width. The pocket for the spreader graft should extend up to the nasal dorsum, otherwise, the graft can increase obstruction. The grafts are secured in place with two 25 gauge needles piercing all the five layers consisting of the upper lateral cartilage, the spreader graft, the septum, spreader graft, and opposite upper lateral cartilage. The caudal part is sutured first with 5-0 PDS usually in three layers, i.e., the spreader grafts and the septum, whereas the cephalic suture unites all five layers.

In case of overly rotated tip, longer spreader grafts are placed extending caudally to enclose a columellar strut which makes the tip derotated. If the spreader graft extends beyond the anterior septal angle, it is called extended spreader graft.

Depending on the deformity of the nose, spreader grafts can have the following effects: Prevention of collapse of the middle vault, prevention of narrowing of the nasal valve area, straightening of the caudal part of the septum, straightening of the cartilaginous nasal dorsum, correction of asymmetric cartilaginous dorsum, straightening of the caudal part of the septum and establishing connection between septum and columella.

Spreader grafts may be contraindicated in patients with borderline or excess middle vault width. Spreader graft placement also should be avoided in some revision rhinoplasty cases as dense scarring and previous cartilage excision may complicate the surgical procedure.

When a spreader graft is placed on the concave side of a C-shaped deviated septum, it can serve both to improve the nasal airway and to correct the brow-tip aesthetic lines. Here, the spreader graft acts as a splint on the dorsal septum while exerting lateral pressure on the upper lateral cartilages.[7]

Instead of placing spreader graft, septal crossbar graft can be inserted between the two incisions at the dorsal part of the L-shaped structure of the septum on the concave side. Once the crossbar graft is in position, it should be secured with sutures of 5-0 PDS. The crossbar graft can be considered as an intraseptal spreader graft in that it is placed between the two parallel incisions in the dorsal septum. By the crossbar graft, twice as much space is obtained at the internal nasal valve as with a single spreader graft.

Gurlek et al. (2006) studied custom-made high-density porous polyethylene extended spreader grafts. The patients had good results with no report of extrusion.[8] Mendelsohn (2005) reported acceptable results in a study with 40 patients. More studies are needed to understand the usefulness of synthetic materials.[9]

External rhinoplasty is a better approach where tip plasty is required along with crooked nose correction. In external approach, septal deviation at dorsal part can be corrected more precisely and spreader graft placement can be done accurately. Nasal blockage along with middle vault or bony deviation can be corrected by endonasal technique.

A proper evaluation of the bony upper-third region of the nose should be done. If the bony dorsum is severely deviated, it should be treated first, as this becomes the base on which the middle-third region is set.

STEPS OF CROOKED NOSE SURGERY

1. Incisions for either external or endonasal approach
2. Mobilization of soft tissues (skeletonization)
3. Hump removal, if required. In presence of a large hump, the hump should be excised obliquely, removing more at the broad concave side to cause symmetry of the bony lateral walls.
4. *Septoplasty:* Septal mucoperichondrium is elevated and septal cartilage is freed from surrounding structures. Final septal correction is done later on, when the deviated external nose has been mobilized.
5. Upper lateral cartilages may be separated from the dorsal border of septal cartilage and unilateral or bilateral (symmetrical or asymmetrical) spreader grafts are placed in the space. If the upper lateral cartilages are unequal, the medial borders of the upper lateral cartilages near the dorsal border of the septum should be trimmed to make them symmetrical.
6. *Osteotomies:* Medial, lateral, transverse and root osteotomies (if required) are done. Multiple osteotomies may be needed in the convex side (in developmental crooked nose).
7. Tip plasty
8. Camouflaging or placement of dorsal onlay grafts.

The advantages of endonasal approach include decreased operative time, rapid recovery, and less scar contracture. However, there is limited exposure in this approach.[10]

The lateral osteotomy should begin at the piriform aperture near the attachment of the inferior turbinate, 3-4 mm above the floor of the nose and should preserve the most caudal part of the piriform crest (Webster triangle) to avoid too much narrowing at the area[11] **(Figs. 3 to 21)**.

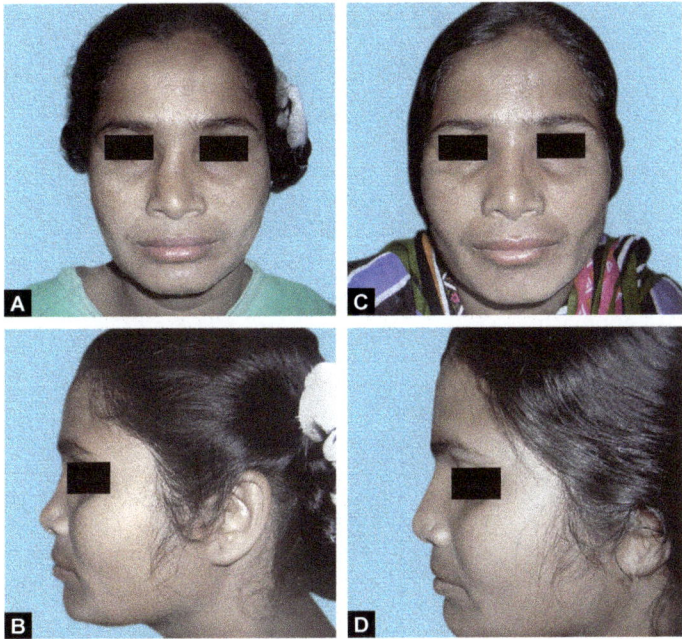

Figs. 3A to D: (A and B) Preoperative; and (C and D) Postoperative views of a case of crooked nose with saddle deformity. Septoplasty and osteotomies were done. Dorsal augmentation was done with layered conchal cartilage.

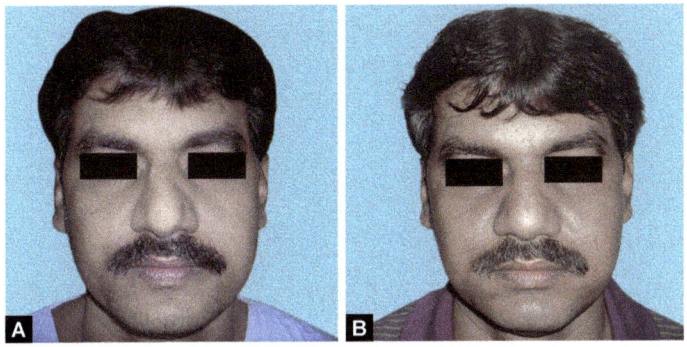

Figs. 4A and B: (A) Preoperative; and (B) Postoperative views of a case of crooked nose with deviated nasal septum (DNS). Septoplasty and osteotomies were done.

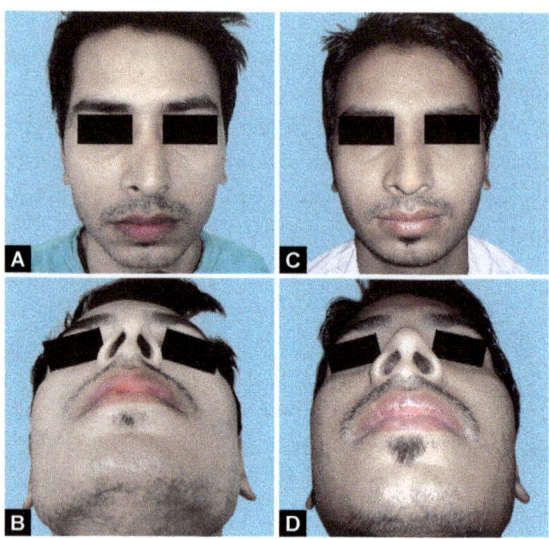

Figs. 5A to D: (A and B) Preoperative; and (C and D) Postoperative views of a crooked nose with gross deviated nasal septum (DNS). Septoplasty and osteotomies were done by endonasal approach.

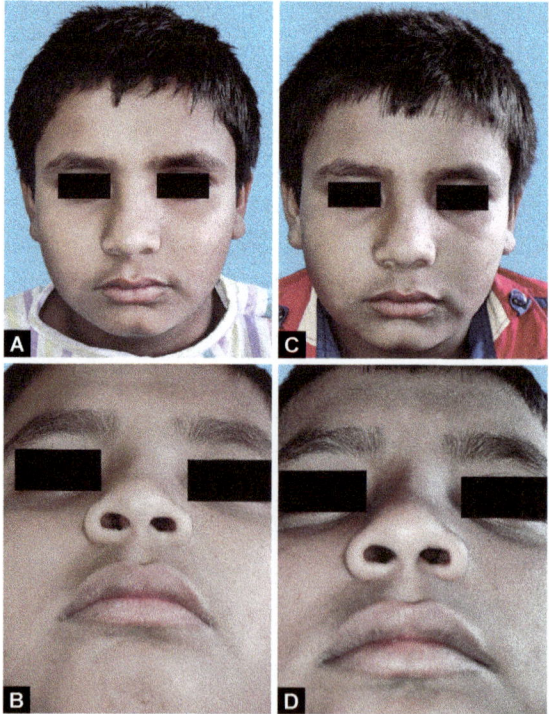

Figs. 6A to D: (A and B) Preoperative; and (C and D) Postoperative views of DNS to right with mild crooked nose in a 9-year-old child, corrected by septoplasty, percutaneous transverse and intranasal lateral osteotomies.

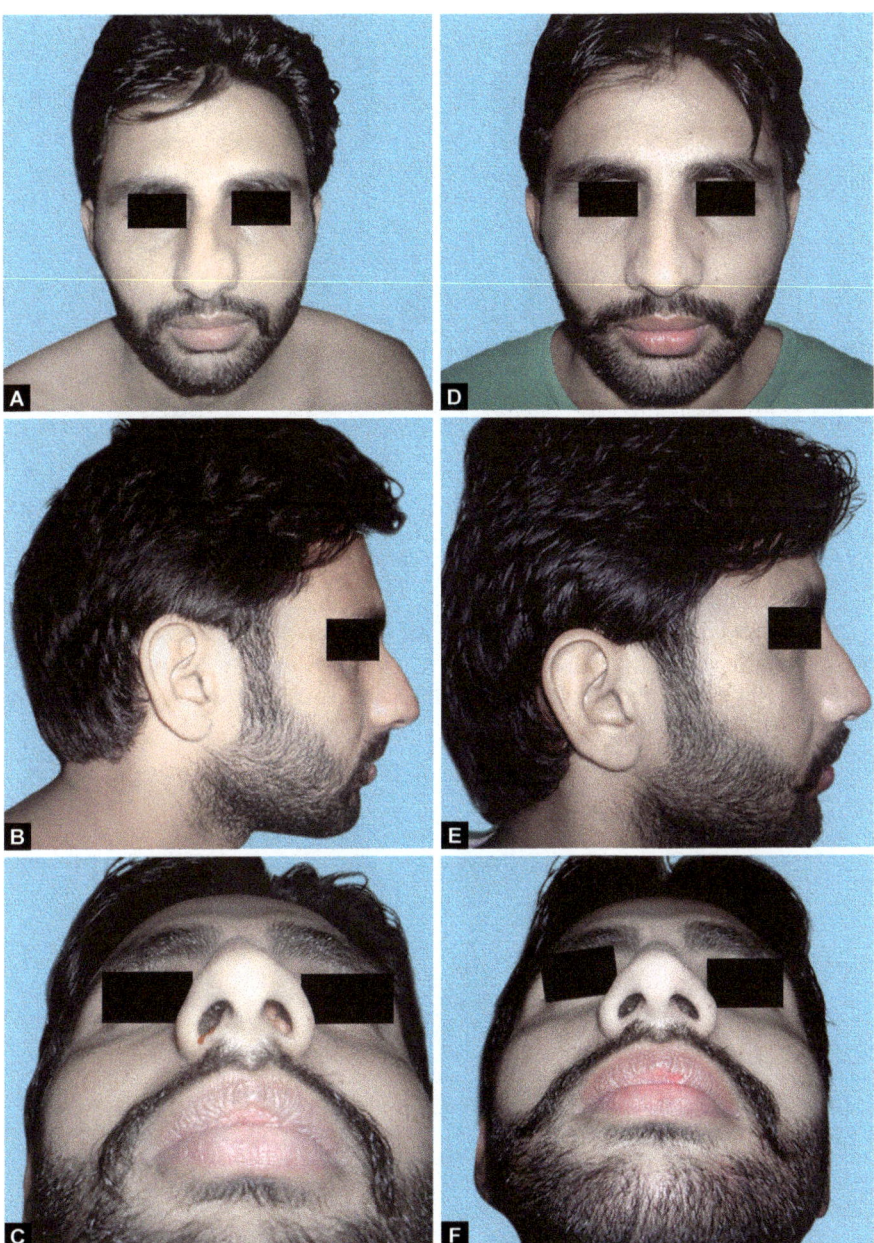

Figs. 7A to F: (A to C) Preoperative; and (D to F) Postoperative views of crooked nose with gross deviated nasal septum (DNS). The patient had a past history of nasal trauma. Septoplasty, bilateral osteotomies, and rasping of the mild bony hump were done by endonasal approach.

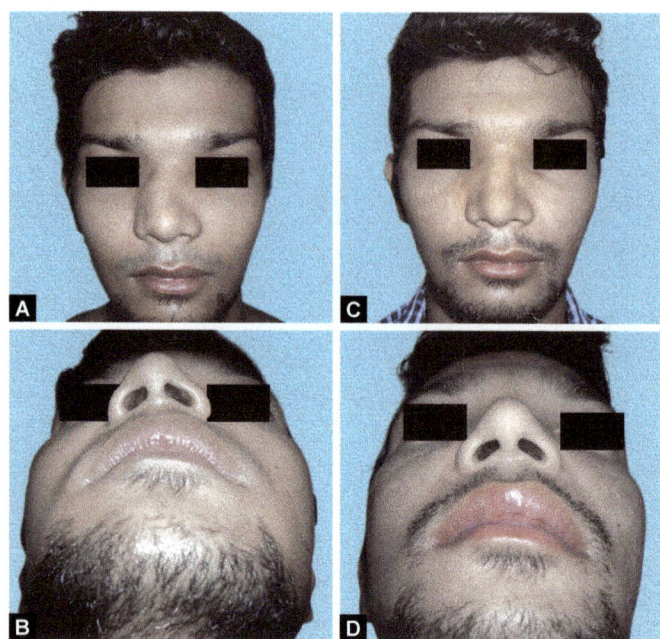

Figs. 8A to D: (A and B) Preoperative; and (C and D) Postoperative views of a crooked nose with gross deviated nasal septum (DNS). Septoplasty and osteotomies were done by endonasal approach.

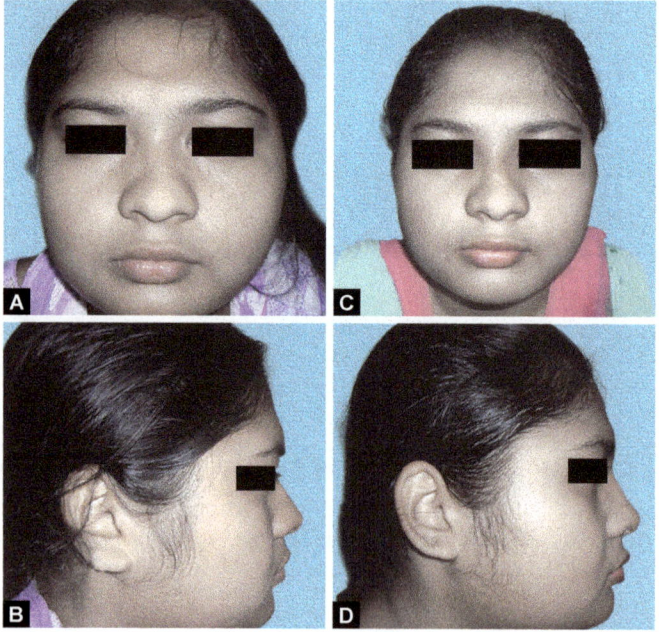

Figs. 9A to D: (A and B) Preoperative; and (C and D) Postoperative views of a deviated nose with deviated nasal septum (DNS). Osteotomies and septoplasty were done by endonasal approach.

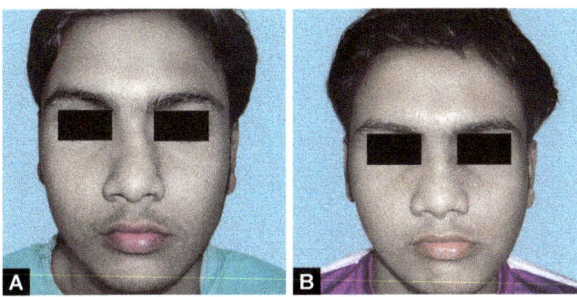

Figs. 10A and B: (A) Preoperative; and (B) Postoperative views of a crooked nose with deviated nasal septum (DNS). Septoplasty and medial, lateral, and transverse osteotomies were done by intranasal approach.

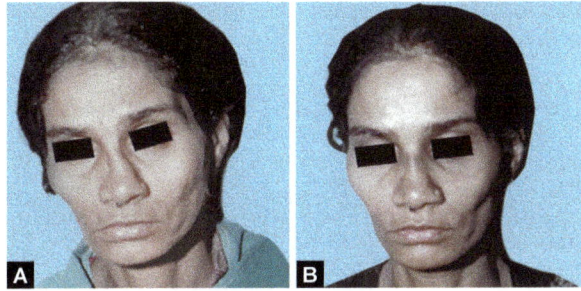

Figs. 11A and B: (A) Preoperative; and (B) Postoperative views of a crooked nose with deviated nasal septum (DNS). Septoplasty and medial and curved lateral osteotomies were done by intranasal approach.

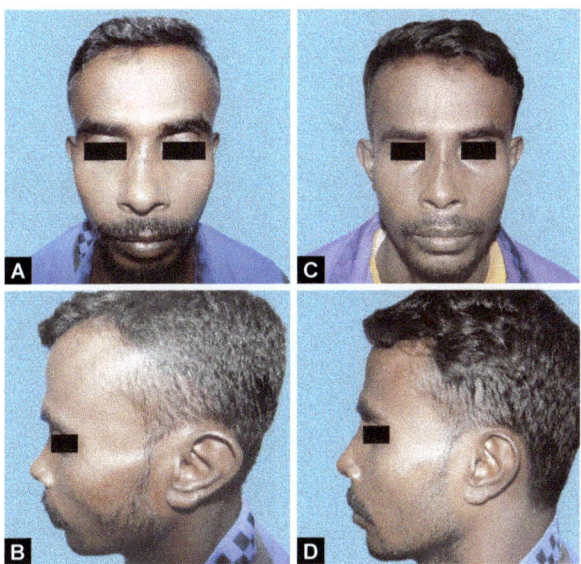

Figs. 12A to D: (A and B) Preoperative; and (C and D) Postoperative views of a crooked nose with deviated nasal septum (DNS). Septoplasty and medial, lateral, and transverse osteotomies were done by endonasal approach.

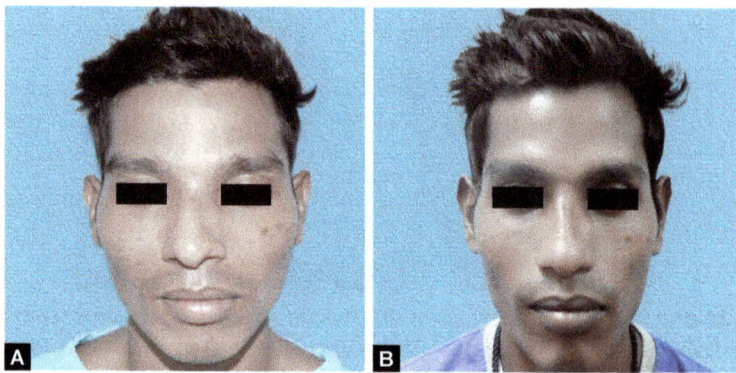

Figs. 13A and B: (A) Preoperative; and (B) Postoperative views of a crooked nose with deviated nasal septum (DNS). Septoplasty, medial, lateral and transverse osteotomies were done by endonasal approach.

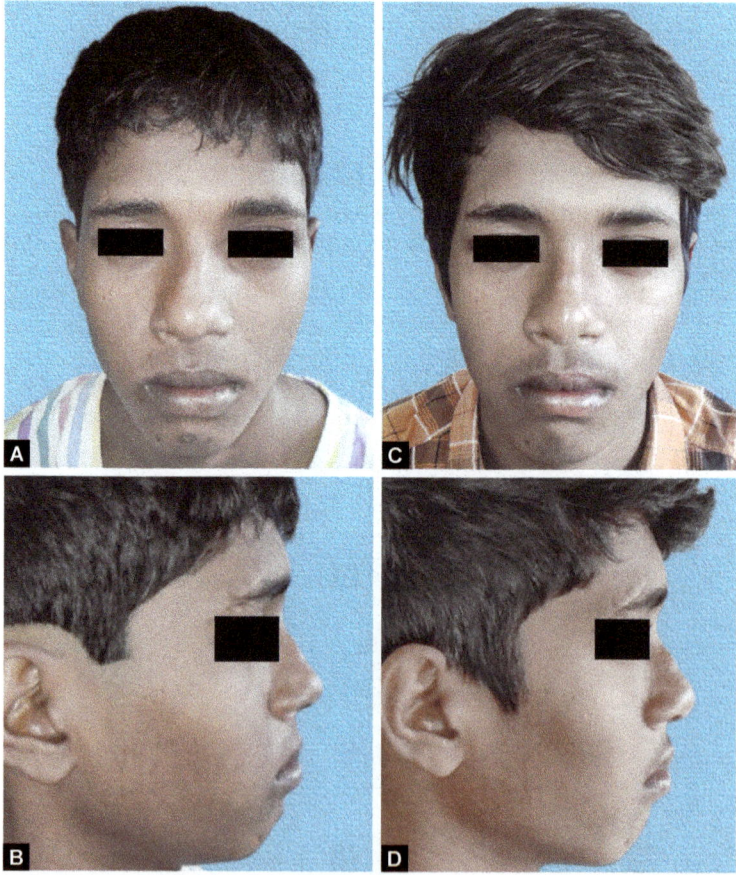

Figs. 14A to D: (A and B) Preoperative; and (C and D) Postoperative views of a case of crooked nose with dorsal depression. Septoplasty, osteotomies, and dorsal augmentation by septal cartilage was done by external approach.

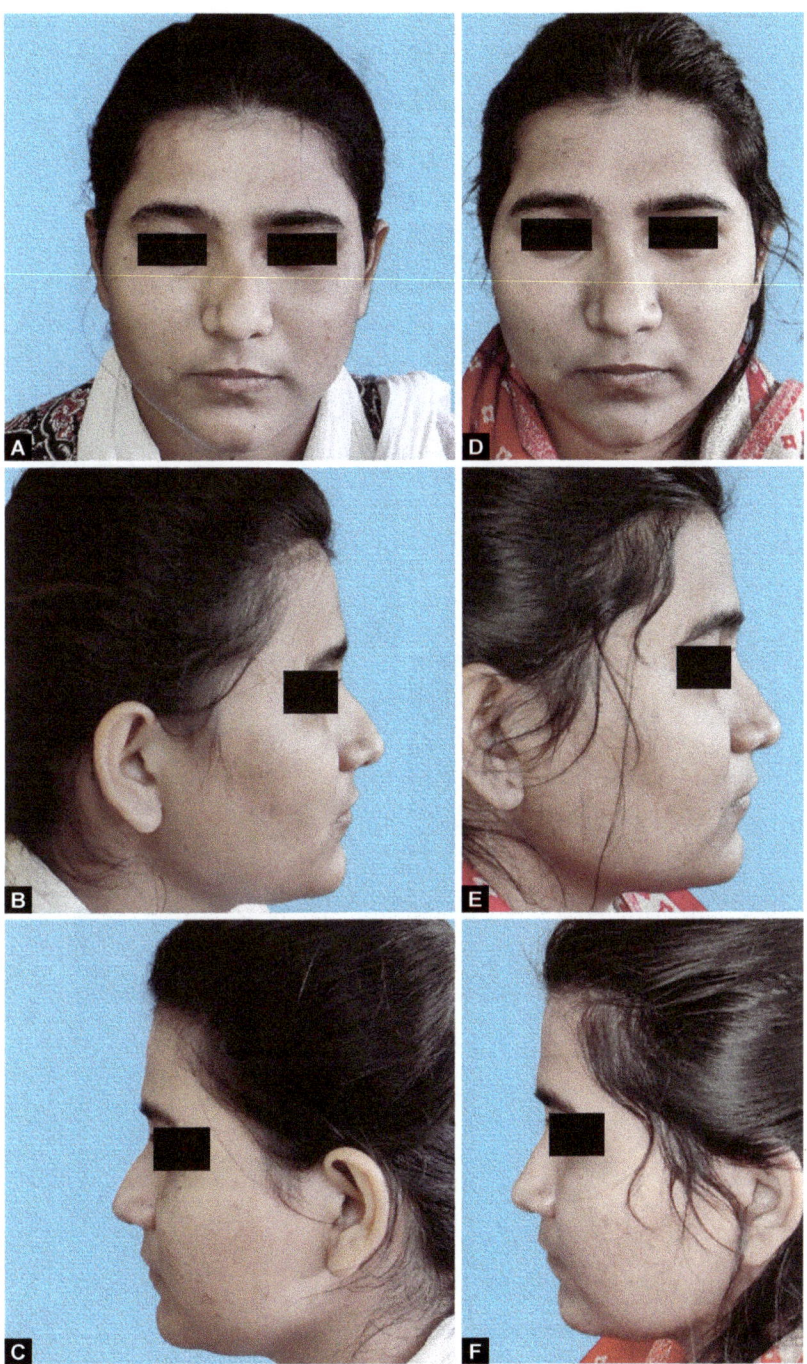

Figs. 15A to F: (A to C) Preoperative; and (D to F) Postoperative views of a crooked nose with deviated nasal septum (DNS), mild hump, and dorsal depression. Septoplasty, osteotomies, rasping of the hump, augmentation with conchal cartilage, cephalic trimming and tip plasty by domal equalization suture were done by external approach.

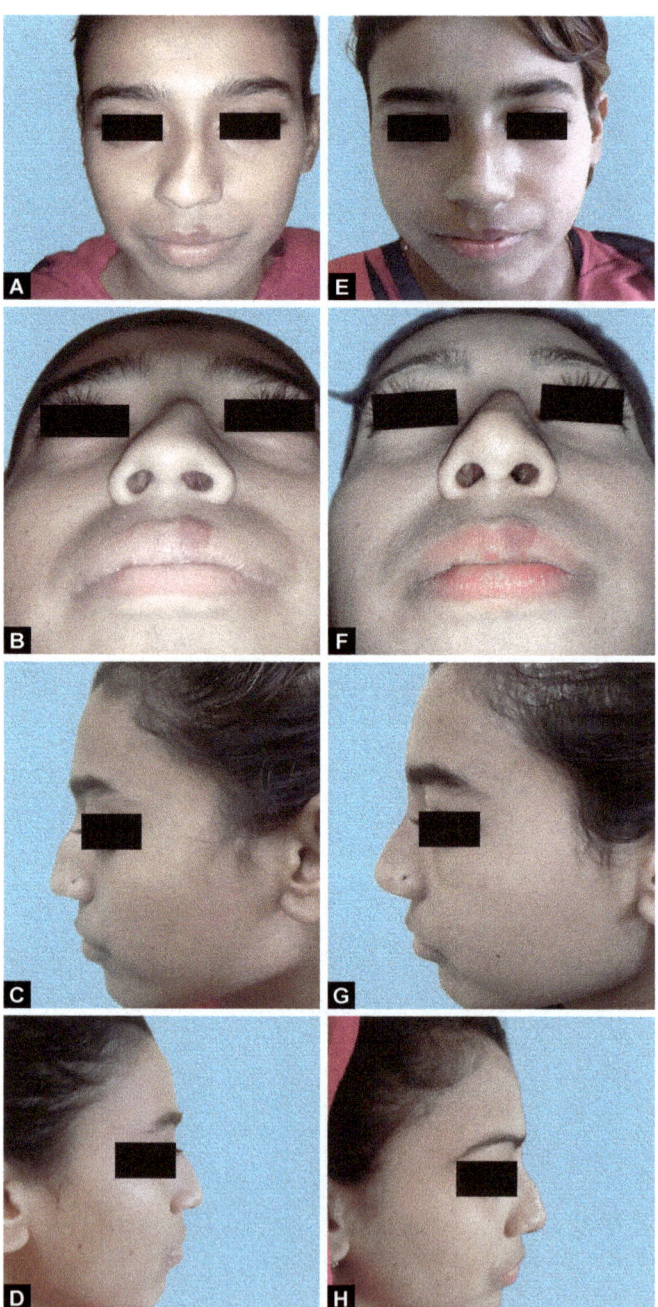

Figs. 16A to H: (A to D) Preoperative; and (E to H) Postoperative views of a case of crooked nose, DNS and depressed cartilaginous dorsum with underprojection of nasal tip. Septoplasty, osteotomies, placement of spreader grafts, and columellar strut were done by external approach. Tip plasty was done by cephalic trimming, domal equalization (interdomal) suture and tip graft. Dorsal augmentation was done with layered conchal cartilage.

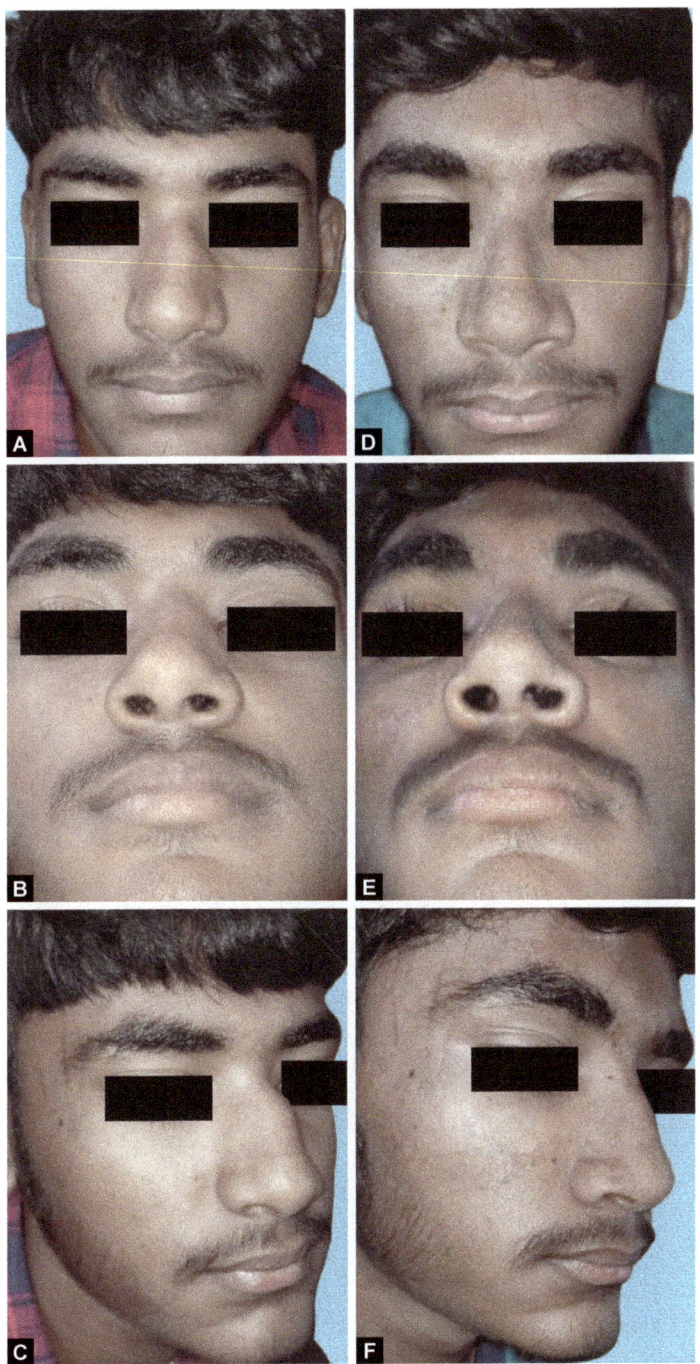

Figs. 17A to F: (A to C) Preoperative; and (D to F) early postoperative views of a crooked nose with mild bony hump. Septoplasty, intranasal medial and low-to-low lateral osteotomies, percutaneous transverse osteotomies, and rasping of the bony hump done by endonasal approach. Supratip augmentation was done with septal cartilage.

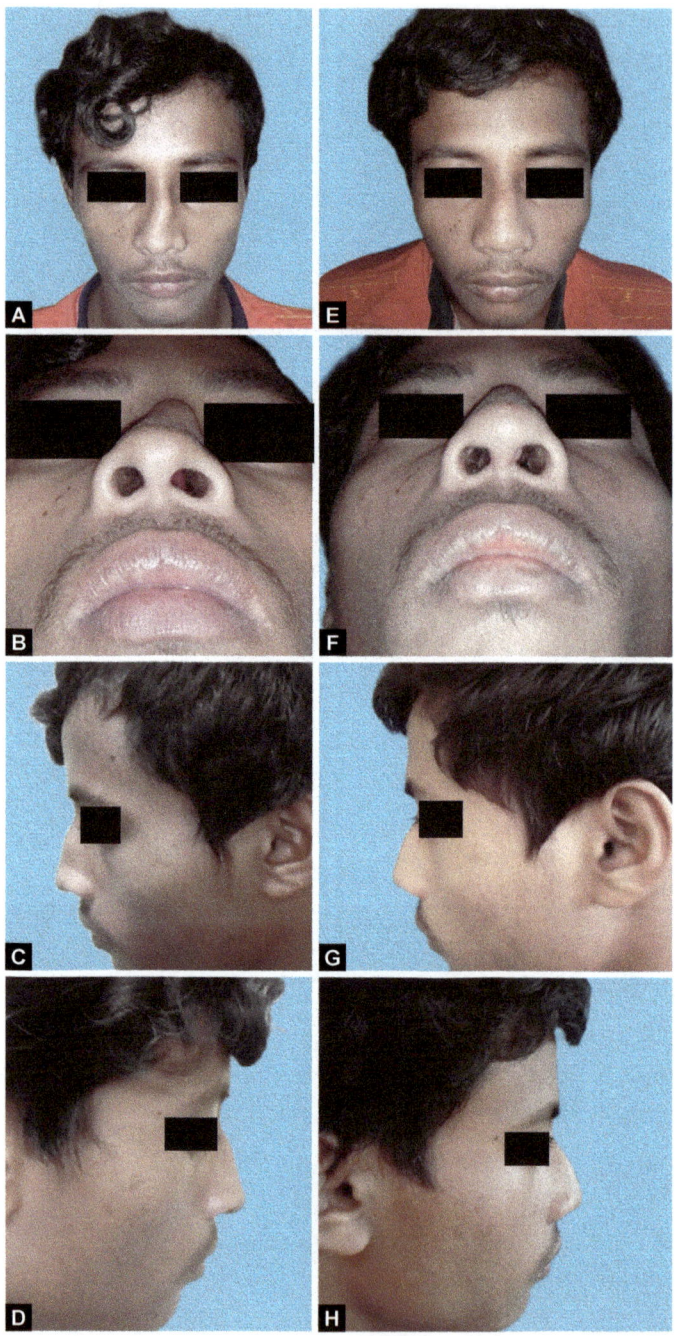

Figs. 18A to H: (A to D) Preoperative; and (E to H) Postoperative views of a case of crooked nose with depressed cartilaginous dorsum and underprojection of nasal tip. Septoplasty, osteotomies, placement of spreader grafts, and columellar strut and dorsal augmentation with layered septal and conchal cartilages were done by external approach. Domal equalization suture was done at the tip.

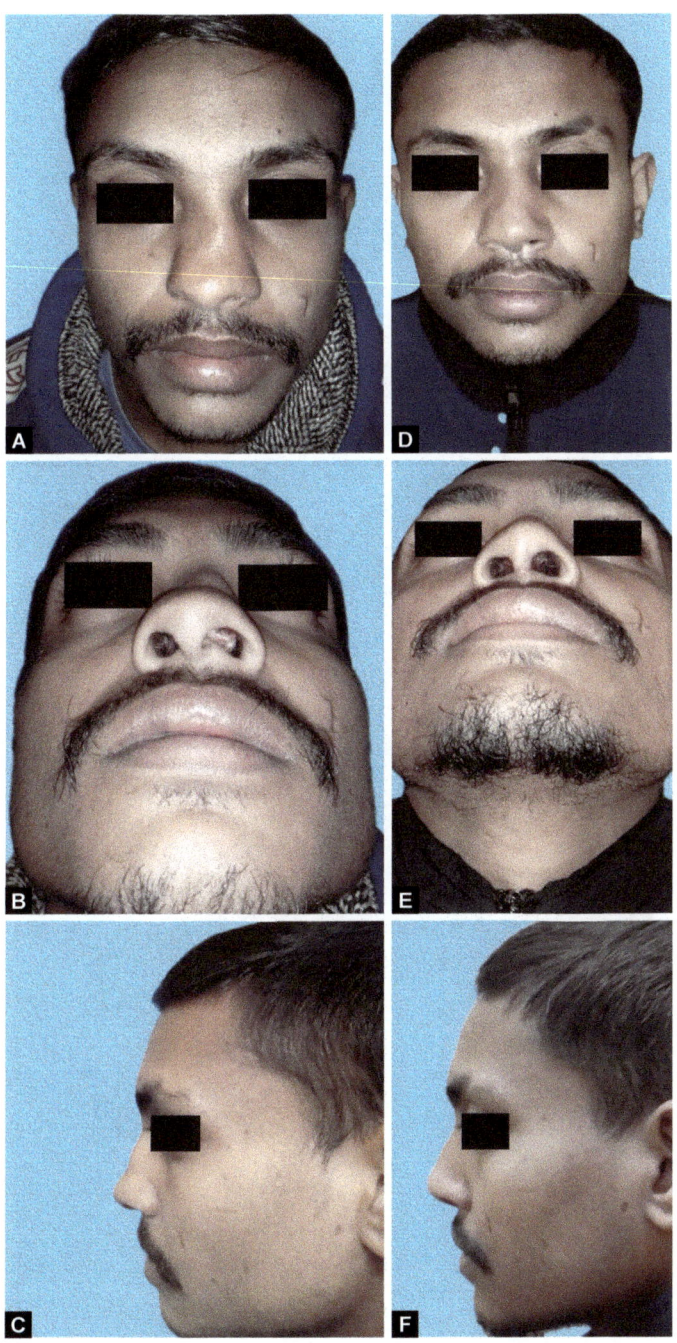

Figs. 19A to F: (A to C) Preoperative; and (D to F) Postoperative views of a crooked nose with gross caudal deviation and dorsal depression. Septoplasty and osteotomies were done by external approach. Caudal deviation was corrected by tongue in groove technique. Dorsal augmentation was done with layered conchal cartilage. Tip plasty was done by interdomal suture.

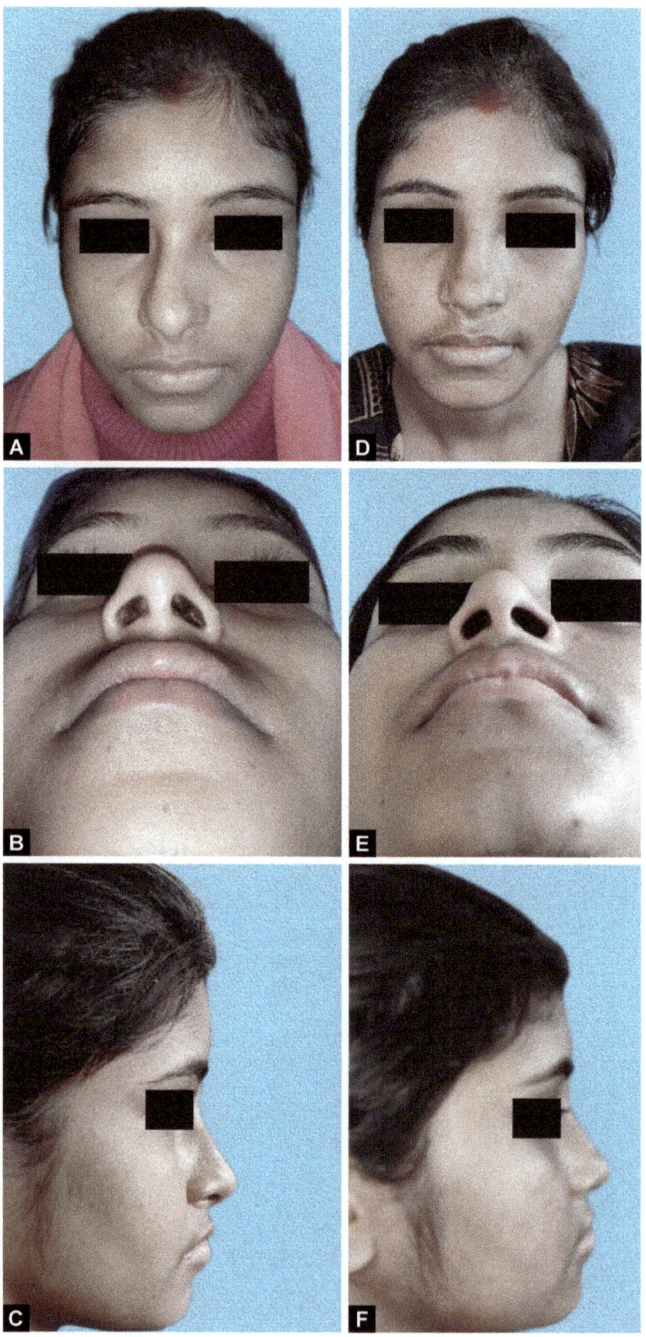

Figs. 20A to F: Preoperative; and (D to F) Postoperative views of a crooked nose with acute nasolabial angle. Septoplasty, intranasal medial and lateral osteotomies, and percutaneous transverse osteotomy were done. To rotate the tip, excision of a triangular piece of caudal septal cartilage (with the base of the triangle toward the dorsum) and cephalic trimming were done. Tip plasty was done by domal equalization suture.

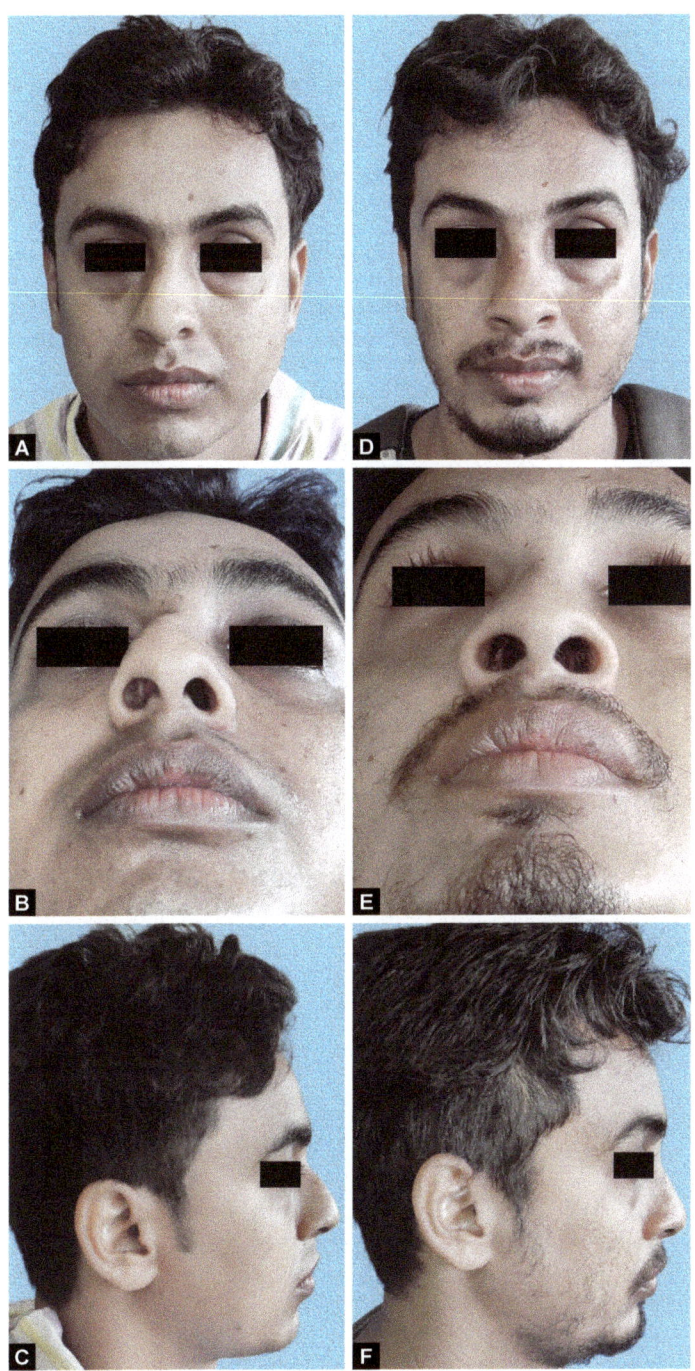

Figs. 21A to F: (A to C) Preoperative; and (D to F) Postoperative views of a crooked nose with DNS to right side. Septoplasty, intranasal medial and lateral osteotomies and percutaneous transverse osteotomy were done by endonasal approach. Mild bony hump was corrected by rasping.

REFERENCES

1. Vuyk HD. A review of practical guidelines for correction of the deviated, asymmetric nose. Rhinology. 2000;38(2):72-8.
2. Nolst Trenite GJ. Rhinoplasty: A practical guide to functional and aesthetic surgery of the nose. Netherlands: Kugler Publications, The Hague; 2005.
3. Allison TP, Joseph LL. New techniques for management of the crooked nose. Arch Facial Plast Surg. 2004;6:263-6.
4. Rohrich RJ, Ahmad J. Rhinoplasty. Plast Reconstr Surg. 2011;128:49e-73e.
5. Rohrich RJ, Adams WP. Nasal fracture management: minimizing secondary nasal deformities. Plast Reconstr Surg. 2000;106:266-73.
6. Tasman AJ, Helbig M. Sonography of nasal tip anatomy and surgical tip refinement. Plast Reconstr Surg. 2000;105(7):2573-9.
7. Toriumi DM, Ries WR. Innovative surgical management of the crooked nose. Facial Plast Clin North Am. 1993;1:63-78.
8. Gurlek A, Ersoz-Ozturk A, Celik M, Firat C, Aslan S, Aydogan H. Correction of the crooked nose using custom-made high-density porous polyethylene extended spreader grafts. Aesthetic Plast Surg. 2006;30(2):141-9.
9. Mendelsohn M. Straightening the crooked middle third of the nose: using porous polyethylene extended spreader grafts. Arch Facial Plast Surg. 2005;7(2):74-80.
10. Shah AR, Miller PJ. Structural approach to endonasal rhinoplasty. Facial Plast Surg. 2006;22(1): 55-60.
11. Webster RC, Davidson TM, Smith RC. Curved lateral osteotomy for airway protection in rhinoplasty. Arch Otolaryngol. 1977;103:454.

CHAPTER 19

Surgery of Alar, Columellar Deformity, and Vestibular Stenosis

INTRODUCTION

On frontal view, the ala and columella look like a gentle "gull-in-flight" where the columella makes the body of the gull and the alar margins make the wings of the gull **(Fig. 1)**. On profile view, the alar margin has a gentle S-shaped appearance.[1] Before correction of the alar deformity, following parts are inspected:

On the basal view:
- Alar base width
- Thickness of the alar lobule
- Thickness of the alar wall
- Flare of the alar wall

On the lateral view:
- Size of the alar lobule
- Alar-columellar relations.

Normally in profile view, columella should be visible about 3–4 mm caudal to alar margin. A line from the apex of the nostril to its lowest point divides the nostril into two equal parts **(Fig. 2)**. The resulting bisection is described as follows: (1) Ideal with 2 mm on either side; (2) excesses >2 mm denoting a

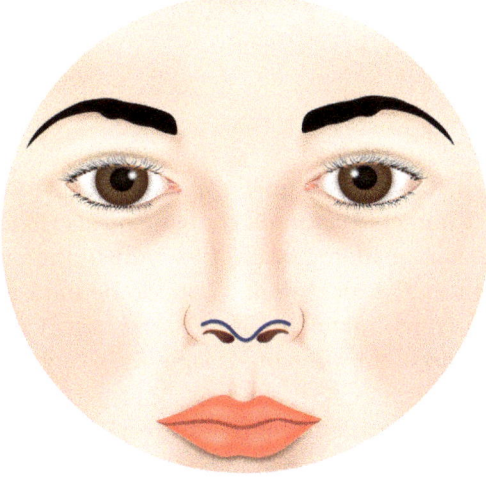

Fig. 1: Gull-wing appearance of the nasal base and columella.

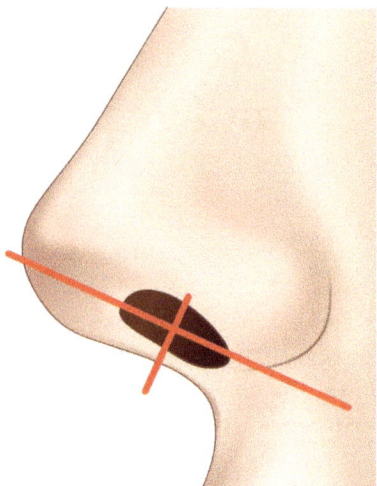

Fig. 2: A line connecting the apex of the nostril to its lowest point divides the nostril into equal halves.

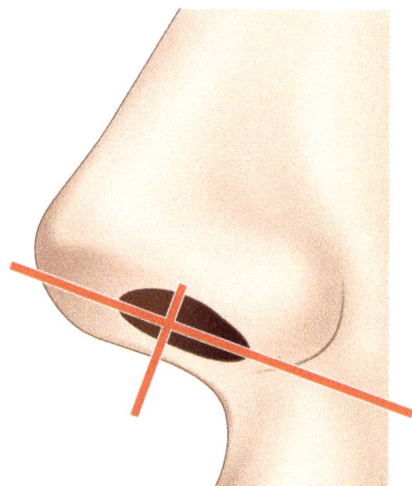

Fig. 3: Retracted ala.

retracted ala **(Fig. 3)**, hanging columella or both; and (3) reductions of 1.5 mm or less indicating a retracted columella or hanging ala **(Fig. 4)**.

The alar base is considered wide if its widest dimension exceeds the intercanthal distance. The alar lobule is said to be thick if it is greater than one-fifth of the horizontal diameter of the nasal base. Excessive alar flare is described when a part of the ala extends laterally, past the alar attachment to the cheek.

Measurement of alar width is done at the level of the alar crease, whereas measurement of alar flare is done at the level of the widest point of the ala, usually 3–4 mm above the alar crease.

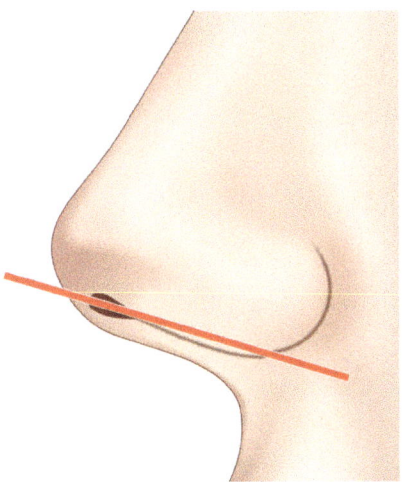

Fig. 4: Hanging ala.

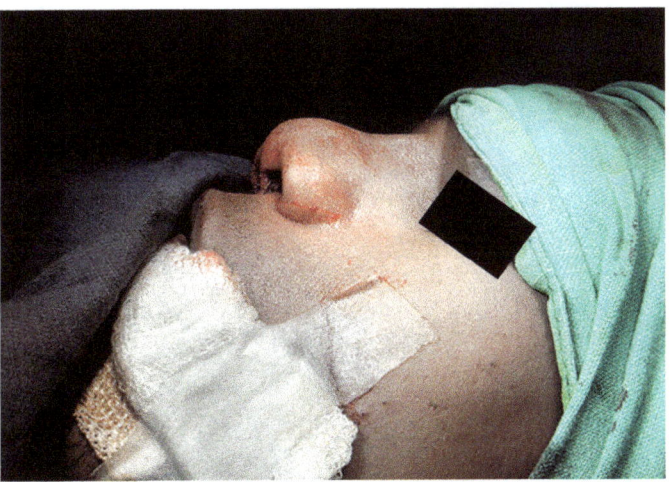

Fig. 5: Incision for alar resection.

The alar base can be divided into thirds. The upper third corresponds to the lobule and the lower two-thirds correspond to the columella. A line transecting the columella at the area of medial crural footplate diversion divides the alar base into two halves.

ALAR FLARE

Alar wedge excision is usually done when isolated alar flare is present.

Alar wedge excision should be the last procedure in rhinoplasty operation.[2] Care is taken to stay just above the alar facial crease, preserving the actual crease.[3] Incision is usually made 1 mm above the alar facial junction, which helps in precise closure and avoids suturing across a concavity **(Figs. 5 to 7)**.

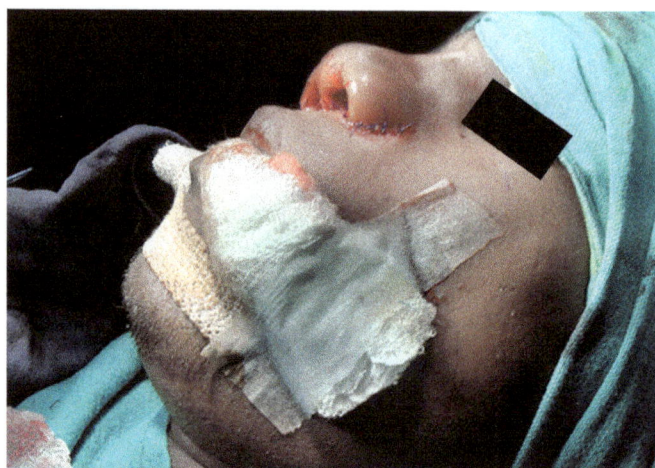

Fig. 6: Suturing after alar resection.

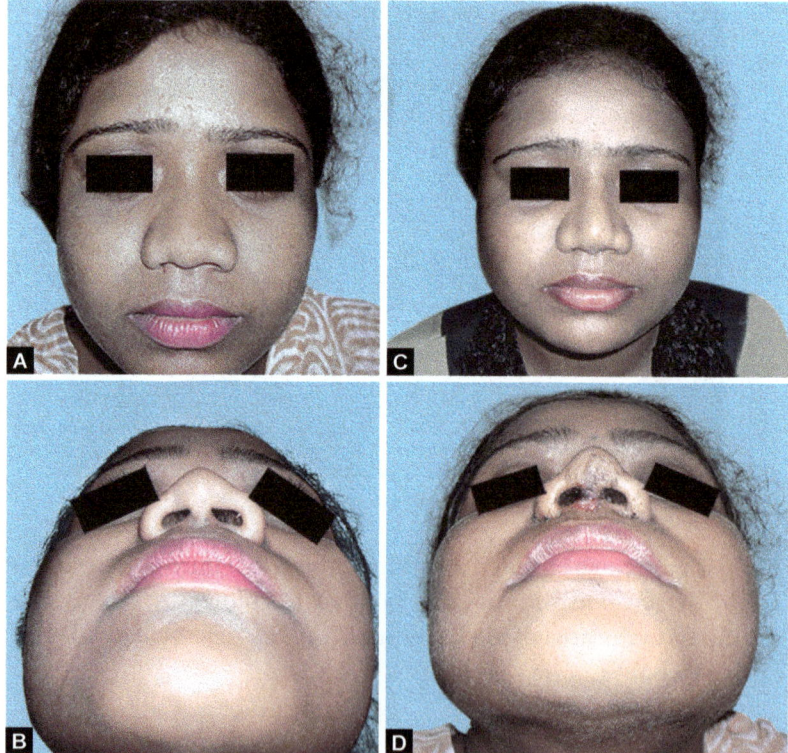

Figs. 7A to D: (A and B) Preoperative; and (C and D) Postoperative views of low dorsum, broad and underprojected nasal tip, and alar flaring. Dorsal augmentation was done with layered conchal cartilage by external approach. Cephalic trimming, transection of the lower lateral cartilages medial to dome, posteriorly based chondral flaps, placement of columellar strut and suturing of the medial crura were done. Alar wedge resection was done on both sides.

Incision placed within the crease may lead to suture marks or distortion of the alar facial junction. Marking of the line of excision is done using a caliper (2.5–4 mm average). Using a fresh 15 number blade, a V-shaped wedge excision is done without damaging the underlying vestibular skin. Closure is done from each end toward the center with the knots tied on the lower side using 6-0 nylon.

Minimal alar reduction can be done by excision of a wedge of skin and subcutaneous tissue from the nostril floor. It will diminish the slight alar flare by diminishing the dimension of the internal border of ala. If the nostril sill is not cut, the scar will be hidden within the nostril floor.

Alar flare can be reduced further by carrying the incision across the sill into the alar-facial junction. By this method, reduction of the alar bulk along with reduction of flare occurs.

WIDE ALAR BASE

Sill excisions are done for wide alar bases. Alar flaring may be increased by sill excisions. In these patients, wedge excisions are combined with sill excisions. A number 11 blade is used to perform the sill resection, followed by a number 15 blade for wedge excision. Wedge excisions correct excessive alar flare. These excisions will not narrow the nostril. Sill excisions narrow the alar base along with nostrils. Sill excisions cannot improve alar flare.

For sill excision, a 2.5–3.5-mm wide vertical trapezoid is drawn. The sides of the trapezoid are vertical with equal triangular extensions into the vestibule and the skin surface. The sill/vestibule area is repaired with a horizontal mattress suture of 4-0 Vicryl which causes eversion of the edges preventing a depressed scar. The skin is sutured with 6-0 nylon.

Overexcision of the ala should not be done as it may lead to direct insertion of the ala into the face.

RETRACTED ALA (FIG. 3)

Alar rim retraction (or notching) is a common complication of primary and secondary rhinoplasty.[4,5]

A notched or retracted ala is corrected by placement of an alar rim graft. Alar rim graft is used for caudal advancement of the alar rim by 2 mm or correcting a notched alar rim. After making a small horizontal incision in the vestibule 3–4 mm behind the rim, a subcutaneous pocket is made parallel to the rim. A straight piece of cartilage graft is introduced in the pocket to correct the deformity. A septal, conchal, or rib cartilage graft approximately 2–3 mm wide, 1–1.5 mm thick, and 15–16 mm long is made in a rectangular shape. The ends are rounded and beveled to avoid visible irregularities and for easy insertion. The length or the width of the graft may vary. The wound is then sutured using 5-0 Vicryl **(Figs. 8 and 9)**. The following changes occur after

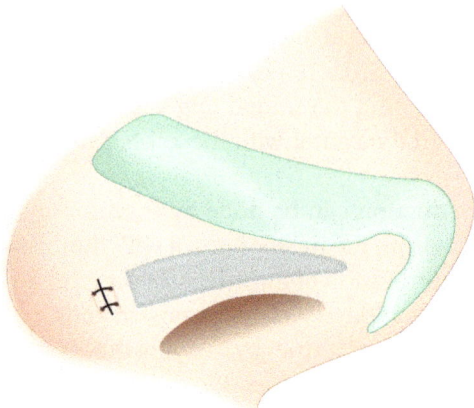

Fig. 8: Alar rim graft.

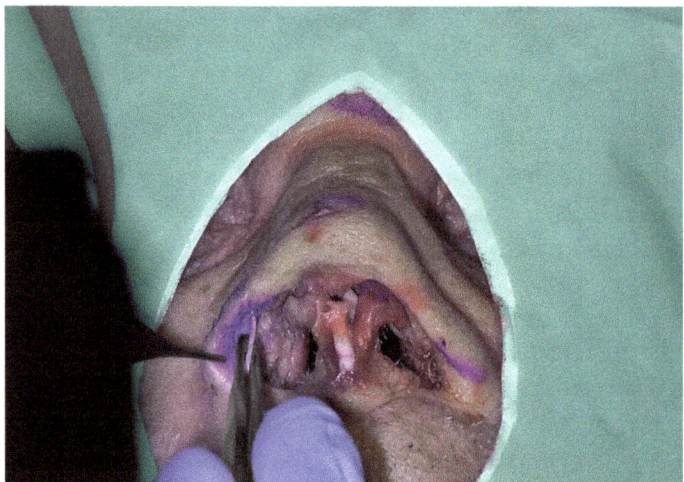

Fig. 9: Placement of alar rim graft in right ala in cadaver.

placement of the graft: (1) Correcting the concavity of the ala; (2) lowering of the alar rim; (3) widening of the nostril; and (4) elongation of the nostril.[6] The potential complications of alar rim graft insertion are visibility of the cartilage, excessive fullness, and warping and stiffening of the alar rim.

The "articulated" alar rim graft is a modified form of the alar rim graft. Here the cephalic and medial edges of the graft are beveled and sutured to the underlying dome cartilage by mattress suture (5-0 PDS) to provide support to the alar margin.

Severe alar retraction (2–4 mm) may need placement of a composite graft to the alar vestibule.[7,8] The composite graft is taken from the cymba concha and consists of cartilage and its overlying skin on one side only. After making an incision 2 mm behind the alar rim, dissection is done over the caudal margin of the lateral crura by scissors. The graft is prepared according to the size of the defect. The graft contains the same amounts of skin and cartilage. During placement of the graft, the skin component will face the nasal vestibule.

Internal V to Y advancement is another effective procedure. A flap is prepared in the subperichondrial plane and is stretched caudally. If the cartilage of the lateral crura is absent, a cartilage graft taken from the septum or pinna can be used. The flap that was incised as a V and dissected is now folded further caudally and Y advancement is done. The flap is then sutured in position using 5-0 Vicryl. Retractions up to 5 mm can be repaired with this procedure.

ALAR COLLAPSE

Alar collapse occurs during inspiratory effort if the lower lateral cartilage is weak, usually due to excessive removal of lateral crus during rhinoplasty. In patients with thin and weak alar sidewalls, cephalic trimming should be avoided as it may cause alar collapse. Alar collapse may also be congenital. This is corrected by placing an alar rim graft in the subcutaneous pocket made at the most caudal aspect of the ala. The graft is fixed by external sutures, which are removed after 1 week.

Alar batten grafts are used to prevent alar retraction and collapse and improve the pinched look found in many postoperative cases. Alar batten grafts are placed in subcutaneous pockets just superior to the lower lateral cartilages **(Figs. 10 and 11)**.

Lateral crural strut grafts are used for reshaping, reconstructing, or repositioning the lateral crura. By an open approach, cephalic trimming of the lateral crus is done and a pocket is created underneath the lateral crura.

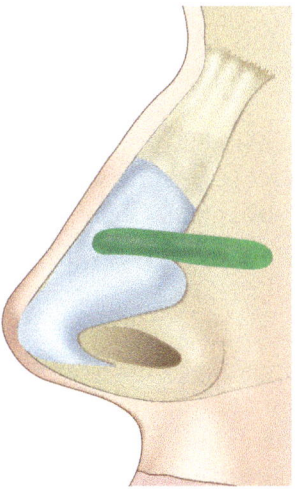

Fig. 10: Alar batten graft.

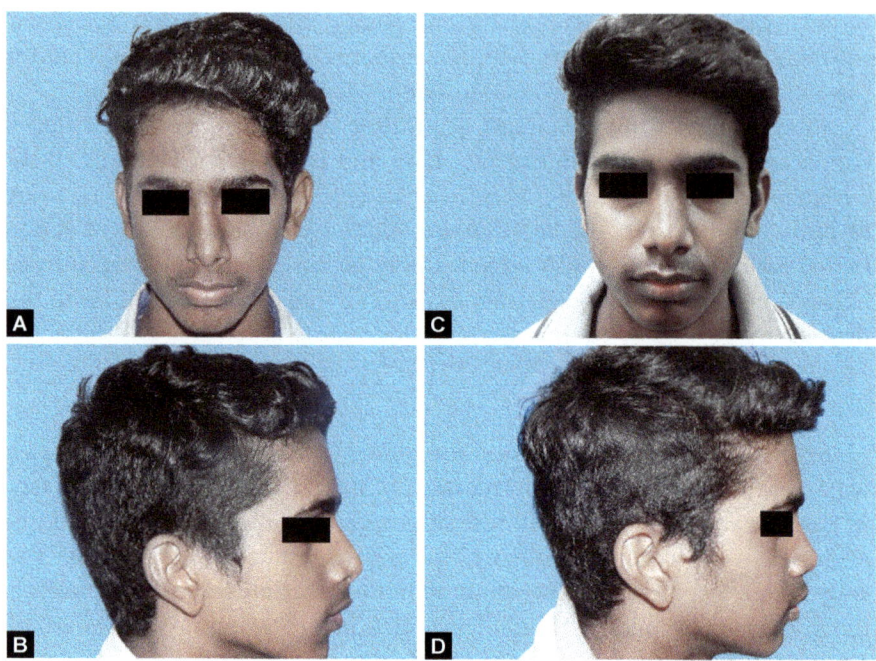

Figs. 11A to D: (A and B) Preoperative; and (C and D) Postoperative views of a patient with alar collapse. Allar batten grafts were placed in both sides.

A cartilage strut, about 3–4 mm wide and 15–25 mm long, is placed deep to the lateral crus in the pocket and secured with 5-0 PDS suture **(Fig. 12)**. The procedure is useful for correction of boxy tips, malpositioned lateral crura, concave lateral crura, and alar rim collapse or retraction.

Lateral crural strut grafts were first described by Guntur (1997).[9] Lateral crural strut grafts are placed in the following three positions: pyriform (Type I), alar base (Type II), and nostril rim (Type III) **(Fig. 13)**. Type I graft supports the alar crease, Type II graft supports the vestibule, and Type III graft supports and reshapes the nostril.

Alar batten graft provides rigidity, but sometimes obscures the alar crease or alters symmetry. In most of the primary cases, alar batten grafts have been replaced by lateral crural strut grafts. Septal or rib cartilage is usually used to make lateral crural strut grafts.

PINCHED NASAL TIP

Pinched nasal tip deformity is due to loss of lateral support and collapse of the lateral crura most commonly due to acquired causes. To correct this deformity, lateral crural spanning graft or interpositional graft can be used. These grafts are bar-shaped or triangular-shaped segments of cartilage placed in between the lower lateral cartilages **(Fig. 14)**.[10]

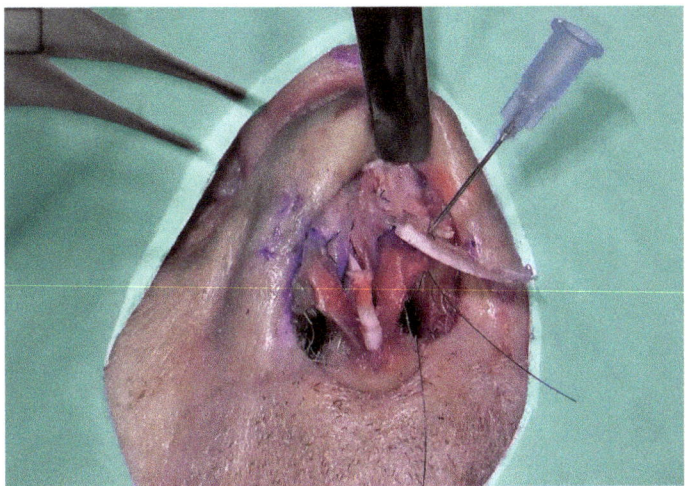

Fig. 12: Suturing of lateral crural strut graft in left side in cadaver.

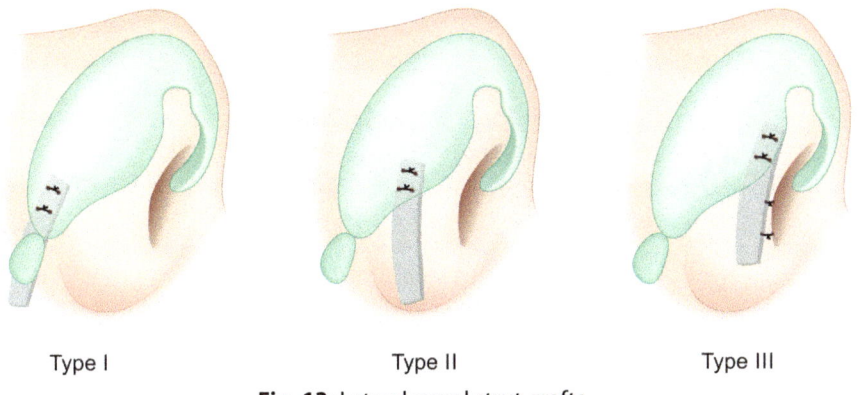

Fig. 13: Lateral crural strut grafts.

INDRAWING OF THE UPPER LATERAL CARTILAGES

Indrawing of the upper lateral cartilages occurs during deep inspiration causing nasal obstruction **(Fig. 15)**. A cartilage onlay graft is inserted in a pocket made superficial to upper lateral cartilage to stiffen the area and prevent indrawing. Beveling the margin of the graft will prevent it from being visible externally. It may also be corrected by placing spreader grafts to increase the area at the internal nasal valve or valve of Minx. Spreader flaps (autospreaders) can also be used instead of spreader grafts. Spreader flaps are made by mucosal elevation, i.e., extramucosally and then infolding the dorsal margins of the upper lateral cartilages and using them as a spreader. Spreader flaps are sutured in a similar fashion as spreader grafts.

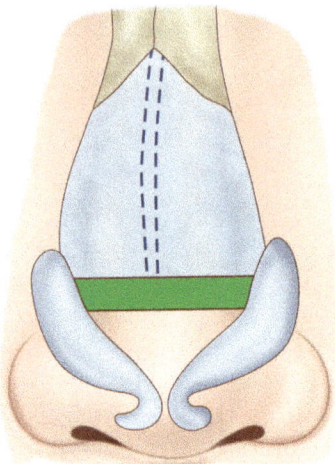

Fig. 14: Lateral crural spanning graft.

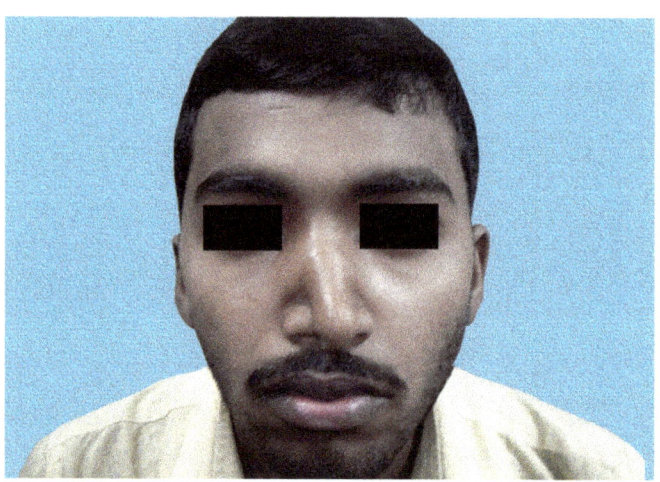

Fig. 15: Collapse of the upper lateral cartilage during inspiration.

Conchal cartilage graft can be used keeping its concave surface down, over the caudal aspect of the upper lateral cartilages as a butterfly graft and fixed with a 5-0 PDS to stiffen the structure of the upper lateral cartilages.

Flaring sutures can also be used to increase the angle of the internal nasal valve. A vertical mattress suture is done by a 5-0 nylon across the caudal part of the upper lateral cartilages and tied across the nasal dorsum, using it as a fulcrum to increase the area of the narrow portion of the internal valve.

THICKNESS OF THE ALA

Excessive thickness of the ala causing convexity of the ala can be corrected by an elliptical incision made over the thick ala near the medial aspect of the

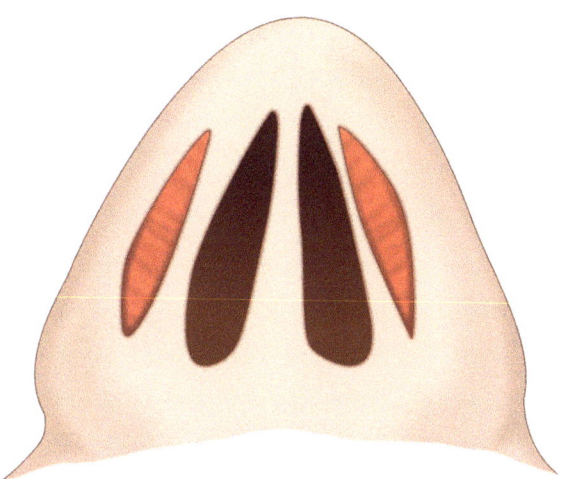

Fig. 16: To correct thick alar margins, symmetrical parts from nostril borders are removed and stitched.

nostril rim. An oval-shaped tissue containing skin and subcutaneous tissue is resected from the nostril border and suturing is done meticulously using 6-0 Vicryl **(Fig. 16)**.[11]

HANGING ALA

The hanging ala **(Fig. 4)** is repaired by excising an elliptical alar skin along with subcutaneous tissue **(Fig. 17)**.[10] A hanging ala can also be corrected by cephalic trimming.

There is limitation of correction of the hanging ala as maximum 2–3 mm of the alar rim can be elevated.

An ellipse is marked 3 mm above the rim and centered at the desired part of maximum elevation. The width of the elliptical area should be twice the desired elevation. Then a full-thickness ellipse of soft tissue is removed at the vestibular side in the same pattern. Closure of the wound is done with 5-0 Vicryl, which usually elevates the alar rim.[11,12]

RETRACTED COLUMELLA

Deficiency of the caudal part of the septal cartilage, underdevelopment of the anterior nasal spine or scarring of columella due to any trauma or surgery may cause retracted columella. It can also be due to an "endorotation" of the nasal septum after mobilization during septoplasty.[13]

Retracted columella can be corrected by placing a strut of septal cartilage inferior to the columella after making a pocket. The cartilage is fixed by a mattress suture. Where tip augmentation is also needed, an extended tip graft with a caudal part can be placed to repair the retracted columella. A columellar

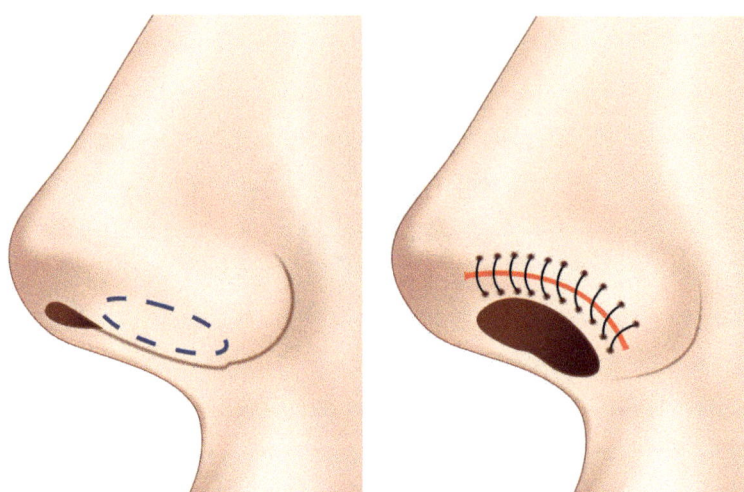

Fig. 17: Correction of the hanging ala by removal of an elliptical piece of tissue.

strut can be positioned in a manner that it will extend beyond the caudal margin of the medial crura. If the caudal septum is weak or absent, a septal extension graft corrects the retracted columella and improves tip support.[14] Septal extension graft acts as a fixed graft to the nasal septum and adds size to the septum.

In severe columellar retraction with inadequate skin cover, V-Y plasty is done to release the soft tissue near the middle portion of columella. Here bilateral V-shaped incisions are made and after elevating the mucoperichondrium segment within the V incisions on both sides of septal cartilage and pulling the triangular flaps caudally, the incisions are closed in a Y fashion forming a new membranous septum. A strip of cartilage is placed caudal to the septal cartilage and fixed to it with 4-0 catgut.

In the case of a retracted columella due to malposition of the septal cartilage following septoplasty, it can be repositioned ("exorotation") and sutured to the nasal spine.

WIDE COLUMELLA

Wide columella may be due to flaring of the medial crura. Correction is done by excising the flaring part of the medial crura along with a strip of excess skin.

HANGING COLUMELLA

Hanging columella may be due to excessive membranous septum, prominent caudal septum, downwardly curved medial crura, overly long lower lateral cartilages, or excessively wide medial crura.[15] To repair the hanging columella, the caudal parts of medial crura along with a strip of skin over it are excised. It may also be corrected by excising a strip of membranous septum or caudal part of septal cartilage. In tongue-in-groove technique, a pocket is created in between the medial crura to position the septal cartilage in the pocket. It can be done either by external or closed approach. The medial crura are then pushed posteriorly and cephalically to keep the septal cartilage in between them in the created pocket. The excess membranous septum is then excised on both sides. To prevent a postoperative wet nasal tip, the excess mucous membrane is excised, instead of excision of the anterior vestibular columellar skin.[16] In case of excessive caudal septum, partial excision of the caudal septum is done first, followed by suturing the caudal septum in between the medial crura by a tongue-in-groove technique.

VESTIBULAR STENOSIS

The correction of vestibular stenosis is a difficult problem. Two parallel incisions are made along the margins of the synechial web, extending from the floor of the nose to the apex of the vestibule. These two incisions are joined at the distal end of the flap by a cut made on the nasal floor. The flap is elevated and the thick scar tissues are dissected from the undersurface of the flap. The dissection and elevation of the flap create a defect in the lateral wall and the floor of the vestibule. The defect is covered with a full-thickness postauricular skin graft and sutured with 5-0 Vicryl. The elevated flap is also sutured with 5-0 Vicryl in its new place at the lateral nasal wall. The vestibule is packed with a small piece of merocele **(Figs. 18 to 21)**.

CONCAVE LATERAL CRUS

Concave lateral crus deformity can be corrected by removing, reversing, and replacing lateral crus with its convex surface outward. This is called lateral crus reversal technique **(Fig. 22)**.

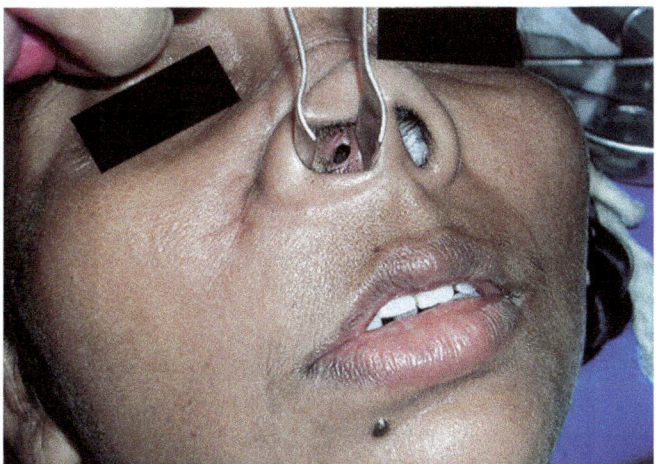

Fig. 18: A case of vestibular stenosis in right side.

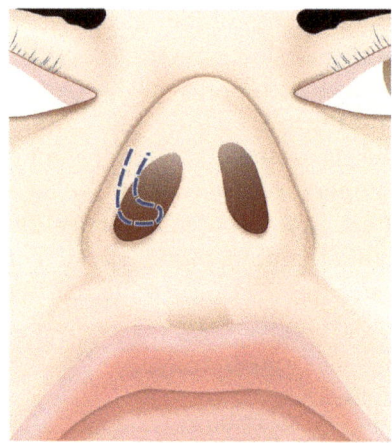

Fig. 19: Parallel cuts made bordering the web in vestibular stenosis (right side).

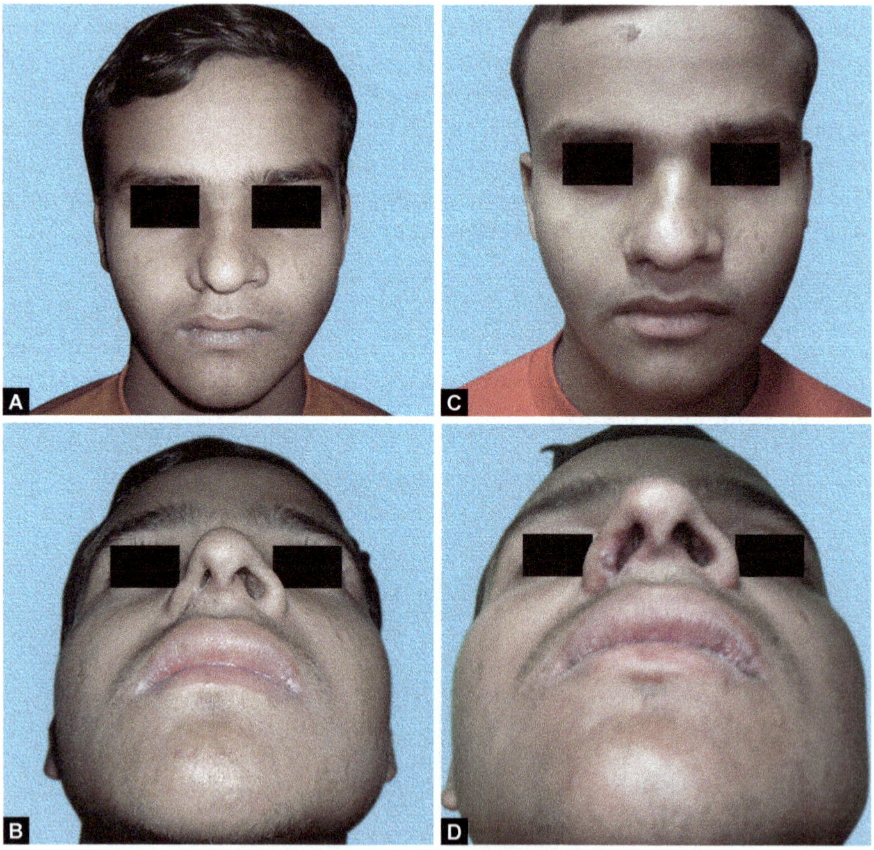

Figs. 20A to D: (A and B) Preoperative; and (C and D) Postoperative views of alar collapse with underdeveloped right ala and vestibular stenosis in right side. Vestibular stenosis was corrected by a full-thickness skin graft placed at the floor of the vestibule. Alar batten graft was placed to correct alar collapse.

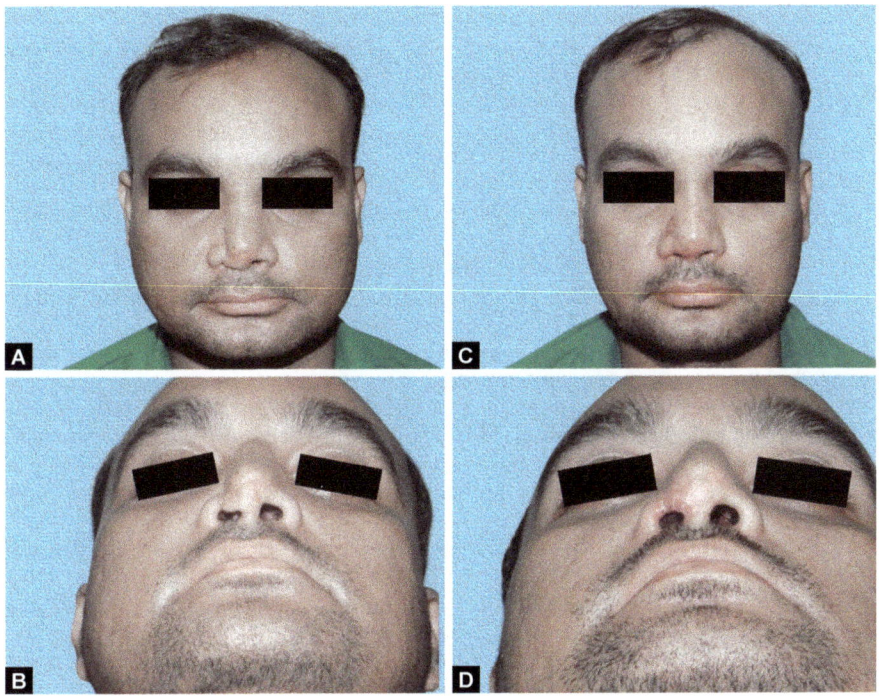

Figs. 21A to D: (A and B) Preoperative; and (C and D) Postoperative views of a case of alar collapse with mild vestibular stenosis in right side. Alar batten graft and rim graft were placed by endonasal approach.

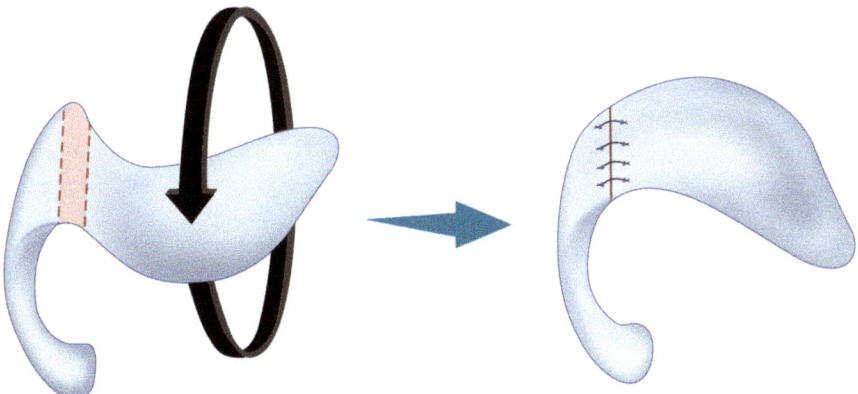

Fig. 22: Lateral crural reversal technique.

REFERENCES

1. Tardy ME, Genack SH, Murrell GI. Aesthetic correction of alar-columellar disproportion. Facial Plast Surg Clin North Am. 1995;3:395-406.
2. Hossam MT Foda. Nasal base narrowing. The combined alar base excision technique. Arch Facial Plast Surg. 2007;9:30-4.

3. Silver WE, Sajjadian A. Nasal base surgery. Otolaryngol Clin North Am. 1999;32:653-68.
4. Alexander AJ, Shah AR, Constantinides MS. Alar retraction: aetiology, treatment and prevention. JAMA Facial Plast Surg. 2013;15(4):268-74.
5. Losquadro WD, Bared A, Toriumi DM. Correction of the retracted alar base. Facial Plast Surg. 2012;28(2):218-24.
6. Guyuron B, Bigdeli Y, Sajjadian A. Dynamics of the alar rim graft. Plast Reconstr Surg. 2015;135(4):981-6.
7. Tardy ME Jr, Toriumi D. Alar retraction: composite graft correction. Facial Plast Surg. 1989;6(2):101-7.
8. Ellenbogen R. Alar rim lowering. Plast Reconstr Surg. 1987;79:50.
9. Guntur JP, Friedman RM. The lateral crural strut graft: technique and clinical applications in rhinoplasty. Plast Reconstr Surg. 1997;99:943.
10. Gunter JP, Rohrich RJ. Correction of the pinched nasal tip with alar spreader grafts. Plast Reconstr Surg. 1992;90(5):821-29.
11. Bahman Guyuron. Alar rim deformities. Plast Reconstr Surg. 2001;107: 856.
12. Gunter JP, Rohrich RJ, Friedman RM. Classification and correction of alar-columellar discrepancies in rhinoplasty. Plast Reconstr Surg. 1996;97:643.
13. Rettinger G. Aktuelle Aspekte der Septorhinoplastik. Otorhinolaryngologio Nova. 1992;2:70-9.
14. Russell WH Kridel, Robert J Chiu. The management of alar columellar disproportion in revision rhinoplasty. Facial Plast Surg Clin N Am. 2006;14:313-29.
15. Joseph EM, Glasgold AI. Anatomical considerations in the management of the hanging columella. Arch Facial Plast Surg. 2000;2:173-77.
16. Kridel RWH, Scott BA, Foda HM. The tongue-in-groove technique in septorhinoplasty. Arch Facial Plast Surg. 1999;1:246-56.

CHAPTER 20

Nasal Reconstruction

INTRODUCTION

Reconstruction of the nose is not easy. It has both convex and concave surfaces and the skin texture and color are difficult to match. The purpose of nasal reconstruction is to recover the lost function and to make the reconstructed part as normal in appearance as possible.

Following are the different options for nasal reconstruction:
- Direct closure by suturing
- Secondary healing
- Repair with skin grafts
- Local flaps
- Regional flaps

DIRECT CLOSURE

As there is limited amount of extra skin on the nose, only small defects <4–5 mm in the upper nose can be closed by suturing without affecting the shape of the remaining nose.

SECONDARY HEALING

Wounds healed by secondary intention do not always produce an unpleasant scar.[1] Small defects on the flat or concave surfaces of the nose can be corrected by secondary healing. Defects near the convex tip or alar rim are not corrected by this method to avoid distortion of the tip or nostril margins by scar contracture. The final scar is usually flat and shiny. The redness of the scar is temporary and fades away after a few months. The problems of secondary healing are infection, delayed healing, hypertrophic scar, hypopigmentation, and contracture of the surrounding area.

SKIN GRAFTS

If direct closure is not possible, a small and superficial defect can be repaired with a skin graft. A split-thickness skin graft contains the epidermis along with part of the dermis. Its thickness varies with the donor site and the need of the patient. The rate of autorejection of the split-thickness grafts is low and it can be taken from the same site again after 6 weeks. The donor site heals by re-epithelialization from the dermis and surrounding skin. A full-thickness skin graft contains the epidermis and the whole dermis. The donor site is either closed directly or overlayed with a split-thickness graft. Cutaneous defect over nasal tip produces bad result if it is repaired with a skin graft, and instead, a local flap or a forehead flap should be used for a better result. Skin grafting can be done in the upper third of nose where skin is thinner. For better cosmetic results, full-thickness skin (Wolfe graft) is better than split skin and is usually taken from postauricular area **(Figs. 1A to C)**. The graft can also be taken from preauricular area and it usually resembles the skin of the upper two thirds of the nose in color, texture, and thickness. After taking a graft of 2 × 3 cm size, primary closure can be done. The graft is immobilized by keeping some of the sutures long and tying over the damp cotton wool placed over the graft. Contraction of the split-thickness skin grafts is more than full-thickness skin grafts during postoperative period and their color, texture and thickness may not resemble the surrounding skin.

Unlike flaps, free grafts do not have their own blood supply. Grafts heal in three stages.[2]

During the initial 24–48 hours, fluid enters the graft by capillary action, which draws the plasma into the skin graft. Normally fibrin is deposited in between the graft and the recipient bed, provided no clot or serum accumulates beneath the graft, separating it from the recipient bed.

In the second stage, blood circulation begins in the skin graft as the vessels from the recipient bed start to connect with vessels in the graft.

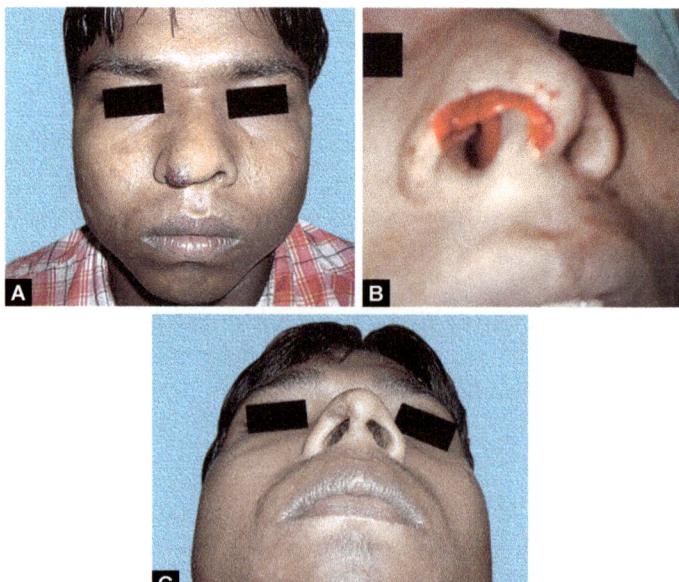

Figs. 1A to C: (A) Preoperative view of nasal hemangioma; (B) Excision of the lesion; and (C) Postoperative view after reconstruction done by postauricular full-thickness skin graft.

In the third stage, a network of blood vessels develops in the graft. If the graft is accepted in the recipient bed, true blood circulation begins within the graft.

A direct interface between the recipient bed and the graft should be maintained during the first week.[3]

LOCAL FLAPS

Local flaps have good blood supply. So, they have a high healing rate and minimal postoperative contraction. Depending on the vascularity, local flaps can be divided into random and axial flaps. The size and length of random local flaps are limited because they have random blood supply but axial flaps based on named blood vessels can be made larger.[4] Wide undermining below the level of SMAS is required to lessen tension and make the flap movable. Based on their movement, local flaps are classified into advancement flaps, rotation flaps, transposition flaps, and interpolation flaps.

Advancement Flap

The advancement flap is first undermined and then advanced in a straight line in the same axis as the defect. Examples of these flaps are the rectangular flap, the cheek advancement flap and the V-Y advancement flap **(Figs. 2 to 8)**.[5]

The length of the advancement flap can be increased by using a "Z"-plasty and/or a back cut. In a V-Y flap, the flap is made twice the size of the defect. For closing a defect of the nasal dorsum, a bipedicled advancement flap can be done.

Rotation Flap/Pivot Flap

A small defect (<1.5 cm) on one side of the nose can be repaired by a rotation flap. Its axis rotates around a pivot. The entire flap is undermined in all directions to avoid too much tension during repair and compromised vascularity.[5] If the flap rotates skin through an arc of >110°, it may produce a dog ear. A bilobed flap is a rotation flap.

Transposition Flap

Transposition flaps are adjacent to the defect and allow movement in more than one plane. They do not have to cross an intact bridge of skin. "Note flap" and rhomboid flap are examples of transposition flaps.

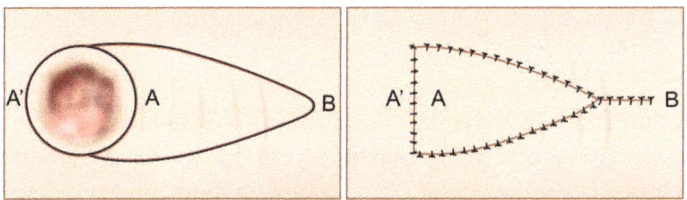

Fig. 2: V-Y advancement flap.

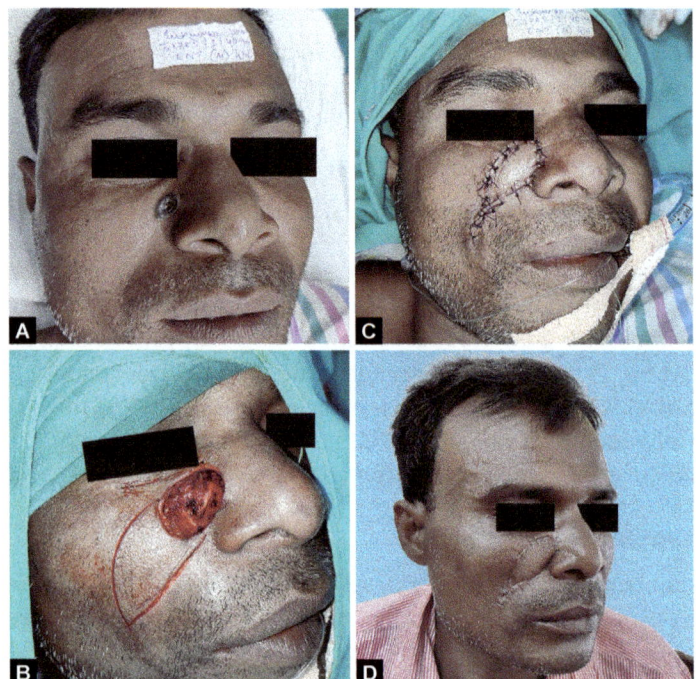

Figs. 3A to D: (A) Preoperatiive view; and (B to D) Operative steps of reconstruction by V-Y advancement flap in a case of basal cell carcinoma of face.

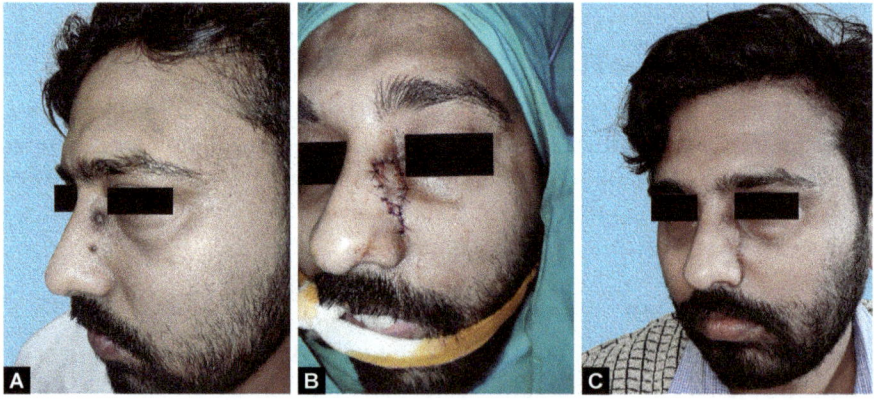

Figs. 4A to C: (A) Preoperative; and (B and C) Postoperative views of seborrheic keratosis of lateral wall of nose, excised and repaired by V-Y advancement flap along the nasofacial sulcus.

Interpolation Flap

Interpolation flaps cross an intact bridge of skin because they are not adjacent to the defect. A second stage is required to cut the pedicle once the flap has developed sufficient vascularity. Nasolabial and paramedian flaps are examples of interpolation flaps.

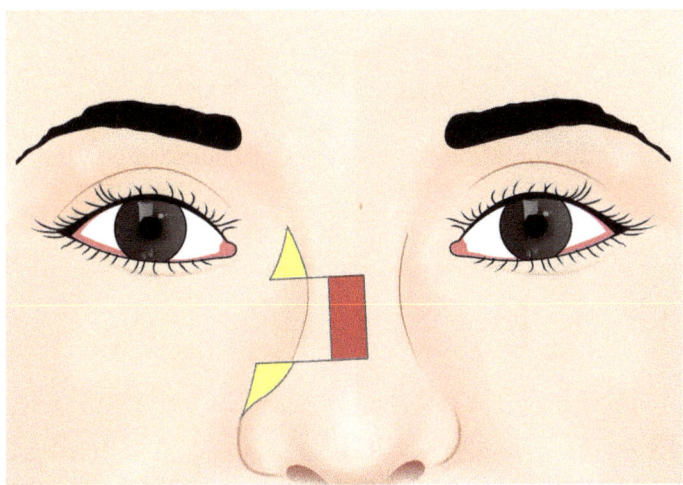

Fig. 5: Lateral nasal advancement flap. Two Burow's triangles (yellow) are excised at the alar groove and nasofacial sulcus.

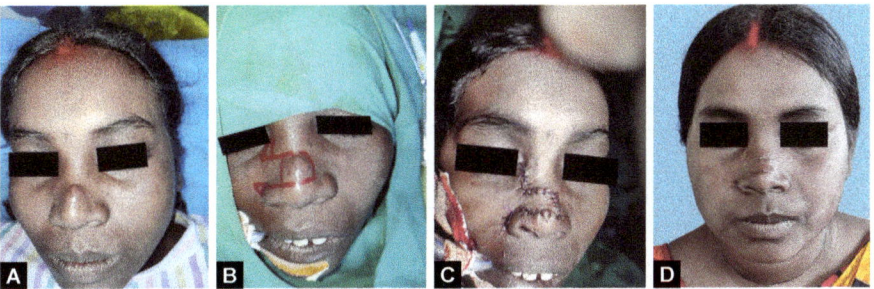

Figs. 6A to D: (A and B) Preoperative; and (C and D) Postoperative views of dermatofibroma of nose, excised and repaired by lateral nasal advancement flap. Two Burow's triangles have been removed along the alar groove and nasofacial sulcus.

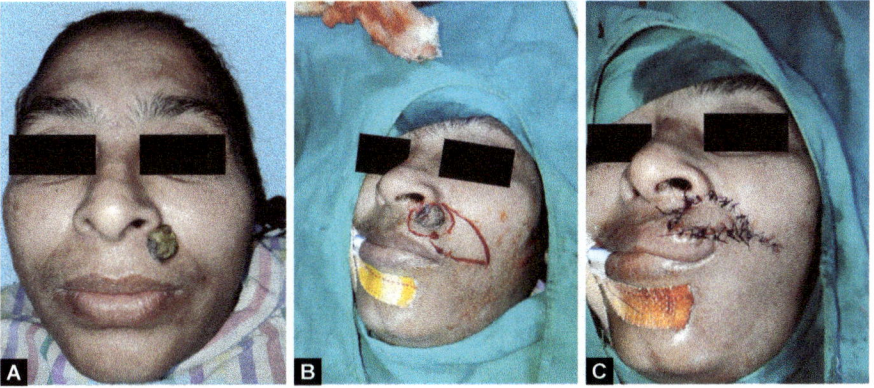

Figs. 7A to C: (A and B) Preoperative; and (C) Postoperative views of basal cell carcinoma of face, excised and repaired by nasolabial V-Y advancement flap.

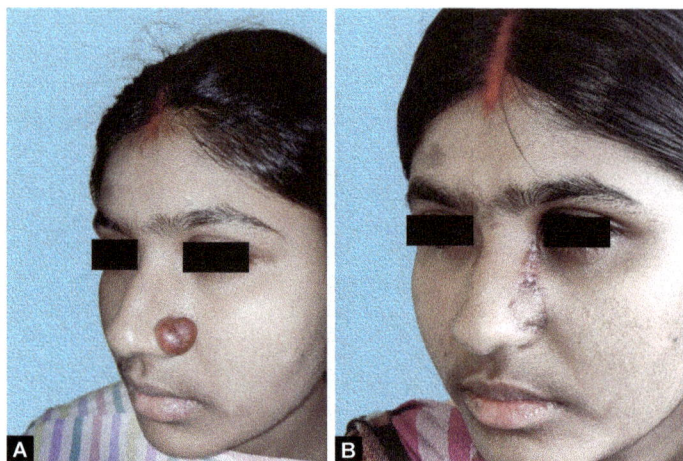

Figs. 8A and B: Preoperative; and (B) Early postoperative views of a case of broad-based keloid at left ala, excised and repaired by V-Y advancement flap.

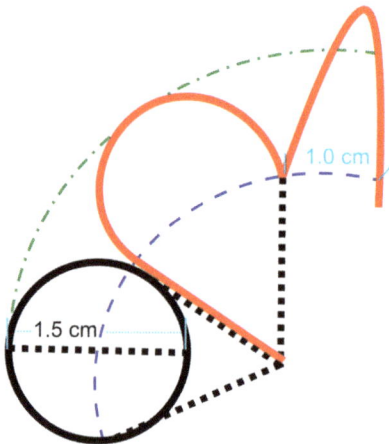

Fig. 9: Zitelli's Bilobed flap.

BILOBED FLAP (ZITELLI'S)

Small defects at the lower third of nose (<1.5 cm) can be repaired with the bilobed flap. The rotation of each lobe should not be >50°. To prevent a dog ear, a small part of skin in between the defect and pivotal point of the flap is removed. The pivotal point is placed some distance away from the edge of the defect. The distance should be equal to the radius of the defect. It is never situated near the medial canthus or margin of the ala. The diameter of the first lobe should be equal to the defect and the second lobe should be smaller but large enough to repair the donor defect adequately **(Fig. 9)**.

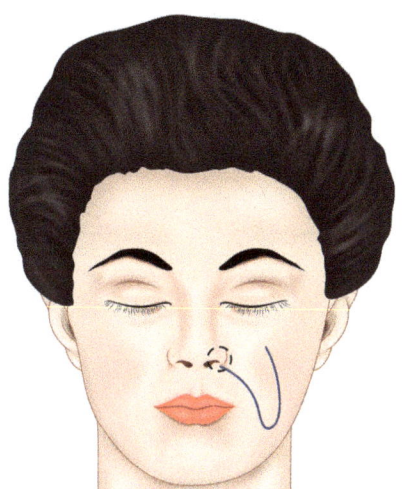

Fig. 10: Nasolabial flap for alar defect (left).

NASOLABIAL FLAP

The nasolabial flap can be used to repair limited alar defects but the size of the flap is limited and it is less vascular, thicker, and hair bearing in males. In full-thickness alar defect, the flap is infolded to make the lining of the nostril. The nasolabial flap is based either inferiorly or superiorly and the pedicle is cut later on. This is based on the perforating branches of facial and angular arteries **(Fig. 10)**.

The nasolabial sulcus is formed by the crease extending from lateral alar rim to the corner of the mouth. The facial artery appears on the face at the anteroinferior border of masseter by turning around the lower border of mandible and then runs anterosuperiorly up to 1.5 cm from the angle of mouth and then vertically to end near the medial canthus of the eye.[6] The flap is commonly made 2–3 mm lateral to the nasolabial fold with the superior limit of the flap is kept inferior to the medial canthus while the inferior limit depends on the nature of the defect. Plane of dissection is kept between subcutaneous tissue and the muscle. The relative ease of harvesting and ability to carry out dissection under local anesthesia along with the benefit of relatively minimal scar makes it one of the most widely used flaps.

GLABELLAR FLAP

Defects of the upper third of nose and medial canthus are usually repaired by a glabellar rotation flap. Excess skin from glabellar region is rotated down to the defect. The flap is pivoted on the medial end of the opposite eyebrow. Forehead defect is closed after undermining **(Figs. 11 to 13)**.

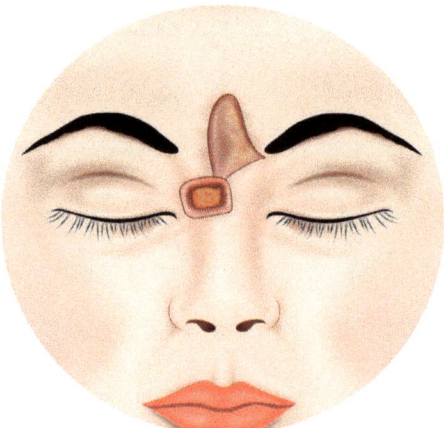

Fig. 11: Glabellar flap.

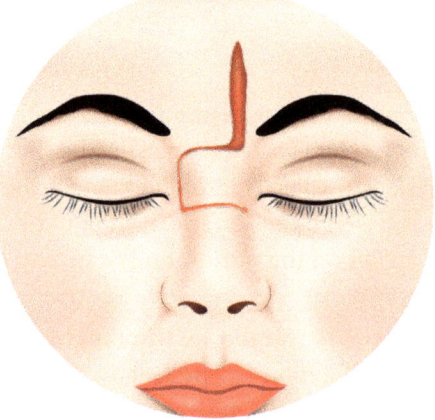

Fig. 12: Glabellar flap is transposed into the defect.

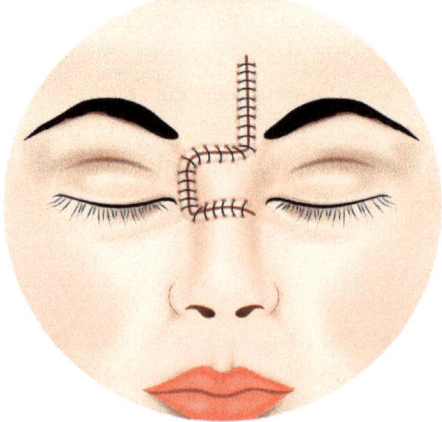

Fig. 13: Glabellar flap-closure of the defect.

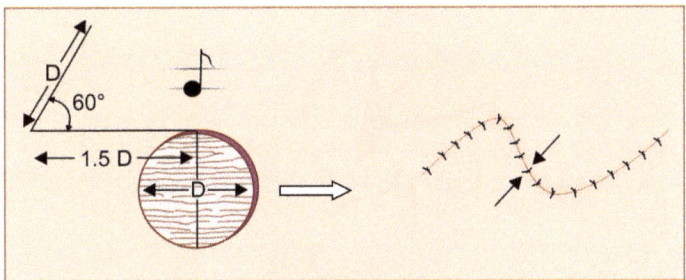

Fig. 14: Note flap.

NOTE FLAP

The note flap and adjoining defect look like a musical note and hence the name. It is like a superiorly based nasolabial flap. A dog ear is removed and the flap moved to repair the area of the defect. No second stage is needed **(Fig. 14)**.

REGIONAL FLAPS

Regional flaps are made from the excess tissue of the facial areas adjacent to the nose like the forehead. These areas can provide tissue for larger defects and for more complex repairs producing a reliable and better result. Large full-thickness tissue defects usually need regional flaps. The midline and paramedian forehead flaps are most commonly used in reconstruction of nose.

COMPOSITE GRAFT

In 1902, Konig described nasal reconstruction by using composite grafts from the pinna.

If the defect at the columella or alar margin is <1 cm in depth the auricular chondrocutaneous composite graft is the method of choice. A wedge-shaped part of composite graft is removed from the auricle. The graft is then shaped to fit the defect of the ala or columella. The apex of the wedge is carried down into the conchal hollow to prevent dog ear **(Fig. 15)**. A composite graft >1 cm is not suitable for the reconstruction because of the limited blood flow, leading to subsequent necrosis of the graft. The auricular composite graft is superior in many aspects. The pinna is considerably similar to the ala and columella in shape, curve, texture, and color. As the ear has parts with various shapes and curves, the graft that is the most similar to the recipient site can be taken. Because of the inclusion of the cartilage in the graft, there is minimal contracture after the healing of the graft. During the surgery, care is taken to remove all devitalized tissue. Incisions should be beveled to increase the contact surface of the recipient site for the graft and if necessary, bipolar diathermy is used with normal saline. During harvesting of the graft, adrenaline

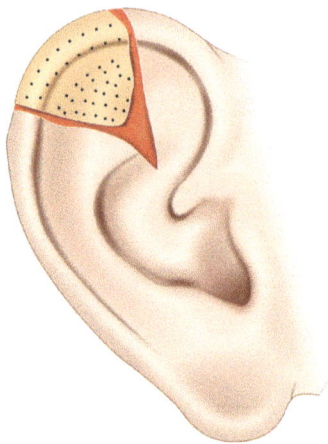

Fig. 15: Composite graft taken from pinna.

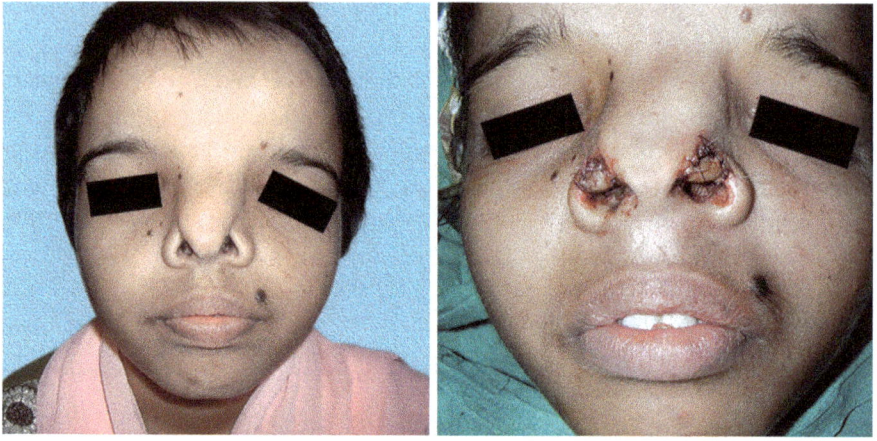

Fig. 16: Congenital alar defect repaired by composite graft taken from pinna.

is not used to prevent constriction of the vessels. Up to 1.5 cm of helix rim can be harvested without creating any deformity. Accurate approximation of the graft to the recipient site is done without tension with interrupted 6/0 Vicryl. Merocele is used in the nostril for the immobilization of the graft. No dressing is applied **(Figs. 16 and 17)**. An elliptical shaped composite graft can also be taken from the outer surface of the cymba concha. Entire conchal bowl can be taken as a composite graft and the defect is repaired with a full-thickness skin graft. This conchal composite graft can be used for lining the inner surface of the paramedian forehead flap.[7]

The vascularization of the composite graft is vulnerable and depends on the limited surface contact along the margin of the graft and the stability of the graft on its bed.[8,9]

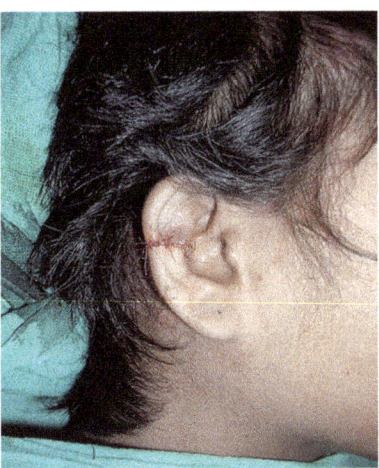

Fig. 17: Suturing of pinna after harvesting composite graft from pinna.

FOREHEAD FLAP

Nasal tip defect is usually corrected by a local flap or a forehead flap. Nasal defects >1.5 cm are better repaired with forehead flap. Nasal defects are usually caused by excision of cutaneous malignancies or by trauma, burns, or sepsis. When the defect needs replacement of support or lining, or if it is located within the infratip or columella, a forehead flap can be used. The forehead flap has very good blood supply. So, free cartilage or bone grafts can be incorporated during the reconstruction.

The forehead flap is the ideal flap because of its size, color, texture, vascularity, and thickness. As it is an axial flap with a pedicle supplied by its dominant vessel, the pedicle can be made as narrow as 1.0–1.2 cm. A narrower pedicle of the forehead flap increases the length and rotation of the flap.[10,11] Forehead flaps are based on the supratrochlear, and terminal branches of the angular and dorsal nasal vessels. There are anastomoses between the supratrochlear, supraorbital, angular, and superficial temporal arteries. The supratrochlear artery comes out from the superior medial part of orbit about 1.7–2.2 cm lateral to the midline at the medial portion of the eyebrow and runs vertically about 2 cm lateral to the midline. The main axial blood supply of midforehead flaps is the supratrochlear artery.[12] The supratrochlear pedicle is located 3 mm lateral to the medial canthus.[13]

The end arterioles of the supratrochlear vessels are situated superficial to the frontalis muscle in the upper third of the flap. So, the surgeon can make the flap thin to gain proper shape of the various nasal subunits.[14]

TYPES OF FOREHEAD FLAPS

There are four types of forehead flaps: (1) Median; (2) paramedian; (3) midline; and (4) oblique flaps.

The median forehead flap having a wide pedicle and based on both supratrochlear vessels was described in the United States by Kazanjian in 1947. The median forehead flap is taken from the center of the forehead, but the flap is not long enough **(Fig. 18)**.

The paramedian forehead flap is based on the ipsilateral or contralateral supratrochlear vessels. It is the ideal flap because having a low turning point it can reach the defect easily and primary closure of the donor area can be done. Donor site morbidity in the glabellar region becomes less due to the narrow pedicle.[15] If a second repair is needed because of recurrence of cancer, then the paramedian flap can be taken from the contralateral forehead **(Figs. 19 and 20)**.

The midline forehead flap is the combination of paramedian and median flaps. Here, the skin flap is taken from the mid forehead. The pedicle is based

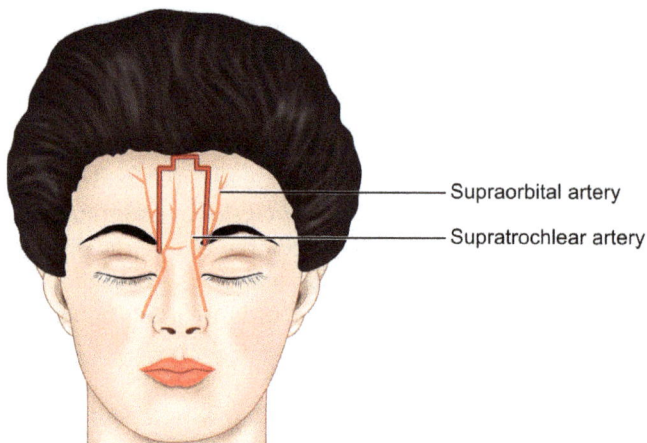

Fig. 18: Median forehead flap.

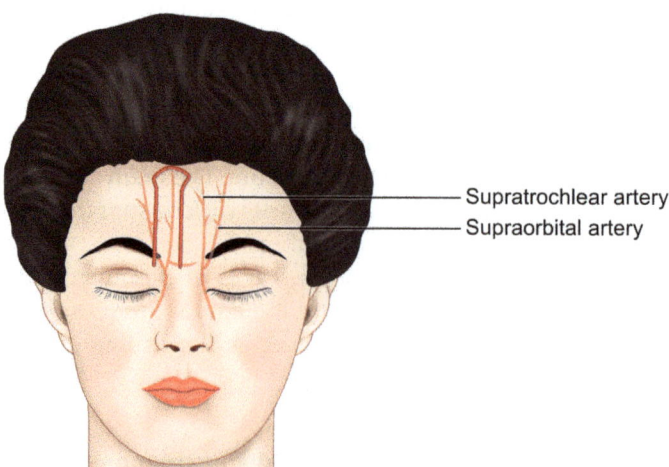

Fig. 19: Paramedian forehead flap.

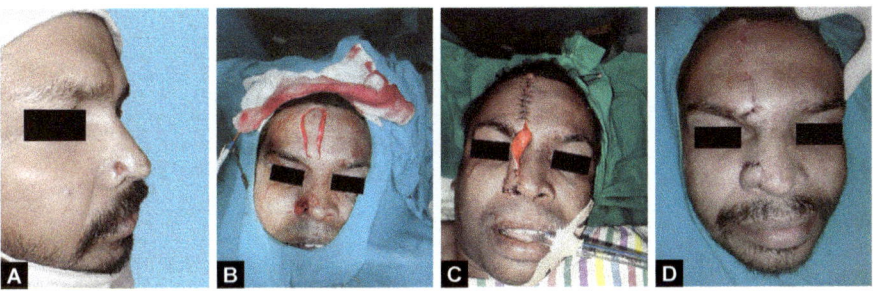

Figs. 20A to D: (A) Preoperative; view and (B to D) Operative steps of nasal reconstruction by paramedian forehead flap in a case of basal cell carcinoma of nose.

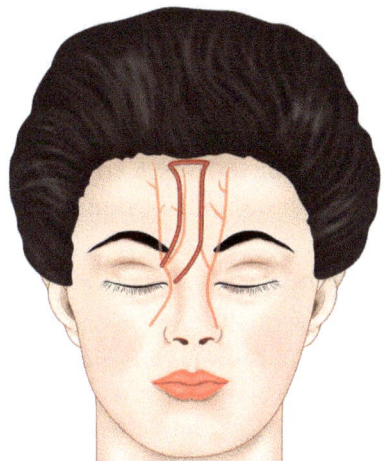

Fig. 21: Midline forehead flap.

on a unilateral supratrochlear vessel and collateral vessels from the medial eyebrow area and runs in an oblique line. There will be a less conspicuous midline donor scar. The midline location gives greater length to the flap and allows for resurfacing of a more caudal nasal defect **(Fig. 21)**.[16]

AESTHETIC UNITS

The principle of aesthetic units is now incorporated as an important step in preoperative planning.[17] The principle is that the human eye captures images only as a series of blocks. These snap shots are then put together into a single image. By completing the aesthetic unit, the surgeon can allow the final scars to stay between two adjacent subunits making them inconspicuous. Each aesthetic subunit is defined by reflections of light, or a change in surface contour.[18] Nine subunits are present on the nose.[19] Out of these following five subunits are convex: the dorsum, tip, columella, and paired alar-nostril sill. Four subunits are concave: the paired lateral walls and paired soft triangles **(Fig. 22)**. During repair of nasal defects, scars should be placed in between

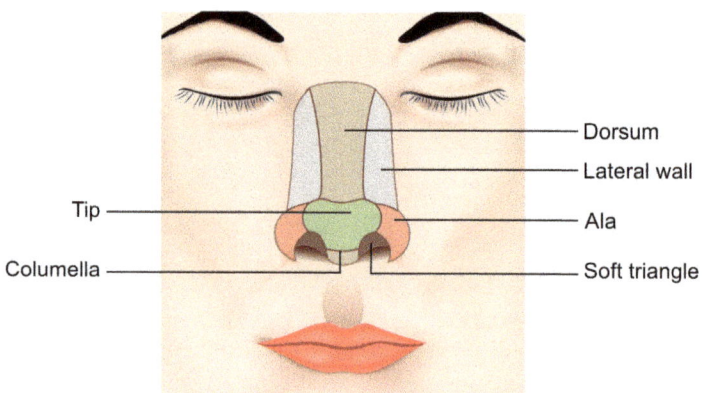

Fig. 22: Aesthetic subunits of the nose.

nasal subunits. For better repair, normal tissue within the subunit can be safely removed.

In the presence of defect of >50% of a convex nasal subunit (tip, ala), repair of the entire nasal subunit should be done.

OPERATIVE PROCEDURE

The repair by forehead flap is usually done in two stages.

A template of the affected nasal subunit is made from the foil of the pack of a suture material. The length of the flap is measured with a silk thread from the tip of the template near the hairline to the base of the pedicle. Now, the silk thread is held at the base of the pedicle and the other end of the thread is rotated down to the distal affected area on the nose. If the thread fails to reach this area, the template is to be placed at a higher site on the forehead or the base of the pedicle is to be repositioned below the level of the eyebrow. The outline of the flap is then marked on the forehead by a marker.

Xylocaine (1%) with 1 in 1,00,000 adrenaline is injected around the affected area and in the soft tissue of the forehead, except near the base of the pedicle. Debridement of the affected area is done. The flap along with the frontalis muscle is dissected superficial to the periosteum from superior to inferior direction. When the elevation reaches 1–2 cm above the eyebrow, blunt dissection is done to prevent injury to the supratrochlear artery. Once the vessel has been detected, elevation is continued up to the root of the nose. After the flap is elevated, it is made thin by removing the distal frontalis muscle and subcutaneous tissue to make the size similar to the defect of the nose. The donor area is repaired after undermining the forehead in a submuscular plane in two layers. The defect is covered with the flap using 5-0 Vicryl for the deep layers, and 5-0 prolene for the skin layer.

The raw undersurface of the pedicle is left open or gently covered. In the second stage, i.e., about 3 weeks following the first stage, the pedicle is divided, the lower part of the forehead is reopened and medial brow area is repaired with the proximal pedicle to achieve a normal inter eyebrow distance. The proximal part of the flap is made thin and shaped to repair the nasal subunit. Any revision surgery like thinning of the flap, is usually done after 3–6 months. The requirement for revision surgery to debulk the flap is reduced if thinning of the flap is done beforehand. Depending on the laxity of the patient's skin, flaps as wide as 4.5 cm can be taken and the donor site repaired primarily.[20,21] Acceptable cosmetic result is obtained if part of the donor site is allowed to heal by secondary intention. In patients with low hairlines, oblique forehead flap can be taken or the flap can be extended into hair-bearing scalp.[22] When the flap is taken with hair-bearing skin, thinning of the flap is done to remove the hair follicles. The distal part of the forehead flap can be hinged on itself 180° (Hinged flap). The inner part represents the most distal aspect of the flap and after it is hinged, may have reduced vascularity.

The alar rim may look bulky and often needs additional revisions **(Figs. 23 to 26)**.

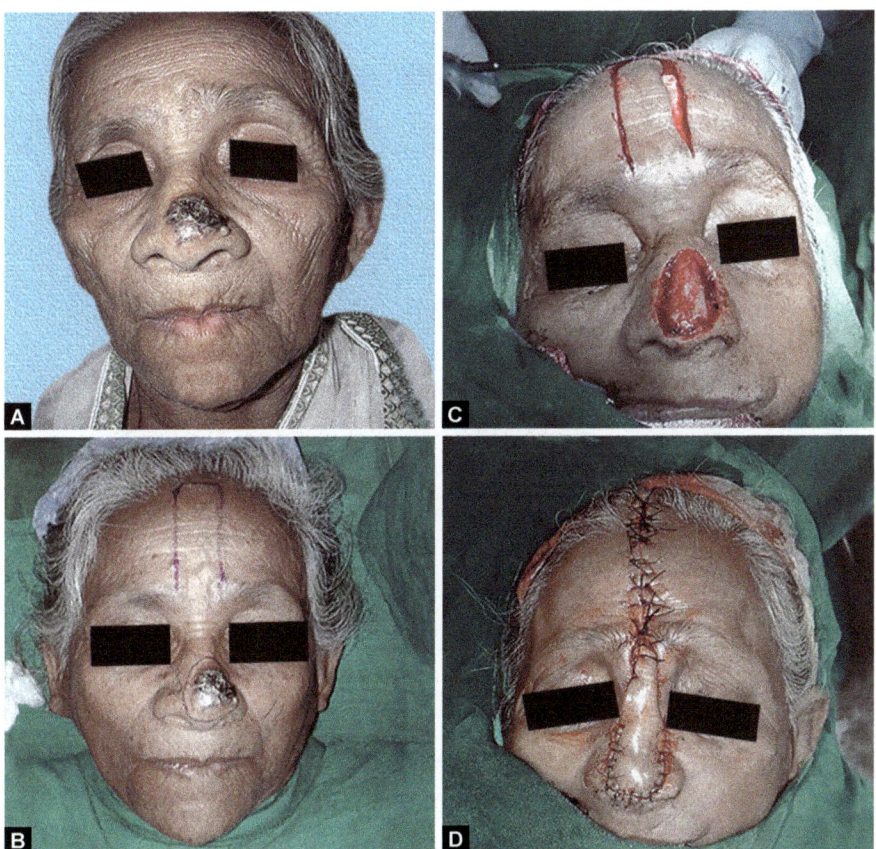

Figs. 23A to D: (A) Preoperative; view and (B to D) Operative steps of nasal reconstruction by median forehead flap in a case of basal cell carcinoma of nose.

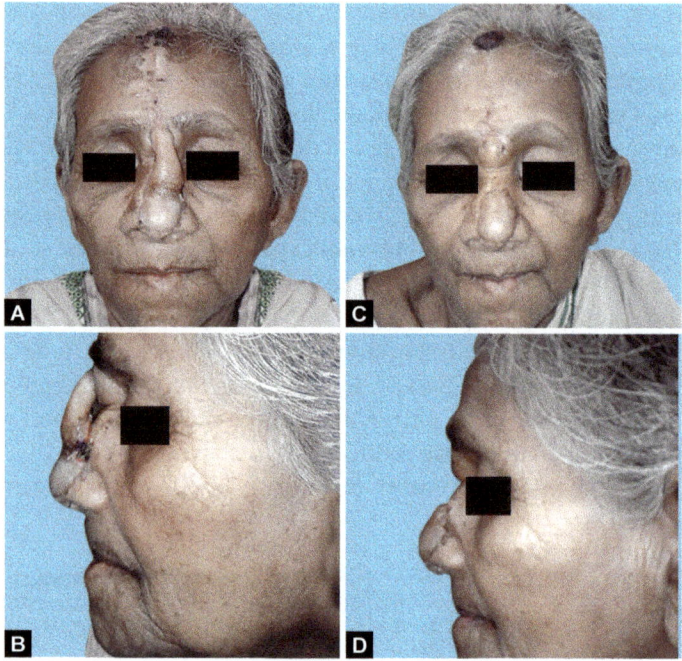

Figs. 24A to D: (A and B) Postoperative views of the first stage; and (C and D) Second stage of nasal reconstruction by median forehead flap in a case of basal cell carcinoma of nose.

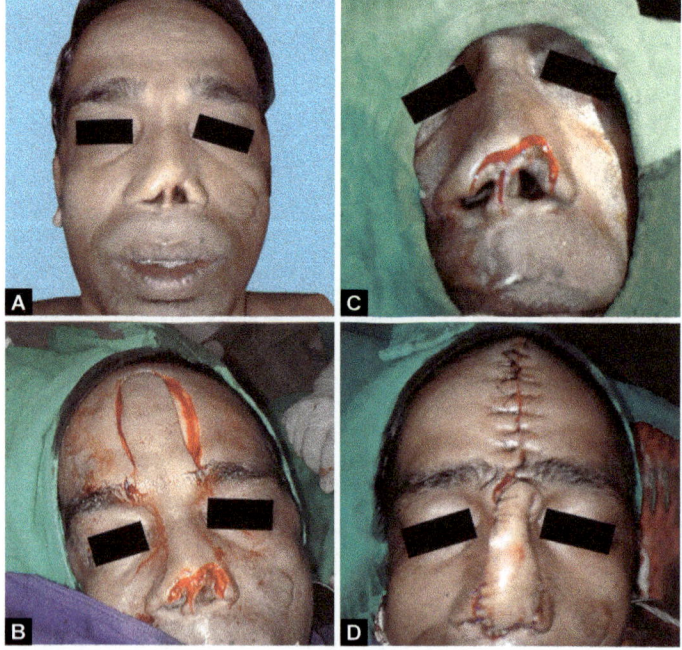

Figs. 25A to D: (A) Preoperative view; and (B to D) Operative steps of nasal reconstruction by midline forehead flap in a case of traumatic nasal deformity.

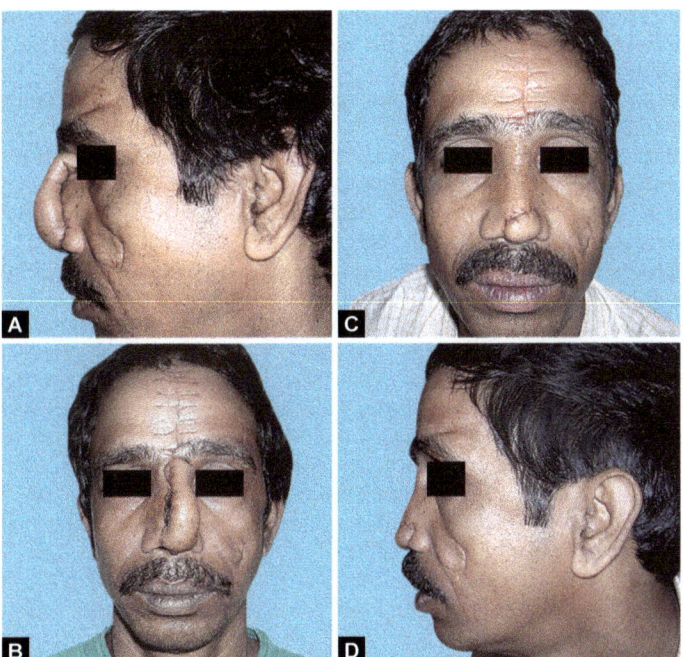

Figs. 26A to D: (A and B) Postoperative views of the first stage; and (C and D) Second stage of nasal reconstruction by midline forehead flap in a case of traumatic nasal deformity.

REFERENCES

1. Ariyan S, Krizek TJ. In defense of the open wound. Arch Surg. 1976;111:293-6.
2. Thomas JR. Skin grafts. In: Thomas JR, Roller J (Eds). Cutaneous facial surgery. New York: Thieme Medical Publishers; 1992. pp. 72-80.
3. Branham GH, Thomas JR. Skin grafts. Otolaryngol Clin North Am. 1990;23:889-97.
4. Hollier HJ, Stucker FJ. Local flaps for nasal reconstruction. Facial Plast Surg. 1994;10:337-48.
5. Thomas JR. Local skin flap. In: Thomas JR, Roller J (Eds). Cutaneous facial surgery. New York: Thieme Medical Publishers. 1992. pp. 77-90.
6. Cunningham DJ, Romanes GJ. Cunningham's manual of practical anatomy (Ed). Fifteenth. Head and Neck and Brain (vol. 3); 14th edition. Oxford, United Kingdom: Oxford University Press; 1979. pp. 96-7.
7. Raghavan U, Jones NS. Use of auricular composite graft in nasal reconstruction. J Laryngol Otol. 2001;115:885-93.
8. Gillies H. New free graft applied to reconstruction of the nostril. Br J Surg. 1943;30:305-9.
9. Maves MD, Yessenow RS. The use of composite auricular grafts in nasal reconstruction. J. Dermatol Surg Oncol. 1988;14:994-9.
10. Burget GC, Menick FJ. Aesthetic reconstruction of the nose. St Louis, Mo, USA: Mosby-Year Book Inc; 1994.
11. Menick FJ. Aesthetic refinements in use of forehead for nasal reconstruction: the paramedian forehead flap. Clin Plast Surg. 1990;17:607-22.
12. Shumrick KA, Smith TL. The anatomic basis for the design of forehead flaps in nasal reconstruction. Arch Otolaryngol Head Neck Surg. 1992;118:373-9.

13. Ugur MB, Savranlar A, Uzun L, Kucuker H, Cinar F. A reliable surface landmark for localizing supratrochlear artery: medial canthus. Otolaryngol Head Neck Surg. 2008;138(2):162-5.
14. Baker SR, Swanson NA. Local flaps in facial reconstruction. St Louis, Mo: Mosby-Year Book Inc; 1995.
15. Boyd CM, Baker SR, Fader DJ, Wang TS, Johnson TM. The forehead flap for nasal reconstruction. Arch Dermatol. 2000;136(11):1365-70.
16. Quatela VC, Sherris DA, Rounds MF. Esthetic refinements in forehead flap nasal reconstruction. Arch Otolaryngol Head Neck Surg. 1995;121(10):1106-13.
17. Burget GC, Menick FJ. The subunit principle in nasal reconstruction. Plast Reconstr Surg. 1985;76(2):239-47.
18. Park SS. Nasal reconstruction in the 21st Century: a contemporary Review. Clin Exp Otorhinolaryngol. 2008;1(1):1-9.
19. Burget GC. Aesthetic restoration of the nose. Clin Plast Surg. 1985;12463-80.
20. Burget GC, Mansor M, Marsh JL (Eds). Surgical restoration of the nose. Current therapy in plastic and reconstructive surgery. Phildelphia, PA: BC Decker; 1989. pp. 400-12.
21. Alford EL, Baker SR, Shumrick KA, Hurley R (Eds). Midforehead flaps. Local flaps in Facial Reconstruction. St. LouisMo: Mosby-Year Book Inc.; 1995. pp. 197-223.
22. Hoffman HT, Baker SR. Nasal reconstruction with the rapidly expanded forehead flap. Laryngoscope. 1989;99:1096-8.

Revision Rhinoplasty

INTRODUCTION

Revision rhinoplasty, also known as redo rhinoplasty, is one of the most difficult procedures in plastic surgery. In general, a rate of revision rhinoplasties between 5 and 10% is to be expected.[1] Though surgeons do not enjoy performing revision rhinoplasty as they consider it as their failure to achieve the goal, they should do revision surgeries and become more experienced. Patients with minor deformities usually return to the primary surgeon. But the patients with major deformities tend to consult a second surgeon.[2] When the primary rhinoplasty was performed by another surgeon, it is a secondary rhinoplasty. Revision rhinoplasty is called when one reoperates on his own primary case.

All secondary rhinoplasties are difficult because the surgeon does not know what has been done before in a secondary case until he performs the surgery.

Revision rhinoplasty is more commonly performed in females.[3] Revision rhinoplasty is one of the most challenging problems in aesthetic surgery. The emotional impact of an improper rhinoplasty can be devastating. A proper preoperative assessment and conservative and precise surgery should be done to avoid the patient's dissatisfaction and medicolegal implication.

Unfavorable results as a consequence of unpredictable healing are usually called "complications," which are beyond the surgeon's control. However, inadequate primary procedure necessitating a revision surgery is called a "mistake," In this situation, the patient blames the surgeon for the bad result.[4] Of all the revision cases, the frequency of having more than one revision lies between 20% and 23%.[2]

Preoperative assessment in revision rhinoplasty is more complicated because of prior surgery, with subsequent changes in the preexisting anatomy. The surgeon must be careful to analyze the deformity, decide how to repair it, and have other alternatives available to him if his diagnosis is not correct. Patients should possess pre- and postoperative photographs for each operation and the operative notes of the previous surgery. The previous surgeon's operative notes may be insufficient and should only be used as a rough guide.[5] The thickness and quality of the skin-soft tissue envelope should be assessed. The skin-soft tissue envelope is palpated to feel the extent of fibrosis and mobility of the skin, which may limit the amount of surgical improvement possible. The nose is examined for the presence of any grafts or implants.

The bony vault is palpated for any irregularities. It is examined to see its height, width, and any deviation. The nasal dorsum should follow a gentle curving line from the medial end of the eyebrow to the nasal tip.[6] The middle vault width and presence of any deviation are assessed. It is palpated to see whether the dorsal septum near the anterior septal angle has been under-resected, resulting in a pollybeak deformity. Tip is examined to assess tip symmetry, rotation, projection, and any alar or columellar deformity. Tip support and presence of any grafts are assessed by palpation. Status of the caudal septum is seen. The patient is observed during normal and deep inspiration to diagnose collapse of the nasal valve. A "modified" Cottle maneuver, in which the lateral wall of the nose is held up by a probe, can diagnose nasal valve collapse if there is subjective improvement in nasal breathing. The position of the nasal tip can also contribute to nasal obstruction. The dropping tip is manually elevated to see whether there is any improvement of nasal airflow. Any residual septal deviation and its contribution to dorsal deviation should be assessed and septum is also examined for any perforation. The septum may be palpated with a probe to see the amount of residual cartilage present.[5] Physical and radiological examinations can never make the exact assessment of the damage done in the previous operations. External approach provides better exposure to see and define the damage and accordingly reconstruct the deformity.[7]

Correct preoperative diagnosis, minimal dissection, use of autogenous graft when required, and a proper preoperative plan are the basis of revision rhinoplasty.[8]

An interval of at least 1 year should be allowed before revision for resolution of scar and swelling.[9] To preserve nasal blood supply and reduce postoperative edema dissection is done in the proper tissue plane (i.e., sub-SMAS). During revision rhinoplasty, the normal tissue planes are absent. So, there is greater risk of damage to skin-soft tissue envelope, in comparison with primary rhinoplasty. Restoration of skin-soft tissue envelope is difficult if it is damaged. The damaged skin causes an aesthetically bad appearance.[10,11] Scarred thin skin is a problem during secondary rhinoplasty surgery. In thin-skin noses, the dissection is done just above the underlying cartilage. The dissection should be done with extra care to avoid buttonhole formation. Repeated injection of local anesthesia is done to have hydrodissection. If any skin perforation occurs, it is repaired meticulously with sutures. Sometimes, additional soft-tissue covering is done with layered deep temporal fascia. The temporal fascia is folded, and sutured along its free edge, and then placed under the skin of the nasal dorsum. The fascia is fixed by direct sutures at the caudal area and by percutaneous sutures in the radix. When the skin over the tip area is very thin, then a "fascial blanket" is placed underneath the dorsal skin and over the entire tip. One should assess the residual L-shaped strut to avoid the risk of septal collapse if reduction of the cartilaginous vault is planned. If the surgeon encounters loss of both the dorsal and caudal portions of the L-shaped strut, without any available septal grafts, he should place both a dorsal graft and a columellar strut from either costal or conchal cartilage.

Most of the revision cases require osteotomies, though it was performed during the primary rhinoplasty. The osteotomies are done mainly due to excessive dorsal width, asymmetries, and crooked nose. In the case of a very wide dorsum, transverse, medial, and low-to-low lateral osteotomies are done. Micro-osteotomies can be done with a 2-mm osteotome to correct small bony asymmetries near the keystone area. Convex lateral walls are made straight by performing "double osteotomies."

Failure to insert spreader grafts during primary rhinoplasty results in collapsed internal nasal valve and an asymmetric or pinched middle part of dorsum. Spreader graft insertion is done after all osteotomies and mobilization of the lateral walls are completed. If septal cartilage is not available, conchal cartilage can be used for spreader grafts. In revision cases, spreader grafts should be wider, longer, and placed higher within the bony vault.

Autogenous material should be used as a graft. Cartilage graft survives better in areas of scarring and diminished vascularity. Alloplastic materials should not be used as grafts in secondary rhinoplasty because the incidence of rejection, infection, or late extrusion of the graft is very high. Septal cartilage, if available, is a better graft than conchal cartilage. For major augmentation, rib cartilage can be used.

A study of complications associated with autologous rib cartilage reports the rate of warping at 3.0%, reabsorption at 0.2%, infection at 0.5%, migration at 0.3%, unfavorable chest scar at 3.0%, and pneumothorax at 0%.[12] Irradiated rib is also another good option given the lack of donor-site morbidity. Kridel et al., evaluated 1,025 irradiated rib grafts and described the incidence of warping of cartilage in 3.25%, infection in 0.9%, and reabsorption of graft in 1.2% of cases.[13]

The common deformities, requiring revision rhinoplasty are pollybeaks, drooping tips, broad nasal tips, dorsal irregularities, supratip depression, uncorrected crooked nose, deformities of columella, etc.[14] **(Figs. 1 to 4)**.

A study on alloplastic graft use in primary rhinoplasty showed a 3.1% removal rate for both Medpore and Gore-Tex implants and 6.5% removal rate for silicone implants.[15]

If loss of tip support occurs due to surgery, usually within a few months, *pollybeak deformity* develops.[16] In pollybeak, the supratip is the highest point of the nose. This deformity has a relatively high cartilaginous dorsum in comparison with the position of the tip with or without a relatively low bony dorsum. Excessive soft-tissue scar formation at the supratip area can be another cause of pollybeak. To correct this deformity, tip projection is increased

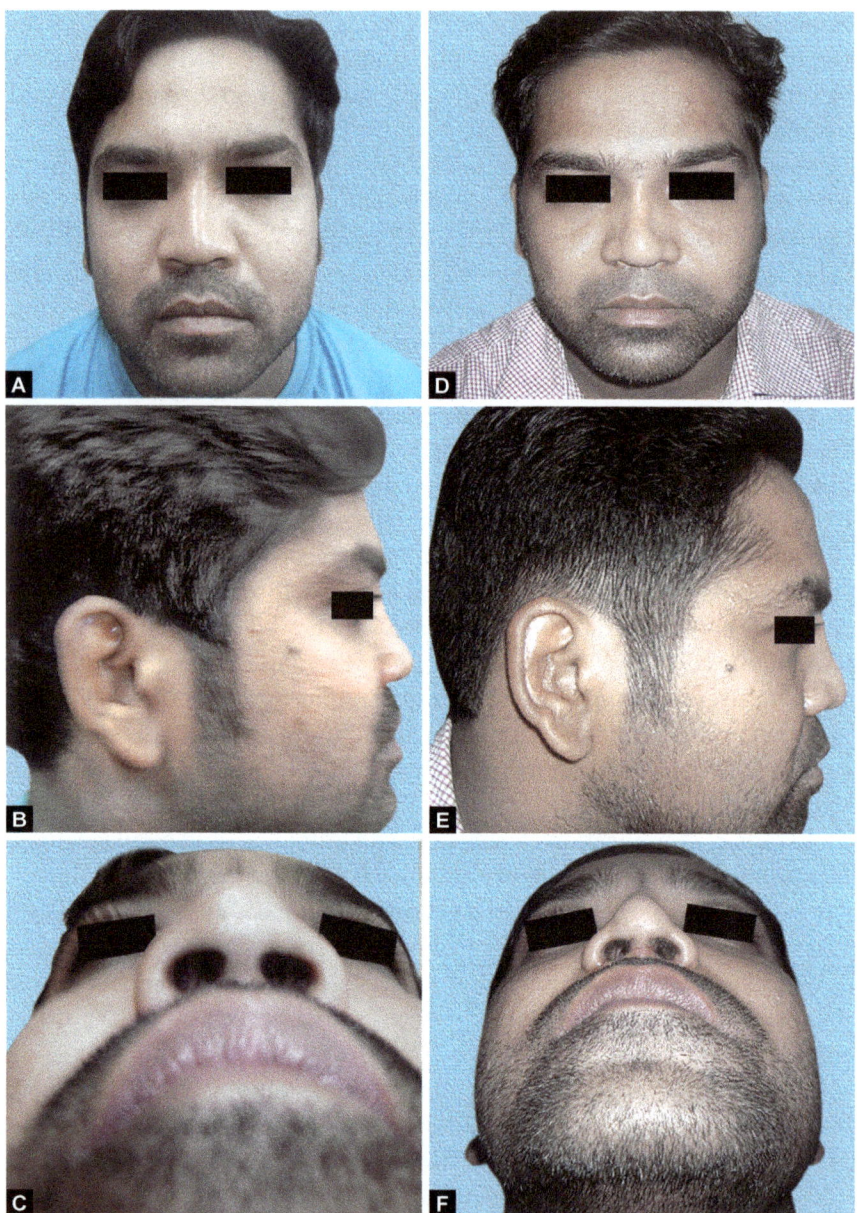

Figs. 1A to F: (A to C) Preoperative; and (D to F) Postoperative views of revision rhinoplasty. The patient had a history of nasal trauma and undergone augmentation rhinoplasty with rib cartilage before. The patient came with a low dorsum, alar flaring, columellar retraction, and broad and underprojected tip. External rhinoplasty was done. Dorsal augmentation was done with layered pinna cartilage. Bilateral cephalic trimming, transection of lower lateral cartilage medial to dome with posteriorly based bilateral chondral flaps and suturing of the medial crura were done to augment tip. A columellar strut was placed in between the medial crura and a tip graft was sutured with it. Alar wedge resection was done.

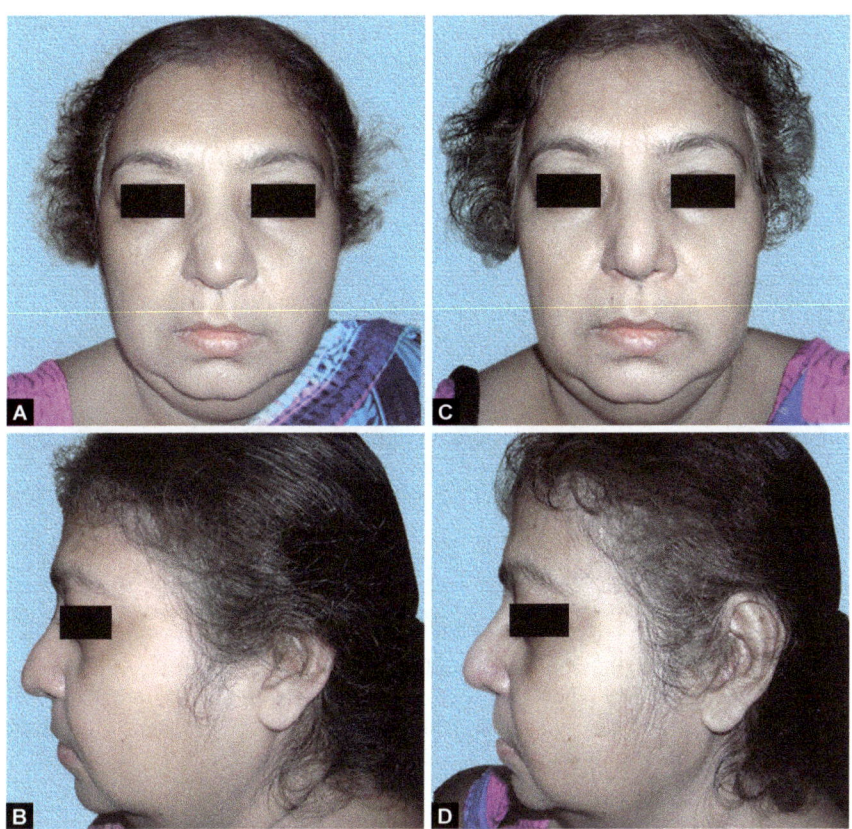

Figs. 2A to D: (A and B) Preoperative; and (C and D) Postoperative views of revision rhinoplasty. The patient had undergone septorhinoplasty before. The patient came with a broad dorsum, bulbous tip, and vestibular stenosis in left side. External rhinoplasty was done. Excess soft tissue was removed from dorsum, sidewalls, and tip. Limited cephalic trimming, and interdomal suturing was done with 5-0 PDS suture to augment tip. Columellar strut was placed and a tip shield graft was sutured with the strut. The dorsal margins of the upper lateral cartilages were sutured. Vestibular stenosis was corrected.

by a columellar cartilage strut using an external approach.[17] Reduction of cartilaginous dorsum may be done if required.

To perform a clean and precise bony hump resection during revision rhinoplasty, sharp osteotomes are required. When the osteotome is not so sharp, asymmetric resection or overresection of the bony hump may occur. Dorsal irregularities may occur after improper hump removal and rasping. To correct this deformity rasping, camouflage or placement of autogenous graft may be done. Crushed cartilages are sometimes used to fill up minor depressions at the side of the nasal dorsum that give the impression of a deviated nose.

Columellar retraction may occur due to excessive resection or abnormal position of the caudal septum and removal of the nasal spine. Upward rotation

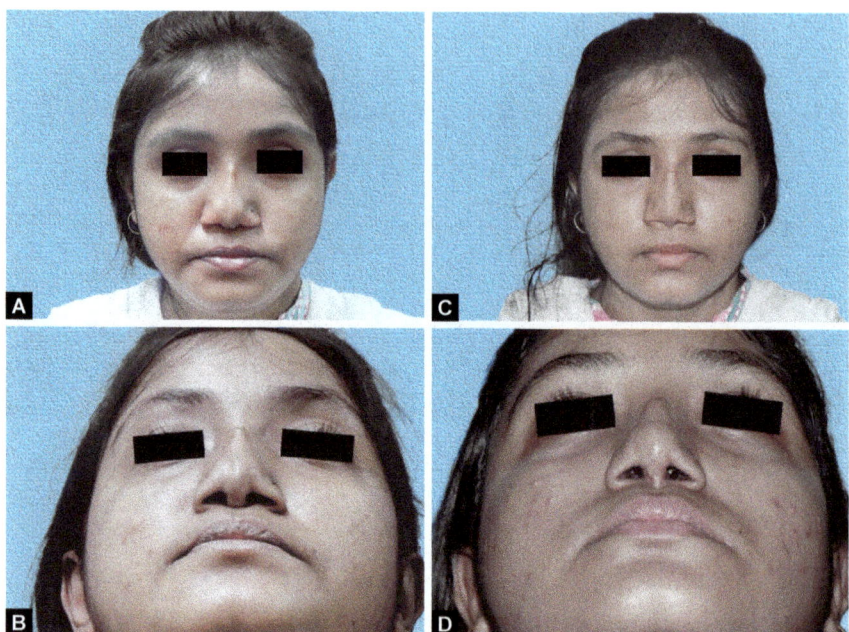

Figs. 3A to D: (A and B) Preoperative; and (C and D) Postoperative views of a case of revision rhinoplasty. Skin-soft tissue envelope was very thin and scarred. Columellar retraction was corrected by columellar strut. Tipplasty was done with tip graft and tip suturing. Augmentation was done by layered conchal cartilage by external approach.

(endorotation) of the nasal septum after mobilization during septorhinoplasty may result in columellar retraction.[18] A cartilage strut may be placed in between the medial crura. If there is malposition of the septal cartilage after septoplasty, the septal cartilage can be repositioned ("exorotation") and sutured to the anterior nasal spine. The "tongue-in-groove" technique during septoplasty results in projection and rotation of the nasal tip but there is a possibility of rigidity and lack of mobility of the tip. To avoid columellar retraction and overrotation of the nasal tip, a septal extension graft is a better choice.

Overshortened noses may give rise to medicolegal problems. The combination of wide nasolabial angle and an overrotated tip looks very bad. Revision is very difficult in some cases, where the mucosal lining is scarred and only limited lengthening of the dorsum and downward rotation of the tip can be done. This deformity can be corrected by the following grafts: Spreader graft, columellar graft, septal extension graft, tip grafts, dorsal grafts, and interposition grafts placed in between upper and lower lateral cartilages.[19] For major lengthening of the nose, a caudal septal extension graft or extended columellar strut along with extended spreader grafts can be used. The extended spreader grafts increase nasal length by pushing the nasal tip down. Overshortened nose can be improved by revision surgery, but accurate reconstruction of all the deformities may not occur.

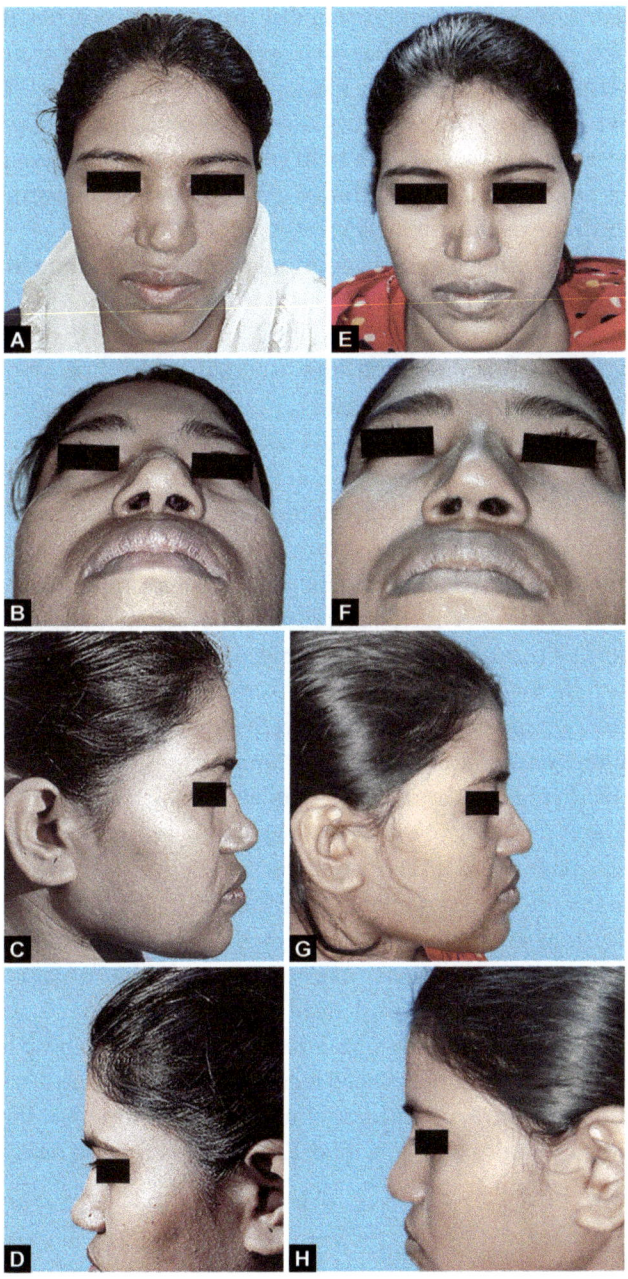

Figs. 4A to H: (A to D) Preoperative; and (E to H) Postoperative views of a case of saddle nose with septal perforation and alar collapse at right side. The patient had past history of septorhinoplasty operations twice. Spreader grafts made from conchal cartilage were placed between dorsal parts of upper lateral cartilages and dorsal septal remnants and sutured with 4-0 PDS. Columellar strut was sutured with spreader graft. Dorsal augmentation was done with conchal cartilage. Cephalic trimming was done at left side and alar batten graft was placed at right side. Tipplasty was done with interdomal suture.

The upward rotated nose may occur due to over resection of anterior septal angle or improper placement of a shield graft. Too much suturing may result in the "snarl tip" and the superiorly rotated tip. The surgeon should remember that instead of tight suturing in every case, he should tighten the suture until the correct result is achieved. The tight transdomal suture beneath the skin can produce sharp points rather than a delicate curve. Tip position suture if not properly done, can result in over rotation of the tip.

The downward rotated nose is commonly due to inadequate support of the medial crura. The tip deformity may result from displacement of the tip graft, asymmetric excision, or suturing. *Tension nose* occurs when the underprojected nose displays inadequate tip definition in thick-skinned or scarred patients and is led by the anterior septal angle.

Inverted V deformity occurs due to collapse of the upper lateral cartilages below the junction of the nasal bones at the keystone area. Here, the middle part of the nose is pinched and the caudal edge of the bony nasal pyramid is visible. Sometimes, dorsal hump removal may result in inadequate support of the upper lateral cartilages and an inverted-V deformity.[20] The deformity is corrected by osteotomies with infracture of the nasal bones and spreader grafts.

Deviation of the bony nasal pyramid may persist due to incomplete fractures or defective osteotomies.[21,22] Asymmetry of tip may occur due to unequal resection of lateral crura or defective placement of columellar strut.

Sometimes, overresection of the lateral crus occurs during cephalic trimming in primary rhinoplasty. This results in retracted ala, bossae, asymmetry, and pinching of tip. *Bossae* usually occurs in persons having thin skin, thick cartilages, and bifid tip. Contracture of the weakened lower lateral cartilages at the nasal tip (knuckling) may occur during healing process.

Cephalic trimming should be avoided in patients with thin alar rim to lessen the risk of retracted ala or collapse of external nasal valve.[23] Alar batten graft is placed to correct retracted ala and nasal valve collapse.

Extrusion of synthetic nasal implant is usually preceded by local area of redness and later ulceration. Delayed reconstruction may cause a severe nasal deformity due to contracture of skin-soft tissue envelope. So, the implant is removed and antibiotics are continued. Early reconstruction can be done after 7 days in a fresh wound.

REFERENCES

1. Parkes ML, Kanodia R, Machida BK. Revision rhinoplasty. An analysis of aesthetic deformities. Arch Otolaryngol Head Neck Surg. 1992;118:695-701.
2. Kamer FM, McQuown SA. Revision rhinoplasty. Analysis and treatment. Arch Otolaryngol Head Neck Surg. 1988;114:257-66.
3. Vuyk HD, Watts SJ, Vindayak B. Revision rhinoplasty: review of deformities, aetiology and treatment strategies. Clin Otolaryngol Allied Sci. 2000;25:476-81.
4. Rettinger G. Foreword in complications of septorhinoplasty. Facial Plast Surg. 1997;1:1.

5. Shah AR. (2010). Anatomy of the nose. Rhinoplasty Information. [online] Available from: https://www.shahfacialplastics.com/blog/rhinoplasty-articles/anatomy-nose-rhinoplasty-information. [Last accessed May, 2023].
6. Tardy ME. Rhinoplasty: the art and the science. Philadelphia: WB Saunders; 1997.
7. Shubailat G. Secondary rhinoplasty. Indian J Plast Surg. 2008;41:80-7.
8. Sheen JH. Secondary rhinoplasty. Plastic and reconstructive surgery. 1975;56:137-45.
9. Webster RC. Revisional rhinoplasty. Otolaryngologic Clinics of North America. 1975;8:753-82.
10. Rettinger G, Zenkel M. Skin and soft tissue complications. Facial Plastic Surgery. 1997;13:51-59.
11. Toriumi DM, Mueller RA, Grosch T, Bhattacharyya TK, Larrabee WF. Vascular anatomy of the nose and the external rhinoplasty approach. Arch Otolaryngol Head Neck Surg. 1996;122:24-34.
12. Wee JH, Park MH, Oh S, Jin HR. Complications associated with autologous rib cartilage use in rhinoplasty: a meta-analysis. JAMA Facial Plast Surg. 2015;17(1):49-55.
13. Kridel RW, Ashoori F, Liu ES, Hart CG. Long-term use and follow-up of irradiated homologous costal cartilage grafts in the nose. Arch Facial Plast Surg. 2009;11(6):378-94.
14. Stucker FJ. Revision rhinoplasty. Trans Pa Acad Ophthalmol Otolaryngol. Spring. 1974;27(1):42-4.
15. Peled ZM, Warren AG, Johnston P, Yaremchuk MJ. The use of alloplastic materials in rhinoplasty surgery: a meta-analysis. Plast Reconstr Surg. 2008;121(3):85-92.
16. Hewell TS, Tardy ME. Nasal tip refinement. Facial Plas Surg. 1984;1:87-124.
17. Vuyk HD, Oakenfull C, Plaat RE. A quantitative appraisal of change in nasal tip projection after open rhinoplasty. Rhinology. 1997;35:124-8.
18. Rettinger G. Aktuelle Aspekte der Septorhinoplastik. Otorhinolaryngol Nova. 1992;2:70-9.
19. Naficy S, Baker SR. Lengthening the short nose. Arch Otolaryngol Head Neck Surg. 1998;124:809-13.
20. Toriumi DM. Management of the middle nasal vault. Operative Techniques in Plas Reconstr Surg. 1995;2:16-30.
21. Larrabee WF Jr. Open rhinoplasty and the upper third of the nose. Facial Plast Surg Clin North Am. 1993;1:23-38.
22. Toriumi DM, Ries WR. Innovative surgical management of the crooked nose. Facial Plast Surg Clin North Am. 1993;1:63-78.
23. Becker DG, Weinberger MS, Greene BA, Tardy ME Jr. Clinical study of alar anatomy and surgery of the alar base. Arch Otolaryngol Head Neck Surg. 1997;123:789-95.

CHAPTER 22

Preservation Rhinoplasty

INTRODUCTION

The aim of preservation rhinoplasty is to maintain and to reshape the present nasal anatomy. Preservation rhinoplasty is not the answer for all nasal defects, but preserving nasal structures results in a more natural appearance.

The principle of preservation has been accepted in rhinoplasty and most surgeons consider preservation rhinoplasty as a better technique, especially in deformities of nasal dorsum. They believe that preservation of nasal structures is better than resection and it produces a more natural result.[1] Dorsum can be modified without disturbing the keystone area, dorsal aesthetic lines, and patency of internal nasal valve, while avoiding dorsal reconstruction.

Osteotomies to close open-roof deformity following standard hump resection can cause irregularities over dorsum. Dorsal preservation technique prevents these irregularities and thus midvault reconstruction is not needed.

Cadaveric dissections have shown us that the bony hump can be easily removed while preserving the cartilaginous dorsum. The keystone area is actually a semimobile osseocartilaginous "joint" and its convexity can be corrected by removing the subdorsal septal cartilage.[2]

HISTORY

The concept of dorsal preservation was first described by the otolaryngologist Goodale in 1899.[3,4] In 1914, Lothrop performed dorsal preservation by subdorsal septal resection, transverse osteotomy, and wedge resections at the nasomaxillary sutures to lower the height of the dorsum.[5] Later on, many surgeons in France performed dorsal preservation following the same techniques.[6,7]

Cottle in 1954 performed dorsal preservation by a different method of septal excision. He removed (1) a vertical 4-mm wide strip of septal cartilage at the junction of septal cartilage and perpendicular plate of ethmoid, and (2) a triangular part of the perpendicular plate beneath the nasal bones. Then, he removed (3) a horizontal strip of septal cartilage from its inferior border, according to the requirement for dorsal lowering **(Fig. 1)**.[8]

Gola in 1989 and Saban in 2006 described dorsal preservation by subdorsal septal resection after making two cuts by sharp scissors, 1 cm cephalic to the anterior septal angle. After removing the strip of septal cartilage, a wedge-shaped part of ethmoid bone was removed by a straight Blakesley forceps[9,10] **(Fig. 2)**.

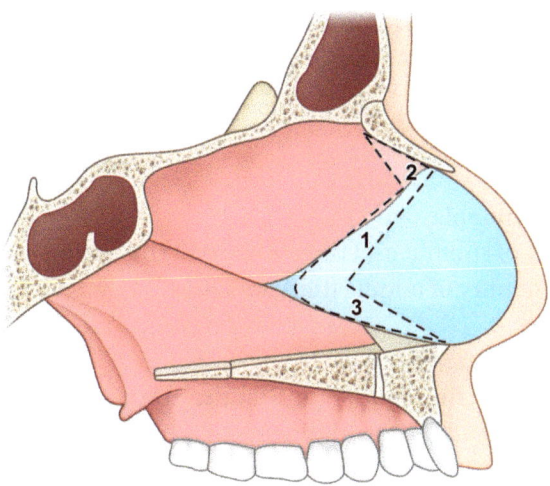

Fig. 1: Cottle's method of dorsal preservation by septal resection at three sites.

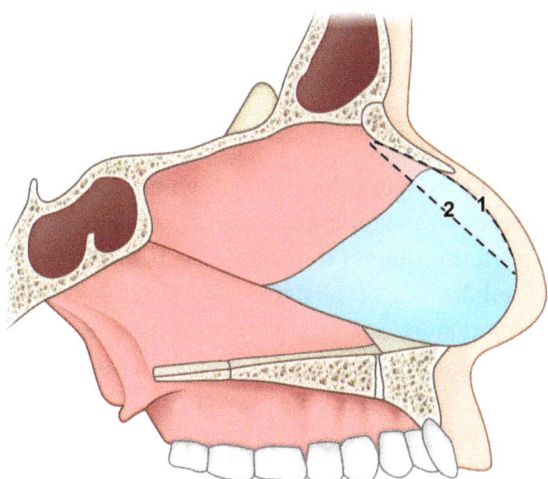

Fig. 2: Dorsal preservation by subdorsal septal resection after making two cuts.

Finnochi (2019) described the modified Cottle procedure, where instead of excision of a vertical strip of septal cartilage, he made a vertical cut in the septum.[11] This procedure is useful in high septal deviation and in deviated noses.

INDICATIONS OF PRESERVATION RHINOPLASTY

- Overprojected nose (tension nose) with straight septum
- Cartilaginous hump with normal radix
- Dorsal hump in an elderly patient with thin skin.

The need for septoplasty along with dorsal realignment is a relative indication of preservation rhinoplasty. The height of the dorsum is dependent on the dorsal septum and a stable septum is required for the push-down or let-down procedure.

CONTRAINDICATIONS

- Secondary rhinoplasty
- Past history of submucosal resection (SMR) operation
- Gross asymmetry of middle third dorsum
- Saddle nose
- Extreme dorsal convexity.

In preservation rhinoplasty, at first the soft tissue is mobilized in the subperichondrial-subperiosteal plane while preserving the scroll area and then surgery of nasal dorsum is done without creating an open-roof deformity. Alar cartilages are preserved and suture tip plasty is done avoiding excision of any cartilage. After elevation of perichondrium from the alar cartilages, the cartilages become more malleable and can be easily shaped with various sutures. Alar malposition can be corrected by simple suturing and fixing the domes to a septal extension graft instead of performing lateral crural transposition.

Mobilization of soft tissue is normally done below the superficial musculoaponeurotic system (SMAS) level which is relatively avascular. But this dissection leads to postoperative numbness, swelling, induration, and fibrosis. Long-term thinning of the soft tissue is also seen.[12] To lessen these complications, mobilization of soft tissue is done in preservation rhinoplasty by a continuous subperichondrial-subperiosteal dissection.[13] With this technique, preservation and/or restoration of the nasal ligaments like Pitanguy's, the intercrural ligament, and the scroll area can be done. Tip projection is improved by preservation of Pitanguy's ligament. It also accentuates supratip break.[14] Ultrasound assessment of the composition of the soft tissue can be done preoperatively and postoperatively over a sequential period with the help of a 25-MHz transducer.[15,16]

In dorsal preservation, limited dorsal skin dissection can be done as wide exposure is not necessary. In patients with an overprojected nose with minimal or no hump, skin undermining of the nasal dorsum may not be needed. In this case, by an open approach, a high subdorsal septal strip is excised and osteotomies are performed to release the osseocartilaginous vault from the midface. External approach provides a good exposure of the septum and removal of septal strips becomes easy.

Mobilization and lowering of the bony nasal vault can be done with either a *push-down or let-down technique* (**Figs. 3 and 4**).

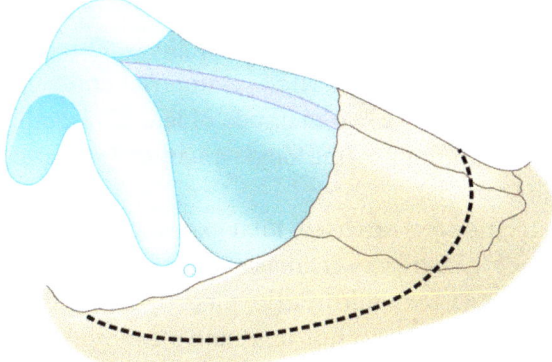

Fig. 3: Push-down technique.

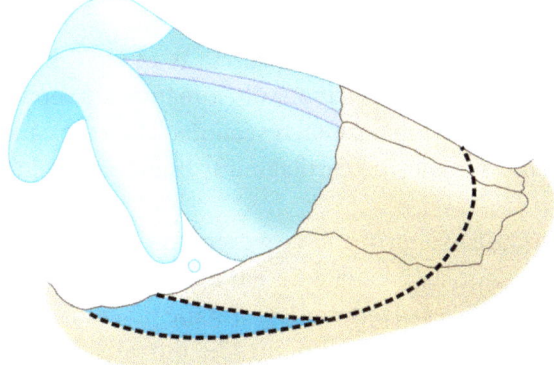

Fig. 4: Let-down technique.

Push-down technique is usually done for lowering of dorsum <4 mm, but let-down technique is done for dorsal lowering of 5–18 mm.[17] The bony pyramid is lowered into the pyriform aperture by the push-down technique following low-to-low lateral osteotomies and transverse osteotomies. Here, the ascending process of the maxilla comes down to lie on the inner side of the pyriform aperture, while the dorsum goes down over the residual septum. Dorsal septal resection is done just below the dorsum without leaving any septal remnant under the keystone area. An excess resection of septal cartilage near the supratip area should be avoided but a slight overcorrection can be done at the keystone area. If mobilization of bony pyramid is incomplete, then osteotomies should be repeated. The radix or root osteotomy is done with 2-mm osteotome to cut through the nasal spine of the frontal bone. It separates the nose from the frontal bone. After complete mobilization, the maneuver of pinching and lowering is done. Pinching of bony pyramid is done with one hand and the other hand will push it downward carefully. After lowering, the surgeon should wait for a few minutes to see if there is any reappearance of the hump.

In a let-down technique, excision of a strip of bone is done laterally at the junction of the nose with the maxilla. Here, the bony pyramid sits on the ascending process of the maxilla. The asymmetric, crooked nose is often corrected by combining these two methods of lateral osteotomies, where a let-down strip excision is done on the longer angulated side and a push-down on the shorter vertical side.

When piezoelectric saws are used, total exposure of the bony dorsum is required. Piezoelectric instruments are useful for osteotomies with minimal damage to soft tissues. Osteotomies and rasping can be done much faster and easier and without unwanted fracture lines and bleeding.

For correction of nasal hump, the osseocartilaginous hump is converted into pure cartilaginous hump by removing the bony hump. In "Spare Roof Technique," Ferreira et al., performed the surgery by either a closed or open approach.[18] They did the surgery in straight Caucasian noses with a hump <5 mm. In this technique, a longitudinal cut is made through the dorsal septum, thus separating the cartilaginous dorsum from the septum. The dorsal hump is reduced by serial 1 mm septal resections. Then the caudal end of the bony hump is removed and the cartilaginous hump is fixed to the septum by sutures.

The subdorsal cartilaginous septal strip excision should start about 6–8 mm cephalic to the anterior septal angle, i.e., at the W-point, where the septum and upper lateral cartilages diverge and end at the junction of septal cartilage and the perpendicular plate of ethmoid. The dorsal strip of bony septum is removed with a 2-mm microtip Rongeur with small cuts. Any twisting movement of the instrument is avoided. Septal strip removal should be done before lateral and transverse osteotomies to avoid unwanted fractures of the perpendicular plate. When adequate dorsal profile is attained, the dorsum is fixed to the underlying septum with 4-0 PDS sutures at three different sites.

In preservation rhinoplasty, tip plasty is done by a combination of a subperichondrial exposure, preservation of ligaments, and an intact lower lateral cartilage.

The "complete technique" of alar preservation consists of suture tip plasty with a columellar strut or, septal extension graft resulting in a symmetrical unified tip complex. Cephalic trimming is not done.[19]

A long-term complication of dorsal preservation technique is recurrence of the hump. Tuncel and Aydogdu, in a study of 520 patients, reported 12% recurrence of dorsal hump.[20] In the subperichondrial dissection, the Pitanguy ligament is preserved and the scroll region is repaired. So, there is much less occurrence of postoperative soft-tissue pollybeak deformity and loss of tip projection. If the dorsal hump is >4 mm, a push-down technique is inadequate and may narrow the internal nasal valve.[21]

REFERENCES

1. Daniel RK, Kosins AM. Current trends in preservation rhinoplasty. Aesth Surg Journ Open Forum; 2020.pp.1-8.
2. Saban Y, Polselli R. Atlas d'Anatomie Chrirurgicale de la Face et du Cou. Florence, Italy: SEE Editrice; 2009.
3. Goodale JL. A new method for the operative correction of the exaggerated Roman nose. Boston Med Surg J. 1899;140:112.
4. Goodale JL. The correction of old lateral displacements of the nasal bones. Boston Med Surg J. 1901;20:538-9.
5. Lothrop O. An operation for correcting the aquiline nasal deformity; the use of new instrument; report of a case. Boston Med Surg J. 1914;170:835-37.
6. G.M. Chirurgie Maxilla-faciale. Paris: Le Francois; 1940. pp. 1127-33.
7. PS, LD. Surgical correction of congenital and acquired deformities of the nasal pyramid. [in French]. Paris: Arnette; 1926. pp. 104-5.
8. Cottle MH. Nasal roof repair and hump removal. AMA Arch Otolaryngol. 1954;60(4):408-14.
9. Gola R, Nerini A, Laurent-Fyon C, Waller PY. Conservative rhinoplasty of the nasal canopy. Ann Chir Plast Esthet. 1989;34(6):465-75.
10. Saban Y, Braccini F, Polselli R. Rhonoplasty: morphodynamic anatomy of rhinoplasty. Interest of conservative rhinoplasty. Rev Laryngol Otol Rhinol (Bord). 2006;127(1-2):15-22.
11. Finnochi V. SPQR technique. Preservation Rhinoplasty Meeting. Rome, Italy; 2019.
12. Toriumi D. Structure Rhinoplasty: Lessons learned in 30 years. Chicago: DMT Solutions; 2019;1645-83.
13. Kosins AM. Subperichondrial dissection and the scroll ligament complex (SLC). Rome, Italy; 2019.
14. Cakir B. Aesthetic septorhinoplasty. Istanbul, Turkey: Springer; 2015.
15. Kosins AM, Obagi ZE. Managing the difficult soft tissue envelope in facial and rhinoplasty surgery. Aesthet Surg J. 2017;37(2):143-57.
16. Kosins AM. Comprehensive diagnosis and management of the difficult rhinoplasty patient: applications in ultrasonography and treatment of the soft-tissue envelope. Facial Plast Surg. 2017;33(5):509-18.
17. Saban Y, Daniel RK, Polselli R, Trapasso M, Palhazi P. Dorsal preservation: the push down technique reassessed. Aesthet Surg J. 2018;38(2):117-31.
18. Ferreira MG, Monteiro D, Reis C, Almeida e Sousa C. Spare roof technique: a middle third new technique. Facial Plast Surg. 2016;32(1):111-6.
19. Regalado-Briz A, Byrd SH. Aesthetic rhinoplasty with maximum preservation of alar cartilages: experience with 52 consecutive cases. Plast Reconstr Surg. 1999;103(2): 671-80; discussion 681-2.
20. Tuncel U, Aydogdu O. The probable reasons for dorsal hump problems following let-down/push-down rhinoplasty and solution proposals. Plast Reconstr Surg. 2019;144(3):378e-85e.
21. Abdelwahab M, Most SP, Patel PN. Impact of dorsal preservation rhinoplasty versus dorsal hump resection on the internal nasal valve: a quantitative radiological study. Aesthetic Plast Surg. 2020;44(3):879-87.

Index

Page numbers followed by *f* refer to figure.

A

Abscess 122
Adrenaline 37, 206
Aesthetic units 205
    principle of 205
Ala 16*f*
    concavity of 182
    in Cadaver, right 182*f*
    notched 181
    retracted 178*f*, 181
    thickness of 186
Alar base
    wide 181
    width 177
Alar batten graft 183, 183*f*, 184, 184*f*, 190*f*, 191*f*
Alar collapse 183, 184*f*
    case of 191*f*
Alar defect 199*f*
    congenital 202*f*
Alar flare 179
Alar groove 8, 197*f*
Alar lobule 7
    size of 177
    thickness of 177
Alar malposition 110
Alar margins, correct thick 187*f*
Alar preservation, complete technique of 224
Alar reduction, minimal 181
Alar resection
    incision for 179*f*
    suturing after 180*f*
Alar retraction severe 182
Alar rim 207
    graft 181, 182, 182*f*
        placement of 182*f*
    lowering of 182
Alar transposition 110, 111*f*
Alar wall
    flare of 177
    thickness of 177

Alar wedge resection 180*f*, 214*f*
Alar width, measurement of 178
Alar-columellar relations 177
Alar-facial groove, level of 92
Allografts 123
Alloplastic
    graft 213
    materials 135
Alloplasts 124
Altered nasal receptor sensitivity 153
Anesthesia 32, 37
    general 36
Anterior septal angle 6, 161
Antihelix, prevent deformity of 129*f*
Areolar tissue 47
Asymmetric bony vaults, correct severely 60
Atrophic rhinitis 49, 152, 156*f*
    primary 152
Auditory canal, upper border of external 6*f*
Aufricht retractor 24
Augment flat nasal bridge 142
Augmentation 138*f*, 140*f*
    dorsal graft for 125*f*
    major 125
    minor 125
    moderate 125
    rhinoplasty 122, 135*f*, 137*f*, 214*f*
Auricular cartilage 107
Auricular composite graft 201
Autografts 123, 125
Autologous cartilage 126
Autologous material 123
Avascular subperichondrial plane 64

B

Bacillus mucosus 152
Balancing procedure 58
Basal cell carcinoma 196*f*

Batten graft 66, 77
Bifid tip 94
Bilobed flap 198
Blakesley forceps 220
Blood
    loss, excessive 132
    vessels and lymphatics 11
Bone
    exposure of 133f
    graft 129, 134
    palatine 19
Bony batten graft 78f
Bony dorsum 13
Bony hump 53
    convexity, degrees of 52
    mild 175f
    rasping of 171f
        mild 165f
    views of 53f
Bony irregularities 54
Bony nasal pyramid, deviation of 218
Bony projection, midline 50
Bony pyramid
    pinching of 223
    wide 85f
Bony vault 13
    soft tissue of 48
Broad nasal tip 100, 213
Brow-tip aesthetic lines 158
Bulbous tip 94, 215f
    case of 109f
Burow's triangles 197f

C

Cadaver
    dissection 40f, 41f, 97f, 106f
    external approach in 67f
    marginal incision in 42f
Cadaveric dissections 220
Calcium hydroxyapatite 148
Calvarial bone 132
    harvesting of 132
Camouflaging 160
    onlay grafts 160
Carbon dioxide, end-tidal 37
Cartilage
    amount of 97, 128
    banking of 132, 133
    caudal edge of upper lateral 5f
    deviated excised 65f
    graft 126, 129, 213
    harvesting of 129f
    incision 129f
    indrawing of upper lateral 185
    lower lateral 15f, 41f, 96f, 105f
    malposition of lower lateral 94
    strip of 64
    upper lateral 96f
Cartilage in cadaver
    lower lateral 14f
    upper lateral 14f
Cartilage splitting
    approach 44, 95
    incision 41, 41f
Cartilage strut 67, 216
    placement of 90
Cartilaginous dorsal integrity, total loss
    of 122
Cartilaginous dorsum 61, 121, 215
    depressed 172f
    narrowing of 91
    reconstruction of 71
Cartilaginous hump 56, 221, 224
Cartilaginous vault
    lower 14
    middle 14
Caudal deviation 76
    correcting 78
    etiology of 76
    types of 76
Caudal margin, expose 33
Caudal nose, deviated 50
Caudal septal
    cartilage, triangular piece of 174f
    deviation, correction of 77
    extension graft 103
Caudal septum 66, 67, 68f, 90
    correct deviation of 2
Cephalic margin 97
Cephalic trimming 44, 45f, 95, 96, 96f,
    97f, 105f, 106, 139f, 170f, 218
    area of 96f
    causes 95
Cleft lip
    and nose 73
    nasal deformity 46, 97, 111f-113f
    nasal tip deformity 94, 110
    unilateral 51
Cocaine nose 114
Coccobacillus foetidus ozaenae 152

Columella 16*f*, 33*f*, 50, 97, 177, 179, 203
  breakpoint 92
  correction of retracted 142
  deformities of 213
  lobular junction 14
  scarring of 187
  wide 188
Columellar cartilage strut 215
Columellar deformity, surgery of 177
Columellar graft 90, 216
Columellar retraction 122, 214*f*, 215, 216
  severe 188
Columellar strut 79, 111, 112, 138*f*, 141*f*, 148*f*, 217*f*
  and suture 98, 99*f*
Columella-septal suture 98
Compression test 73
Compressor naris 11
Concave lateral crus 189
  deformity 189
Conchal cartilage 126, 128, 129*f*, 147*f*, 149*f*, 213, 217*f*
  augmentation with 169*f*
  graft 111, 186
  harvesting of 128, 128*f*
  layered 163*f*, 170*f*, 216*f*
  pieces of 134
  sutured, pieces of 125*f*
Conchal composite graft 202
Conchal hollow 201
Contralateral infiltration 34*f*
Convex
  lateral wall 85
  subunits of 205
Costal cartilage 146*f*, 213
  harvest 130*f*
Cottle's elevator 70
Cottle's maneuver, modified 212
Cottle's method 221*f*
Cottle's procedure, modified 221
Cottle's test, positive 160
Cranial bone grafts 125
Crooked nose 59*f*, 158, 163*f*, 164*f*, 166*f*
  case of 163*f*, 164*f*, 174*f*
  correction of 158, 159
  surgery of 158
    steps of 162
  types of 159
  uncorrected 213

Crural footplate
  diversion, medial 179
  suturing medial 101
Crural strut graft, suturing of lateral 185*f*
Crura-septal suture, medial 101
Cut fragments, overlapping of 110
Cutting and suture technique 79, 79*f*

D

Dacryocystitis, chronic 63
Deep temporal fascia, partial sheet of 58
Deformity 54
  correction of 44
  type of 110
Delivery approach 44, 95
Depressed nasal dorsum, cause of 122
Deviated nasal septum 53*f*, 109*f*, 111*f*, 163*f*, 166*f*-168*f*
Diazepam 32
Digital pressure 143
Dilator naris
  anterior originates 11
  posterior 11
Disease, warping and fear of 123
Dislocation 63
Dog ear, prevent 198, 201
Domal creation suture 99, 100*f*, 107, 146*f*
Domal equalization 100*f*
  suture 58*f*, 100, 170*f*, 174*f*
Domal junction 16
Dome
  scoring 106
  transection of 97
Dorsal aesthetic lines 8, 122, 158*f*
Dorsal augmentation 125*f*, 126, 141*f*, 170*f*, 173*f*
  useful graft for 127
Dorsal cartilage graft 60
Dorsal convexity, extreme 222
Dorsal depression 168*f*
Dorsal deviation 212
Dorsal graft 90, 111, 216
Dorsal hump
  overreduction of 122
  resection of 57
Dorsal septal
  deviation 68*f*
  margin 2

Dorsal septum 93
Dorsum 45
　middle third 222
　parts of 122
　pinched middle part of 213
Drooping tip 90, 213

E

Ecchymosis 121
Empty nose syndrome 39, 60, 153
En bloc hump reduction 54
Endochondral bone 132
Endonasal
　approach 164f, 171f
　cartilage-splitting approach 44
　delivery approach 44
Endoscopic dacryocysto-rhinostomy 63
Endoscopic septoplasty 69, 70
　techniques 69
Endoscopic sinus surgery, functional 63
Epistaxis 63
Estrogen deficiency 152
Ethmoid
　bone, 18-gauze needle 78f
　gross deviations of 20
　perpendicular plate of 20, 220
Extracorporeal septoplasty 70, 71
　modified 71
Extramucosal dissection 71
Extramucosal tunnels 55
Eye, medial canthus of 199
Eyebrow 212
Eyelids
　medial 13
　swelling of 120

F

Face 196f
　basal cell carcinoma of 197f
Facial aesthetics 160
Facial and angular arteries, branches
　of 199
Facial asymmetries 159
Facial proportions guide 25
Fascia 47
　diced cartilage in 127
Fascial blanket 212
Fibrous sling 93
Fix nasal skin 119f

Flap
　advancement 195
　hinged 207
　interpolation 196
　local 193, 195
　regional 193
　V-Y advancement 195f
Flaring sutures 186
Fomon angular scissors 24
Forehead defect 199
Forehead flap 203
　median 204f, 207f
　midline 205f, 209f
　stages of 206
　types of 203
Fractured nasal bones, reduction of 160
Frankfort line 6
Frankfort plane 29
Free-flap graft technique 1
Frontal bone
　nasal process of 21f
　nasal spine of 19
Frontalis muscle 206

G

Gait disturbance 132
Gillies osteotome 24, 55, 86f
Glabella 4
Glabellar flap 199, 200f
Glabellar region 199
Gnathion 6
Goldman's technique 104
Gore-tex 124
Graft
　absorption of 136
　balanced cross section of 155
　bilateral spreader 71, 78
　common problems of 136
　composite 201, 202f
　corrected 216
　displacement of 136
　extrusion of 136
　fixation of 131
　heal, stages of 194
　healing of 201
　immobilization of 202
　interposition 90
　material, source of 133
　placing spreader 162

unilateral spreader 78
used for spreader 213
visibility 136
warping of 136
Gray's struts 74
Greenstick fracture 51
Groove technique, tongue in 173*f*
Gross deviated nasal septum 59*f*, 164*f*, 166*f*
Gull-wing appearance 177*f*

H

Hair follicles 207
Hanging
columella 90, 188
secondary 193
tip 94, 94*f*, 107
Hanging ala 178, 179*f*, 187
correction of 188*f*
Hematoma 136
Hemitransfixion incision 40, 63
Hemostasis 143
Heterologous 124
Homografts 123
Human immunodeficiency virus test 28
Hump 94*f*
amount of 52
chisel for removal of 24
dorsal 221
reduction 52
amount of 55
incremental 56, 57*f*
minimize 58
removal of 38, 52, 60
resection of 52*f*
types of 52
Hyaluronic acid 146
Hydrodissection 212
Hydroxyapatite 124, 132
Hypophysectomy 63
Hypotension, controlled 37

I

Ice packs 144
Iliac crest bone graft 133*f*
harvesting of 131, 133*f*
Implants, types of 123
Inadequate projection, tip with 93, 102

Infection 136
spread of 135
Inflammatory disease, chronic 152
Inframammary fold 129
Infraorbital nerve 13, 32
Infraorbital rim, lower border of 6*f*
Infratip lobular graft 103
Infratip lobule 8
Infratrochlear nerve supplies 13
Instruments 24
Intercartilaginous incision 40, 40*f*, 86*f*
bilateral 95
Intercrural sutures 98
Interdomal fibrous attachment 93
Interdomal suture 98, 100, 100*f*, 141*f*, 145*f*, 170*f*
Internal valve, reconstruction of 38
Intracartilaginous 41, 41*f*
Intranasal needle prick 35*f*

K

Kazanjian technique 135
Keloid, case of broad-based 198*f*
Keystone area 8, 223
Killian incision 40
Kilner alar retractor 24
Klebsiella ozaenae 152

L

Lateral crura 101*f*
cephalic malposition of 107
Lateral crural
mattress suture 98, 101, 102*f*
reversal technique 191*f*
spanning graft 186*f*
steal 98, 101*f*, 102
suture 101
strut graft 111*f*, 183, 185*f*
turn-in flap 96
Lateral crus, over-resection of 218
Laughing strut 107
Left nostril, closure of 154*f*
Leprosy 153
Leptorrhine nose 25
Let-down technique 222, 223*f*, 224
Levator labii superioris alaeque nasi muscle 10
Lignocaine 32
Limen nasi 4

Liquid silicone 148
Lobule 4, 16f
  projection 9
Lower lateral cartilage
  exposure of 107
  medial to dome, transection of 106f
Lupus vulgaris 153
Lymphatic drainage 118
Lymphatics of columella, transection of 45

M

Malinac retractor 24
Marginal incision 41
Marionette septoplasty 79
Mattress suture 182
McIndoe osteotome 55
Medial canthus 27f
Medpore 124
Membranous septum 20
  strip of 188
Merciful anosmia 152
Mersilene 124
Micro-osteotomy 87
Midcolumellar approach 133
Midforehead flaps, axial blood supply of 203
Mouth, angle of 199
Mucoperichondrial elevator 24
Mucoperichondrial flap 65, 65f
  elevation of 64, 70, 71
Mucoperichondrial tunnels 70
Mucosal glands, atrophy of 152
Muscle 47
Musculoaponeurotic system, superficial 222

N

Nasal advancement flap, lateral 197f
Nasal airflow
  improvement of 212
  subjective assessments of 63
Nasal anatomy 4
Nasal base and columella 177f
Nasal blockage 63, 73, 120
Nasal bone 48, 87f, 96f, 220
  fracture 63
    reduction of 63
  fragments 85
    small 60

Nasal breathing
  difficulties in 63
  subjective improvement in 212
Nasal cavity 26, 118
Nasal congestion 63
Nasal crests of maxillary 19
Nasal defects 220
Nasal deformity
  external 28
  traumatic 208f, 209f
Nasal dorsum 34f
  surgery of 222
Nasal endoscopy 28
Nasal height 9
Nasal hemangioma 194f
Nasal hump
  corrected 53f
  perceptual lessening of 142
  removal 55f
Nasal index 9
Nasal injury, traumatic 142
Nasal length 9
Nasal lobule 122
Nasal muscles 47
  layer of 47
Nasal obstruction 63, 153
  complete 73
  symptom evaluation 63
Nasal projection, angle of 6
Nasal reconstruction 193, 207f
  operative steps of 205f
  options for 193
  stages of 209f
Nasal septum 19, 19f
  correction of deviated 2
  examined for deviated 26
  severe deviated 73
Nasal spine 50, 51
  anterior 19, 21f, 50, 64, 65, 142
  prominent 51
  redeviation of 51
Nasal splints 50
Nasal structures, preserving 220
Nasal superficial musculoaponeurotic system 47
Nasal surface 10
Nasal tip 17
  defect 203
  deformity, types of 93
  surgery of 92
  underprojection of 172f

Nasal trauma 73, 159
　history of 214*f*
Nasal valve
　angle of internal 186
　area 5
　diagnose collapse of 212
　external 8
　internal 4, 185
Nasal width 9
Nasalis 11
Nasion 4, 13
Nasoalar crease, formation of 95
Nasofacial
　angle 6, 8*f*
　sulcus 196*f*, 197*f*
Nasofrontal angle 6, 7*f*
Nasolabial angle 6, 7*f*, 90
　acute 174*f*
Nasolabial flap 196, 199, 199*f*
Nasolabial sulcus 199
Nasolacrimal duct system 88
Natural grafts 123
Nonsurgical rhinoplasty 136
Nose
　aesthetic subunits of 206*f*
　basal cell carcinoma of 205*f*, 207*f*, 208*f*
　blood supply of 12*f*
　collapse of right lateral wall of 148*f*
　deformity of 161
　dermatofibroma of 197*f*
　deviations of 26
　downward rotated 218
　inspection of 26
　lateral wall of 196*f*
　middle third of 90
　muscles of 10, 11*f*
　nerve supply of 12, 13*f*
　overprojected 221
　overshortened 90, 216
　palpation of 26
　physiology of 21
　reconstruction of 201
　shortening of 38, 90
　upward rotated 218
Nostril 178*f*
　apex of 177
　borders removed 187*f*
　elongation of 182
　right 33

sill 8
size of 142
widening of 182

O

Olfactory nerves 152
Onlay
　cartilage grafts 113*f*
　grafts, dorsal 160
　tip graft 103, 111, 112
Oozing 39
Open-roof deformity 60
　cause of 60
　close 220
Osteochondral junction 130
Osteotome 36*f*
Osteotomy 35, 82, 162, 163*f*, 166*f*, 220
　double 213
　incomplete 87
　indications for double 85
　instrument for lateral 82
　intermediate 85
　intranasal lateral 75*f*, 82, 83*f*
　lateral 36*f*, 60, 82, 83, 83*f*, 87, 163
　　line of 83
　medial 86, 86*f*
　multiple 162
　oblique 84
　paramedian 86
　percutaneous lateral 83
　percutaneous transverse 75*f*, 164*f*
　perform curved lateral 84
　transverse 86
Overly rotated tip, case of 161

P

Palpebral conjunctiva 13
Parallel cuts 132
Paramedian flap 196
Paramedian forehead flap 201, 202, 204, 204*f*, 205*f*
Parrot beak nose 94*f*
Peck graft 103
Pedestal effect 113
Pediatric septoplasty, indications for 73
Pedicle, raw undersurface of 206
Perichondrium 19*f*, 47
Periosteum 19*f*, 47
Peripheral vascular disease 32

Perpendicular plate 224
    triangular part of 220
Piezo device 48
Piezoelectric instruments 224
Piezoelectric saws 224
Pinched nasal tip 184
    deformity 184
Pinna 202f
    composite graft 202f
Pinocchio nose 112, 113
Piriform crest, caudal part of 163
Pitanguy ligament 224
    preservation of 222
Pivot flap 195
Plaster of Paris 119f
Plaster splint, size of 119
Plumping grafts 91
Plunging tip 94, 107
Polly-beak deformity 60
    develops 213
Polyacrylamide gel 148
Polydioxanone sutures 101
Polyester fiber mesh 124
Polyethylene
    high-density 124
    terephthalate 124
Polymethylmethacrylate 148
Polytetrafluoroethylene 124
Porous polyethylene 124
Postauricular skin graft,
        full-thickness 154f
Postrhinoplasty advice 120
Premaxilla 50
Prepackaged sterile syringe 143
Promethazine 32
Prominent scroll, excision of 91
Pronasale 9
Pupils 27f
Push-down technique 222, 223,
        223f, 224
Pyriform
    aperture 8
        base of 82
        types of 184

R

Radiesse 148
Radix augmentation 58

Regional flaps 201
Residual cartilage, amount of 212
Residual septal deviation 212
Rethi goodman incision 41, 48f
Retracted columella 142f, 178, 187
Revision rhinoplasty 211, 213, 214f, 215f
    preoperative assessment in 211
Rhinomanometry 27
Rhinoplasty 4, 24, 32, 37, 63, 111
    anatomy and physiology 4
    basic technique 38
    complication rates 39
    dissection 12
    end of 87
    external 42f, 48f, 162, 215f
    for crooked nose 159
    history of 1
    in atrophic rhinitis 152
    indications of
        nonsurgical 142
        preservation 221
    instruments used in 24f
    operation 25, 28
    operative steps 38
    preservation 220, 222
    primary 211, 213, 218
    principles 38
    secondary 97, 211, 222
    skin incisions for 43f
    surgical approaches 43
Rhinoscleroma, atrophic stage of 153
Rib cartilage 107, 126, 127, 131, 144f,
        156f, 184, 214f
    graft 71, 126
        harvesting of 128
    harvesting of 131f
    warping of 155
Rifamycin 127
Rim graft 191f
Rocker deformity 60, 87
Root osteotomy 88, 223
Rotation flap 195

S

Saddle deformity 122, 153, 163f
Saddle nose 137f, 222
    case of 142f
    causes of 122

correction of 142
implantation 122
management of 133
Saddle nose deformity 115, 147f
cases of 133
classification of 122
correction of 133
post-traumatic 143f, 149f
Saline, normal 129f
Sandwich grafts, bilateral stenting 65
Scroll region 6
Seborrheic keratosis 196f
Sellion 4
Semimobile osseocartilaginous
joint 220
Septal abscess 146f
Septal cartilage 64, 126, 171f, 184, 213
caudal part of 187
closed technique 140f
concave side of 78f
junction of 224
pieces of 134
removal of 72
strut of 187
triangular piece of 90f
vertical strip of 221
Septal deviation 63
complicated 46, 97
severe 73
types of 62
Septal dislocation, newborns 73
Septal excision,
graft 66f, 79, 90, 216
in Cadaver, suturing of 69f
sutured 68f
method of 220
Septal hematoma 122
Septal perforation, repair of 46, 97
Septal resection 221f
Septal surgery, extensive 122, 153
Septal suturing 118
Septi nasi muscles, depressor 47
Septocolumellar suture 102
technique 104
Septoplast 167f
Septoplasty 35, 38, 62-64, 114f, 162, 163f, 166f-168f
external approach for 67, 68f
Septorhinoplasty 74
operations 217f

Septum 19f, 45
bony part of 88
caudal
deviation of 76, 76f, 77f, 79f, 140f
dislocation of 72f, 76f
part of 72, 90
central part of 159
fracture of 63
function of 21
part of 20
reduction of dislocated 73
spine, redeviation of 51
straight 221
symptomatic deviated 62
Sesamoid cartilages 8
Severe saddle deformity, case of 134, 140f, 156f
Shield graft 103, 111, 112, 149f, 215f
placement of 146f
sutured tip 103f
Silicone 124
Sill excisions 181
Silver nasal chisel 24, 25
firmly 82
Sinus diseases 28
Sinusitis 63
Skeletonization 15f, 47, 162
Skin
full-thickness 194
necrosis of 136
texture 193
vestibular 36f
Skin graft 193
full-thickness 190f, 202
postauricular full-thickness 194f
repair with 193
split-thickness 194
Skin-soft tissue envelope 134, 211
contracture of 218
mobilization of 50
Sleep apnea 73
Sleeping, disturbance in 63
Snarl tip 218
Sodium
biborate 153
bicarbonate 153
chloride 153
Soft tissue 35, 47
envelope 10
exposing, mobilization of 98f

filler agents 146
  mobilization of 38, 47, 48, 48*f*, 162, 222
  undermining of 47
Soft triangle 6
Solid silicone 124
Spare roof technique 224
Sphenoid bone, crest of 19
Splinting 118
Spreader flaps 57, 185
Spreader graft 56*f*, 57, 67, 90, 160, 161, 216
  maintain 55
  placement of 160
Stab incision 82
Staphylococcus 119
  aureus 119
Subcostal approach 130
Subcutaneous tissue 47
  overlying, excision of 91
Subdorsal cartilaginous septal strip excision 224
Subdorsal septal
  cartilage 220
  resection 220, 221*f*
Sublabial lateral osteotomy 84
Submucous resection
  operation 52, 222
  technique 2
Subperichondrial-subperiosteal dissection 222
Supra-alar pinching, postoperative 97
Supramid mesh 124
Supraorbital ridges 4, 158*f*
Supraperiosteal planes 34
Supratip
  area 8, 121
  augmentation 171*f*
  depression 109*f*, 122, 213
Supratrochlear artery 203
Supratrochlear pedicle 203
Supratrochlear vessels, arterioles of 203
Suture
  and dressing 38, 118
  techniques 98
  tip plasty 97
  with remnant cartilage 65*f*
Suturing, direct closure by 193

Swinging door
  method 77
  technique 65, 66*f*, 77*f*
Synthetic grafts 124
Synthetic nasal implant, extrusion of 218
Syphilis 153

T

Teflon 124
Temporal arteries, superficial 203
Temporal fascia 126
  deep 212
Tension nose 113, 221
Tip 4
  anatomy 15*f*
  anchoring suture 101
  asymmetrical 94
  deformities, correction of 102
  diamond 92
  overprojecting 93, 104
  projection 9
  rhinoplasty, difficult 46, 97
  upwardly rotated 110
  volume 17
Tip grafts 90, 170*f*, 216
  shield-shaped 103
Tip plasty 92, 98, 138*f*, 139*f*, 145*f*, 162, 170*f*
  placement of 146*f*
Tip support
  loss of 213
  mechanism 93
  major 93
Tip-defining points 8
Tip-positioning suture 98, 101
Tongue-in-groove technique 69, 79*f*, 114*f*, 189, 216
Toxic shock syndrome 119
Tranquilizers 32
Transcolumellar incision 118
Transdomal suture 98-100
Transfixion incision 40
Transposition flap 195
Triangular columellar strut 110
Trichion 9
Tripod theory 92
  of Anderson 92

Tunnels
　anterior 64*f*
　inferior 64*f*

U

Umbrella graft 104
Upper lateral cartilage, collapse of 186*f*

V

V deformity, inverted 61, 218
Valsalva 131
Valve of Minx 185
V-deformity 54
Venous drainage 118
Vertical wedge, resection of 77
Vestibular stenosis 189, 190*f*
　correction of 189
　left side 215*f*
　mild 191*f*
　right side 189*f*, 190*f*
　surgery of 177

Vicryl purse-string suture 131
V-Y advancement flap 198*f*

W

Webster triangle 8, 82, 163
Wet nasal tip 189
Wolfe graft 194

X

Xenografts 124
Xylocaine 206

Y

Young's operation, left side 156*f*

Z

Zitelli's bilobed flap 198*f*
Zitelli's flap 198

EU GSPR Authorised Reprsentative
Logos Europe, 9 rue Nicolas Poussin
1700, La Rochelle, France
Phone: +33 (0) 6 67 93 73 78
E-mail: contact@logoseurope.eu

www.ingramcontent.com/pod-product-compliance
Ingram Content Group UK Ltd.
Pitfield, Milton Keynes, MK11 3LW, UK
UKHW051559010326
468476UK00022B/21